# Medical Sociology

# Medical Sociology

M. Thamilarasan

RAWAT PUBLICATIONS

Jaipur • New Delhi • Bangalore • Guwahati • Kolkata

ISBN 978-81-316-0755-8





*Published by*
Prem Rawat for **Rawat Publications**
Satyam Apts, Sector 3, Jawahar Nagar, Jaipur 302 004 (India)
Phone: 0141 265 1748/7006 Fax: 0141 265 1748
E-mail: info@rawatbooks.com
Website: www.rawatbooks.com

*New Delhi Office*
4858/24, Ansari Road, Daryaganj, New Delhi 110 002
Phone: 011 2326 3290

Also at *Bangalore, Guwahati* and *Kolkata*

Typeset by Rawat Computers, Jaipur
Printed at Chaman Enterprises, New Delhi

# Contents

# Preface

To some people it appears irrelevant for sociology to involve itself with the study of medicine or health. However, the very core of the field of sociology is the study of society. L.F. Ward has put it this way: 'Sociology is the study of social phenomena'. M. Ginsberg further made it clear by laying out a definition of sociology as 'the study of human interaction and interrelations, their conditions and consequences'.

Medical sociology is a deeper study of sicknesses and diseases, and the treatment and reaction of society towards the sick in the light of sociology, the study of human interaction and interrelations. Medical sociology provides an extensive study of health and health related decisions in a society, finding root causes and, individual and cultural solutions to health problems. The founding father of medical sociology, Talcott Parsons has built a firm theory that proposed a model of behaviour on the part of the sick, the society, and the attending health care professionals. Similarly, the focus of medical sociology centres around the view of health and health related issues with the human welfare in mind. It covers topics as vast as topics of individual behaviour and interests to a state's health policies, governmental schemes and programmes, disparities in access to health care systems and laws pertaining to the health of society. A study of health in a community cannot undermine the importance of medical sociology because the very community that is under study is a collection of humans living together within a limited and defined geographical area in which they carry out most of their day-to-day activities; the very interest of the subject of sociology.

This book presents the concept of medical sociology by tracing its early beginnings, development over time, and its scope of study in today's world. The book clarifies the methods adopted in the field of medical sociology, re-examines the very concept of health, brings to light the disparities in access to health care systems across places, specifically deals with habits for prevention of diseases, presents the nature and treatment of diseases, and layout the social-cultural bearings on health. Occupational diseases, a topic ignored by many corporates and individuals are also dealt with briefly in this book. This book has also been written for health care professionals. Hospitals are viewed as social organization where communication, cooperation and relationships contribute significantly in the treatment of the sick.

The author is privileged to have written this book with the inspiration from venerated pioneers in the field of sociology as well as of medical sociology. The author is genuinely grateful to the professors, research scholars, and students who have encouraged the writing of this book.

The author expresses his gratitude to the professors who have led to the completion of this book: R. Shankar, Senior Professor and Head (Retd.), M. Thavamani, Professor and Head, Department of Sociology, Bharathidasan University, Tiruchirapalli, and A. Karuppiah, Professor and Head, Department of Sociology, University of Madras, Chennai.

Last but not the least, the author offers his heartfelt gratitude to his parents and spouse for their untiring support that has made the publication of the book a reality.

**M. Thamilarasan**

# 1

# Introduction to Medical Sociology

Sociology – 'the scientific study of human behaviour in groups and the social forces that influence behaviour'. Medical sociology is a subfield of sociology that 'encompasses a body of knowledge that places health and disease in a social, cultural and behavioural context'.

Medical sociology has experienced significant growth worldwide in numbers of practitioners. At the centre of medical sociology is the sociological study of the social institution of medicine, its knowledge, practice and effects. Medical sociologists investigate the social organization and production of health and illness, including relevant aspects of the sociology of the profession along with science and technology studies that relate to medicine and health care. They are also interested in lay experiences of health and illness, and some medical sociologists work at the boundaries of health, demography and social gerontology to explore phenomena at the intersection of the social and clinical sciences.

Throughout history, human beings have been interested in and deeply concerned with the effects of the social environment on the health of individuals and the groups to which they belong. Today it is clear that social factors play a critically important role in health, as the greatest threats to the health and well-being of individuals stem largely from unhealthy lifestyles and high risk behaviour. Sociology's interest in medicine as a unique system of human social behaviour and medicine's recognition that sociology can help health practitioners to better understand their patients and provide improved forms of health care have begun to bring about a convergence of mutual interest between the two disciplines.

Medical sociology is concerned with the social causes and consequences of health and illness. Medical sociology brings sociological perspectives, theories and methods to the study of health and medical practice.

Medical sociology is the sociological study of the social institution of medicine, its knowledge, practice and effects. Medical sociologists investigate the social organization and production of health and illness, including relevant aspects of the sociology of the profession and science and technology studies that relate to medicine and health care. They are also interested in lay experiences of health and illness, and some medical sociologists work at the boundaries of health, demography and social gerontology to explore phenomena at the intersection of the social and clinical sciences.

## Medical Sociology: Meaning and Definitions

Medical sociology is concerned with the relationship between social factors and health, and with the application of sociological theory and research techniques to questions related to health and the health care system.

Medical sociology is the study of individual and group behaviours with respect to health and illness. Medical sociology is concerned with individual and group responses aimed at assessing well-being, maintaining health, acting upon real or perceived illness, interacting with health care systems, and maximizing health in the face of physiologic or functional derangement. It also analyses the impact of the psychological conditions resulting from our environment on our health. Medical sociology includes the study of medical professional, as well as the study of human behavioural responses to health and illness

The field of medical sociology is usually taught as part of a wider sociology, clinical psychology or health studies degree course, or on dedicated Master's degree courses where it is sometimes combined with the study of medical ethics/bioethics.

Medical sociology involves the sociological analysis of medical organizations and institutions; the production of knowledge and selection of methods, the actions and interactions of health care professionals, and the social or cultural (rather than clinical or bodily) effects of medical practice. The field commonly interacts with the sociology of knowledge, science and technology studies, and social epistemology. Medical sociologists are also interested in the qualitative experiences of patients, often working at the boundaries of public health, social work, demography and gerontology to explore phenomena at the intersection of the social and clinical sciences. Health disparities commonly relate to typical categories such as class and race. Objective sociological research findings quickly become a normative and political issue.

Early work in medical sociology was conducted by Lawrence J. Henderson whose theoretical interests in the work of Vilfredo Pareto inspired Talcott Parsons' interests in social systems theory. Parsons is one of the founding fathers of medical sociology, and applied social role theory to interactional relations between sick people and others. Key contributors to medical sociology since the 1950s include Howard Becker, Mike Bury, Peter Conrad, Jack Douglas, David Silverman, Phil Strong, Bernice Pescosolido, Carl May, Anne Rogers, Anselm Strauss, Renee Fox, Joseph W. Schneider and Thomas Szasz.

The field of medical sociology is usually taught as part of a wider sociology, clinical psychology or health studies degree course, or on dedicated Master's degree courses where it is sometimes combined with the study of medical ethics/bioethics. In Britain, sociology was introduced into the medical curriculum following the *Good Enough Report* in 1944: 'In medicine, "social explanations" of the aetiology of disease meant for some doctors a redirection of medical thought from the purely clinical and psychological criteria of illness. The introduction of "social" factors into medical explanation was most strongly evidenced in branches of medicine closely related to the community – Social Medicine and, later, General Practice'.

### *Objectives and Principles*

Medical sociology is important and it is the critical role that social factors play in determining the health of individuals, groups and the larger society. Social conditions and situations not only promote the possibility of illness and disability, but they also enhance prospects for disease prevention and health maintenance. Many of the greatest threats to an individual's health and physical well-being today is largely from unhealthy lifestyles and high risk behaviour and this is true for heart disease, cancer, AIDS and a host of modern-day health problem. Healthy lifestyles and the avoidance of high-risk behaviour, on the other hand, advance the individual's potential for a longer and healthier life. The major objectives of medical sociology are as follows:

- Influences on individuals' experience of health and illness.

- Influences on the response to illness (from doctors/medical community).
- Important to understand health seeking behaviour and uptake of services.
- Necessary for planning public health programmes and health services.

Some have argued that medical sociology should be thought of as a loosely connected network of disparate subgroups rather than as a single discipline. Many medical sociologists tend to argue against certain axioms in the biomedical model of health and illness. They reject the reductivist approach of biomedicine, which claims that health and disease are natural phenomena that exist in the individual body rather than in the interaction of the individual and the social world; they reject the doctrine of specific etiology, the vision that disease can be induced by introducing a single specific factor into a healthy animal; and they reject biomedicine's claim to scientific neutrality. Like sociology in general, subgroups within medical sociology vary according to dichotomies such as human agency versus social structure, conflict versus consensus, and idealism versus realism. subgroups also vary according to subject matter, thus the sociology of medicine can be distinguished from the sociology of health and illness, the sociology of healers, and the sociology of the health care system. Medical sociologists also distinguish between the sociology of health, the study of health, illness, and health care to further sociological theory; and sociology in health, the use of sociological insights to complement biomedicine's objectives and priorities. There are four often interrelated areas of research in medical sociology: the social production of health and illness, the social construction of health and illness, postmodern perspectives on health and illness, and the study of the health care system and its constituent parts.

Medical sociology as a discipline became formalized in the 1950s. It was realized that a person's social position affected the person's health. Medical sociology is based on three principles:

- Health is a matter of direct social concerns and society had an obligation to protect it.
- Social and economic conditions have an effect on health and disease.
- Steps must be taken to promote health and combat disease.

### *Scope and Its Relevance to Patient Care*

Recognition of the significance of the complex relationship between social factors and the level of health characteristics of various groups and societies has led to the development of medical sociology as an important substantive area within the general field of sociology. As an academic discipline, sociology is concerned with the social causes and consequences of human behaviour; thus it follows that medical sociology is concerned with the social causes and consequences of health and illness. Medical sociology brings sociological perspectives, theories and methods to the study of health and medical practice. Major areas of investigation include the social facets of health and disease, the social behaviour of health care personnel and people who utilize health care, the social functions of health organizations and institutions, the social pattern of health services, and relationship of health care delivery systems to other systems.

## Difference between Sociology of Medicine and Sociology in Medicine

The relationship between social conditions and factors that influence health and the development of disease has long been a major interest of human kind. Throughout history people have generally tended to view health problems from the perspective of their own particular societies and cultures. As a result, they have usually responded to the threat of disease in predictable ways. Knowledge about norms, values, beliefs, social structures and lifestyles has provided insight not only about the social organization of human resources designed to cope with health hazards, but also about the nature and causes of illness. The recognition therefore, of the significance of the complex relationship between social factors and the level of health characteristic of specific social groups has led to the development of medical sociology as an important substantive area within the general field of sociology. As an academic discipline, sociology is concerned with the function, structure, and the roles of social institutions and social processes and with the social behaviour of persons and groups. Thus, it follows that medical sociology is concerned with the social facets of health and illness, the social functions of health institutions and organizations, the relationship of systems of health care delivery to other social systems, and the social behaviour of health personnel and those people who are consumers of health care.

Robert Straus (1957) has made a significant observation about medical sociology that helps to explain its current orientation. Straus suggested that medical sociology was divided into two separate but closely interrelated areas: 'sociology in medicine' and 'sociology of medicine'.

The sociologist in medicine is a sociologist who collaborates directly with the physician and other health personnel in studying the social factors that are relevant to a particular health disorder. The work of the sociologist in medicine is intended to be directly applicable to patient care or to the solving of a health problem. Some of the tasks of the sociologist in medicine are to analyse the etiology or causes of health disorders, the differences in social attitudes as they relate to health, and the way in which the incidence and prevalence of a specific health disorder is related to such social variables as age, sex, socio-economic status, racial/ethnic group identity, education, and occupation. Such an analysis is then intended to be made available to health practitioners to assist them in treating health problems. Thus, sociology in medicine can be characterized as applied research and analysis primarily motivated by a medical problem rather than a sociological problem. Sociologists in medicine usually work in medical schools, nursing schools, health schools, teaching hospitals, health agencies and other health organizations. They may also work for a governmental agency like the US Department of Health, Education and Welfare in the capacity of bio-statisticians, health planners, administrators and advisers.

The 'sociology of medicine', on the other hand, has a different emphasis. It deals with such factors as the organization, role relationship, norms, values, and beliefs of medical practice as a form of human behaviour. The emphasis is upon the social processes that occur in the medical setting and how these contribute to our understanding of medical sociology in particular and to our understanding of social life in general. With few exceptions, there no unique or special theories that pertain exclusively to the sociology of medicine; instead, the sociology of medicine shares the same goals as all other areas of sociology and may consequently be characterized as research and analysis of the medical environment from a sociological perspective. Although some sociologists of medicine are employed in health institutions, the majority work as professors in the sociology departments of universities and colleges.

## Historical Background of Health and Illness

The study of health and illness within society is not revolutionary, and neither is its research a new feat. Humans have long sought after advice from those with the knowledge or skill in healing. Paleopathology historical records allow an examination of how ancient societies dealt with illness and outbreak. Rulers in Ancient Egypt sponsored physicians that were specialists in specific diseases. Imhotep was the first medical doctor known by name. An Egyptian who lived around 2650 BC, he was an adviser to King Zoser at a time when Egyptians were making progress in medicine. Among his contributions to medicine was a textbook on the treatment of wounds, broken bones, and even tumours.

Stopping the spread of infectious disease was of utmost importance for maintaining a healthy society. The outbreak of disease during the Peloponnesian War was recorded by Thucydides who survived the epidemic. From his account it is shown how factors outside the disease itself can have an impact on society. The Athenians were under siege and concentrated within the city. Major city centres were the hardest hit. This made the outbreak even more deadly and with probable food shortages the fate of Athens was inevitable. Approximately 25 per cent of the population died of the disease. Thucydides stated that the epidemic 'carried away all alike'. The disease attacked people of different ages, sexes and nationalities.

Ancient medical systems stressed the importance of reducing illness through divination and ritual. Other codes of behaviour and dietary protocols were widespread in the ancient world. During the Zhou Dynasty in China, doctors suggested exercise, meditation and temperance to preserve one's health. The Chinese closely link health with spiritual well-being. Health regimes in ancient India focused on oral health as the best method for a healthy life. The Talmudic code created rules for health which stressed ritual cleanliness, connected disease with certain animals and created diets. Other examples include the Mosaic Code and Roman baths and aqueducts.

Those that were most concerned with health, sanitation and illness in the ancient world were those in the elite class. Good health was thought to reduce the risk of spiritual defilement and, therefore, enhanced the social status of the ruling class who saw themselves as the beacon of civilization. During the late Roman Period, sanitation for the lower classes was a concern for the leisured class. Those that had the means would donate to charities that focused on the health of non-elites. After the decline of the Roman Empire, physicians and concern with public health disappeared except in the largest cities. Health and public doctors remained in the Byzantine Empire focusing on preventing the spread of diseases such as small pox that lead to a smaller mortality rate in much of the Western World. Other factors that allowed the modern rise in population includes: better nutrition and environmental reforms (such as getting clean water supplies).

The present-day sense of health being a public concern for the state began in the middle ages. A few state interventions include maintaining clean towns, enforcing quarantines during epidemics and supervising sewer systems. Private corporations also played a role in public health. The funding for research and the institutions for them to work were funded by governments and private firms. Epidemics were the cause of most government interventions. The earlier goal of public health was reactionary, whereas the modern goal is to prevent disease before it becomes a problem. Despite the overall improvement of world health, there still has not been any decrease in the health gap between the affluent and the impoverished. Today, society is more likely to blame health issues on the individual rather than on society as a whole. This was the prevailing view in the late 20th century. In the 1980s, the Black Report, published in the United Kingdom, went against this view and argued that the true root of the problem was material deprivation. This report proposed a comprehensive anti-poverty strategy to address these issues. Since this did not parallel the views of England's conservative government, it did not go into action immediately. The Conservative government was criticized by the Labour Party for not implementing the suggestions that the Black Report listed. This criticism gave the Black Report the exposure it needed and its arguments were considered a valid explanation for health inequality. There is also a debate over whether poverty causes ill-health or if ill-health causes poverty. Arguments by the National Health Services gave considerable emphasis on poverty and lack of access to health care. It has also been found that heredity has more of a bearing on health than social environment, but research has also proved that there is indeed a positive correlation between socio-economic inequalities and illness.

### Historical Development of Medical Sociology

Medical sociology was established as a specialized field initially in the United States during the 1940s. The first use of the term 'medical sociology' has appeared as early as 1894 in an article by Charles McIntire on the importance of social factors in health. Other early work included essays on the relationship between medicine and society in 1902 by Elizabeth Blackwell, the first woman to graduate from medical school in America, and James Warbasse in 1909. However, these early publications were produced by people more concerned with medicine than sociology and it remained for Bernard Stern to publish the first work from a sociological perspective in 1927, titled *Social Factors in Medical Progress*. A few publications followed in the 1930s, such as Lawrence Henderson's 1935 paper on the physician and patient as a social system which subsequently influenced Talcott Parsons's conceptualization of the sick role; but it was not until after the World War II that medical sociology began in earnest as significant amounts of federal funding for socio-medical research became available.

Under the auspices of the National Institute of Mental Health, medical sociology's initial alliance with medicine was in psychiatry. A basis for cooperation between sociologists and psychiatrists existed because of earlier research in 1939 on urban mental health conducted in Chicago by Robert Faris and H. Warrne Dunham. A particularly significant cooperative effort that followed was the publication in 1958 of *Social Class and Mental Illness*, a community study by August Hollingshead and Frederic Redlich. This landmark research, conducted in New Haven, Connecticut, produced important evidence that social factors could be correlated with different types of mental disorders and the manner in which people received psychiatric care. Persons in the most socially and economically disadvantaged segments of society were found to have the highest rates of mental disorder in general and excessively high rates of schizophrenia, the most disabling mental illness in particular. This study attracted international attention and is the best known single study in the world of the relationship between mental disorder and social class. This book played a key role in the debate during the 1960s, leading to the establishment of community mental health centres in the United States, as did other significant joint projects involving sociologists and psychiatrists such as the midtown Manhattan study of Leo Srole and his colleagues (1962).

Funding from federal and private organizations also helped stimulate cooperation between sociologists and physicians in regard to socio-medical research on problems of physical health. The Russell Sage foundations funded a programme in 1949 to improve the utilization of social sciences research in medical practice. One result of this programme was the publication of Social Sciences in Medicine (Simmons and Wolff, 1954). Other work sponsored by the Sage

Foundation came late and included Edward Suchman's book *Sociology and the Field of Health* (1963). Thus, the direction of work in medical sociology in the United States when large scale funding first became available was towards applied or practical problem solving, rather than the development of theory.

This situation had important consequences for the development of medical sociology. Unlike law, religion, politics, economics and other social institutions, medicine was ignored by sociology's founders in the late nineteenth century because it did not shape the structure and nature of society. Emile Durkheim (1951) analysed European suicide rates in 1897 and Karl Mark's collaborator Fredrich Engels (1973) linked the poor health of the English working class to capitalism in a treatise published in 1845. However, Durkheim, Marx, Max Weber, and other major classical theorists did not concern themselves with the role of medicine in society. Medical sociology did not begin until after World War II, nor achieve any significant development until the 1960s. The field, therefore, developed relatively late in the evolution of sociology as and academic subject and lacked major statements on health and illness from the classical theorists. Consequently, medical sociology came of age in an intellectual climate far different from sociology's more traditional specialties with direct roots in nineteenth and early twentieth century social thought. As a result, it faces a set of circumstances in its development different from that of most other major sociological subdisciplines.

The circumstances that most affects medical sociology is the pressure to produce work that can be applied to medical practice and the formulation of health policy. This pressure originates from government agencies and medical sources, both of which either influence or control funding for socio-medical research and have little or no interest in purely theoretical sociology.

Yet the tremendous growth of medical sociology in both the United Stats and Europe in recent years most likely would not have been possible without the substantial financial support for applied studies provided by the respective governments. For example, in the United States, where medical sociology has reached its most extensive development, the emergence of the field was greatly stimulated by the expansion of the National Institutes of Health in the late 1940s. Particularly significant, according to Hollingshead (1973), who participated in some of the early research programmes, was the establishment of the National Institute of Mental Health, which was instrumental in encouraging and funding joint social and medial projects. 'it was through the impetus provided by this injection of money', notes Malcolm Johnson (1975), 'that sociologists and medical men changed their affiliation and embraced the field of medical sociology'. When Alvin Gouldner (1970) discussed the social sciences as a well financed government effort to help cope with the problems of industrial society and the welfare state in the West during the post World War II era, the prototype social science in this regard was medical sociology.

## Sociological Methods in Health

Methodological concerns are critical to sociological research. The great debate in sociology has been on the relative merits and role of quantitative versus qualitative approaches. Both approaches are widely used and play a critical role for health. Sociology has long recognized that the social world comprises both an objective and a subjective reality. For example, the objective reality of having cancer is accompanied by the subjective reality of the experience of cancer by the patient, and the patient's family and friends. Both realities are relevant to the sociological approach. The subjective, qualitative approach is generally discussed in the theory and methods concerned with illness behaviour, but qualitative approaches are equally applicable to the understanding of social policy, world systems, and areas of sociology where statistical measurement is difficult or less relevant.

Within health, surveillance is seen as a key approach to describing the distribution and dynamics of disease. In sociological approaches to health, the role of social and behavioural factors in health and illness is central. Survey methodology has occupied a central place in sociological research since the middle of the twentieth century. The concern has been with the collection, management, analysis, interpretation, and use of large quantities of data obtained by direct interview with respondents. Social surveys are characterized by large random samples, complicated questionnaires and the use of multivariate statistics for analysis. By their very nature, most sociological variables are complex to measure and to analyse. For example, the assessment of socio-economic status of an individual requires the accurate measurement of several variables that sit within a larger social context. Socio-economic status (SES) is regarded as a product of several components, including income, residence, education, and occupation. Determining the relative weight of each of these components is a major analytical problem. Thus, when considering the role of socio-economic status on health care outcomes, there is no easy answer to what mechanism actually works to determine the observed relationship between SES and health.

The Sociology of Health and Illness looks at three areas: the conceptualization, the study of measurement and social distribution, and the justification of patterns in health and illness. By looking at these things researchers can look at different diseases through a sociological lens. The prevalence and response to different diseases varies by culture. By looking at bad health, researchers can see if health affects different social regulations or controls. When measuring the distribution of health and illness, it is useful to look at official statistics and community surveys. Official statistics make it possible to look at people who have been treated. It shows that they are both willing and able to use health services. It also sheds light on the infected person's view of their illness. On the other hand, community surveys look at people's rating of their health. Then, looking at the relation of clinically defined illness and self reports and find that there is often a discrepancy.

A great deal of the time, mortality statistics take the place of morbidity statistics because in many developed societies where people typically die from degenerative conditions, the age in which they die sheds more light on their life-time health. This produces many limitations when looking at the pattern of sickness, but sociologists try to look at various data to analyse the distribution better. Normally, developing societies have lower life-expectancies in comparison to developed countries. They have also found correlations between mortality and sex and age. Very young and old people are more susceptible to sickness and death. On an average, women typically live longer than men, although women are more likely to have bad health.

Disparities in health were also found between people in different social classes and ethnicities within the same society, even though in the medical profession they put more importance in 'health related behaviours' such as alcohol consumption, smoking, diet, and exercise. There is a great deal of data supporting the conclusion that these behaviours affect health more significantly than other factors. Sociologists think that it is more helpful to look at health and illness through a broad lens. Sociologists agree that alcohol consumption, smoking, diet, and exercise are important issues, but they also see the importance of analysing the cultural factors that affect these patterns. Sociologists also look at the effects that the productive process has on health and illness while also looking at things such as industrial pollution, environmental pollution, accidents at work, and stress-related diseases.

Social factors play a significant role in developing health and illness. Studies of epidemiology show that autonomy and control in the workplace are vital factors in the etiology of heart disease. One cause is an effort – reward imbalance. Decreasing career advancement opportunities and major imbalances in control over work have been coupled with various negative health costs. Various studies have shown that pension rights may shed light on mortality differences between retired men and women of different socio-economic statuses. These studies show that there are outside factors that influence health and illness.

## Practical Application versus Theory

The direction taken by medical sociology early in its development is best summarized by Robert Straus (1957). Straus suggested that medical sociology had become divided into two separate but closely interrelated areas: sociology in medicine and sociology of medicine.

The sociologist in medicine is a sociologist who collaborates directly with the physician and other health personnel in studying the social factors that are relevant to a particular health disorder. The work of the sociologist in medicine is intended to be directly applicable to patient care or to the solving of a pubic health problem. Some of the tasks of the sociologist in medicine are to analyse the etiology or causes of health disorders, the differences in social attitudes as they relate to health, and the way in which the incidence and prevalence of a specific health disorder is related to such social variables as age, sex, socio-economic status, racial/ethnic group identity, education and occupation. Such an analysis is then intended to be made available to health practitioners to assist them in treating health problems. Sociologists in medicine usually work in medical schools, nursing schools, health schools, teaching hospitals, health agencies, and other health organizations. They may also work for a governmental agency like the US Department of Health and Human Services or the Centres for Disease Control and Prevention in the capacity of biostatisticians, health planners, administrators and advisers.

The sociology of medicine, on the other hand, has a different emphasis. It deals with such factors as the organization, role relationships, norms, values, and beliefs of medical practice as a form of human behaviour. The emphasis is on the social processes that occur in the medical setting and how these contribute to our understanding of medical sociology in particular and to our understanding of social life in general. The sociology of medicine shares the same goals as all other areas of sociology and may consequently be characterized as research and analysis of the medical environment from a sociological perspective. Most sociologists of medicine are employed as professors in the sociology departments of universities and colleges.

However, the division of work in medical sociology into a 'sociology of medicine' and 'sociology in medicine' eventually created problems. Medical sociologists affiliated with sociology departments in universities were in a stronger position to produce work that satisfied sociologists as good sociology. But sociologists in medical institutions had the advantage of participation in medicine as well as research opportunities unavailable to those outside medical practice. Tension began to develop between medical sociologists. First, an evolution has taken place in medical sociological work toward research relevant to health practitioners and policymakers. This development is largely due to the willingness of governmental agencies and private foundations to only fund health related research which can help solve problems or improve conditions. Regardless of whether a medical sociologists works in a health care or academic setting, most research in the field today deals with topics that have some practical utility.

Second, a growing convergence between medical sociology and the general discipline of sociology is emerging. This situation is aided by the fact that all sociologists share the same training and methodological strategies in their approach to research. Theoretical foundations common throughout sociology are also being increasingly reflected in medical sociological work, while many health issues investigated by medical sociologists call for knowledge of social processes outside of the socio-medical realm. For example, studies of health reform in the United States require consideration of the larger sociological literature on social change, power, the political process, socio-economic factors, and connections between social institutions and research on job-related stress demands familiarity with occupational structure. Therefore as Bernice Pescosolido and Jeanne Kronenfeld point out, medical sociologists need to understand the general nature of social change and social institutions to recognize, describe, and draw from these changes and institutions implications for health, illness and healing. Thus, much of the future success of medical sociology is linked to its ability to utilize the findings and perspectives of the larger discipline in its work and to contribute, in turn, to general sociology.

While the division of medical sociology as outlined by Straus (1957) is losing much of its distinctiveness in the United States, it never really developed elsewhere in the world. In Great Britain, Germany, and the Netherlands, where medical sociology has developed more extensively than elsewhere in Europe, the subdiscipline is concentrated in medical schools (Claus, 1982). In Japan, medical sociologists are found in both health institutions and sociology departments, but the majorities are faculty members in schools of medicine. A major difference worldwide in comparison to the past is that the field has achieved a state of development that allows it to investigate medical problems from an independent sociological perspective. Contemporary medical sociologists are less concerned with whether work is in the 'sociology of medicine' or 'sociology in medicine', but rather with how much it increases our understanding of the complex relationship between social factors and health.

At present, medical sociologists constitute the largest and one of the most active groups of people closing sociological work in the United States and Western Europe. Medical sociologists comprise the second largest section of the American Sociological Association and the largest sections of the British and German Sociological Associations. About one out of every ten American sociologists is a medical sociologist; in Germany, the German Society for Medical Sociology, an organization just for persons working in the field of medical sociology, has more members than the entire German Sociological Association. In Europe, medical sociologists have been identified in twenty-seven different countries (Claus, 1982), and this population provides the basis for the European Society for Health and Medical Sociology established in 1983. Earlier, in 1974, the Japanese Society for Health and Medical Sociology had been established (Sonoda, 1988). Not only have the numbers of medical sociologists continually increased, but as Rene Fox (1985) points out, the scope of matters pertinent to medical sociology has clearly broadened an issue of health, illness and medicines have become a medium through which general issues and concerns about society have been expressed. One result is that numerous books and scientific journals dealing with medical sociology have been and continue to be published in the United States and elsewhere. The future of medical sociology itself is very positive.

## Sociological Perspectives on Health and Illness

Sociology as a discipline developed from theoretical writings of the nineteenth century and the first half of the twentieth century. The predominant theories stem from the work of Karl Marx, Emile Durkheim, Max Weber, Talcott Parsons, Robert Merton and James Coleman. The influence of this rich theoretical foundation has manifested itself in major debates over the role of sociology as a science. European and American perspectives on sociology as a science differ, with the American perspective favouring sociology as a scientific discipline and emphasizing a more quantitative methodological approach than the European approach.

Several key concepts in sociology relate to its role in health. Foremost is the emphasis on society rather than the individual. The individual is viewed as an actor within larger social processes. This distinguishes the field from psychology. The emphasis is on units of analysis at the collective level, such as the family, the group, the neighbourhood, the city, the organization, the state and the world. Of key importance is how the social fabric, or social structure, is maintained and how social processes, such as conflict and resolution, relate to the maintenance and change of social structures. A sociologist studies processes that create, maintain and sustain a social system, such as a health care system in a particular country. The scientific component of this study would be the concern with the processes regulating and shaping the health care system. Sociology assumes that social structure and social processes are very complex. Therefore, its methodology is appropriately complex and often, particularly in American Sociology, dominated by multivariate statistical methods of analysis. The advent of the computer in the second half of the twentieth century presented the field with the opportunity to work with very large bodies of data and complex variables.

Health has been and remains a much applied field. It is also characterized by a population-based approach to health, and statistical methods are deemed the appropriate underlying method for the field. It is viewed as a science that seeks to intervene, control and prevent large-scale processes that negatively affect the public's health. By these criteria, there is a strong logical fit of sociological principles and practices within health. Nonetheless, sociology has not been the key social science discipline in health. That position has gone to psychology, where the emphasis on individual behaviour resonates more with a biomedical model. Despite this, many of the primary concerns of present-day health, with large-scale variables such as social capital, social inequality, social status, and health care organization and financing, remain topics best suited to the sociological perspective and methodology. The emphasis in health is thus shifting towards a sociological perspective.

The Sociology of Health and Illness examines the interaction between society and health. The objective of this topic is to see how social life has an impact on morbidity and mortality rate, and vice versa. This aspect of sociology differs from medical sociology in that this branch of sociology discusses health and illness in relation to social institutions such as family, employment, and school. The sociology of medicine limits its concern to the patient-practitioner relationship and the role of health professionals in society. The sociology of health and illness covers sociological pathology (causes of disease and illness), reasons for seeking particular types of medical aid, and patient compliance or non-compliance with medical regimes.

Health, or lack of health, was once merely attributed to biological or natural conditions. Sociologists have demonstrated that the spread of diseases is heavily influenced by the socio-economic status of individuals, ethnic traditions or beliefs, and other cultural factors. Where medical research might gather statistics on a disease, a sociological perspective on an illness would provide insight on what external factors caused the demographics that contracted the disease to become ill.

This topic requires a global approach of analysis because the influence of societal factors varies throughout the world. This will be demonstrated through discussion of the major diseases of each continent. These diseases are sociologically examined and compared, based on the traditional medicine, economics, religion and culture that is specific to each region. HIV/AIDS serves as a common basis of comparison among regions. While it is extremely problematic in certain areas, in others it has affected a relatively small percentage of the population. Sociological factors can help to explain why these discrepancies exist.

There are obvious differences in patterns of health and illness across societies, over time, and within particular society types. There has historically been a long-term decline in mortality within industrialized societies, and on average, life-expectancies are considerably higher in developed, rather than developing or undeveloped societies. Patterns of global change in health care systems make it more imperative than ever to research and comprehend the sociology of health and illness. Continuous changes in economy, therapy, technology and insurance can affect the way individual communities view and respond to the medical care available. These rapid fluctuations cause the issue of health and illness within social life to be very dynamic in definition. Advancing information is vital because as patterns evolve, the study of the sociology of health and illness constantly needs to be updated.

## International Outlook on Health and Illness

### *Africa*

HIV/AIDS is the leading epidemic that affects the social welfare of Africa. Human Immunodeficiency Virus (HIV) can cause AIDS which is an acronym for Acquired Immunodeficiency Syndrome (AIDS), a condition in humans in which the immune system begins to fail, leading to life-threatening infections. Two-thirds of the world's HIV population is located in Sub-Saharan Africa. Since the epidemic started, more than 15 million Africans have died by complications with HIV/AIDS.

People apart of religious subgroups of Sub-Saharan Africa and those who actively and frequently participate in religious activities are more likely to be at a lower risk of contracting HIV/AIDS. On the opposite end, there are many beliefs that an infected male can be cured of the infection, by having sex with a virgin. These beliefs increase the number of people with the virus and also increase the number of rapes against women.

Herbal treatment is one of the primary medicines used to treat HIV in Africa. It is used more than standard treatment because it is comparatively affordable. Herbal treatment is more affordable but is not researched and is poorly regulated. This lack of research on whether the herbal medicines work and what the medicines consist of is a major flaw in the healing cycle of HIV in Africa.

Economically, HIV is a heavy hitter in tearing down the economy. The labour force in Africa is slowly diminishing, due to HIV-related deaths and illness. In response, government's income declines and so does tax revenue. The government has to spend more money than it is making, in order to care for those affected with HIV/AIDS.

A major social problem in Africa with regard to HIV is the orphan epidemic. The orphan epidemic in Africa is a regional problem. In most cases, both of the parents are affected with HIV. Due to this, the children are usually raised by their grandmother and in extreme cases they are raised by themselves. In order to care for the sick parents the children have to take on more responsibility by working to produce an income. Not only do the children lose their parents but they also lose their childhood as well. Having to provide care for their parents the children also miss out on education which increases the risk of teen pregnancy and people affected with HIV. The most efficient way to diminish the orphan epidemic is prevention – preventing children from acquiring HIV from their mothers at birth, as well as educating them on the disease as they grow older. Also, educating adults about HIV and caring for the infected people adequately, will lower the orphan population.

The HIV/AIDS epidemic is reducing the average life expectancy of people in Africa by twenty years. The age ranges with the highest death rates, due to HIV, are those between the ages of 20 and 49 years. The fact that this age range is when adults acquire most of their income, they cannot afford to send their children to school, due to the high medication costs. It also removes the people who could give aid in responding to the epidemic.

### *Asia*

Asian countries have wide variations of population, wealth, technology and health care, causing attitudes towards health and illness to differ. Japan, for example, has the third highest life expectancy (82 years old), while Afghanistan has the 11th worst (44 years old). Key issues in Asian health include childbirth and maternal health, HIV and AIDS, mental health, and ageing and the elderly. These problems are influenced by the sociological factors of religion or belief systems, attempts to reconcile traditional medicinal practices with modern professionalism and the economic status of the inhabitants of Asia.

Like the rest of the world, Asia is threatened by a possible pandemic of HIV and AIDS. Vietnam is a good example of how society is shaping Asian HIV/AIDS awareness and attitudes towards this disease. Vietnam is a country with feudal, traditional roots, which, due to invasion, wars, technology and travel is becoming increasingly globalized. Globalization has altered traditional viewpoints and values. It is also responsible for the spread of HIV and AIDS in Vietnam. Even early globalization has added to this problem – Chinese influence made Vietnam a Confucian society, in which women are of less importance than men. Men in their superiority have no need to be sexually responsible, and women, generally not well educated, are often unaware of the risk, perpetuating the spread of HIV and AIDS as well as other STIs.

Confucianism has had a strong influence on the belief system in Asia for centuries, particularly in China, Japan, and Korea, and its influence can been seen in the way people chose to seek, or not seek, medical care. An important issue in Asia is societal impact on the ability of disabled individuals to adjust to a disability. Cultural beliefs shape attitudes towards physical and mental disabilities. China exemplifies this problem. According to Chinese Confucian tradition (which is also applicable in other countries where Confucianism has been spread), people should always pursue good health in their life, with an emphasis on health promotion and disease prevention. To the Chinese, having a disability signifies that you have not lead a proper lifestyle and, therefore, there is a lack of opportunities for disabled individuals to explore better ways to accept or adapt to their disability.

Indigenous healing practices are extremely diverse throughout Asia but often follow certain patterns and are still prevalent today. Many traditional healing practices include shamanism and herbal medicines, and may have been passed down orally in small groups or even institutionalized and professionalized. In many developing countries, the only health care available until a few decades ago were those based on traditional medicine and spiritual healing. Now, governments must be careful to create health policies that strike a balance between modernity and tradition. Organizations like the World Health Organization try to create policies that respects tradition without trying to replace it with modern science, instead regulating it to ensure safety but keeping it accessible. India, in particular, tries to make traditional medicines safe but still available to as many people as possible, adapting tradition to match modernization while still considering the economic positions and culture of its citizens.

Mental health issues are gaining an increasing amount of attention in Asian countries. Many of these countries have a preoccupation with modernizing and developing their economies, resulting in cultural changes. In order to reconcile modern techniques with traditional practices, social psychologists in India are in the process of 'indigenizing psychology'. Indigenous psychology is that which is derived from the laws, theories, principals, and ideas of a culture and unique to each society.

In many Asian countries, childbirth is still treated by traditional means and is thought of with regional attitudes. For example, in Pakistan, decisions concerning pregnancy and antenatal care (ANC) are usually made by older women, often the pregnant woman's mother-in-law, while the mother and father to be, are distanced from the process. They may or may not receive professional ANC depending on their education, class, and financial situation. Generally in Asia, childbirth is still a woman's area and male obstetricians are rare. Female midwives and healers are still the norm in most places. Western methods are overtaking the traditional in an attempt to improve maternal health and increase the number of live births.

Asian countries, which are mostly developing nations, are ageing rapidly even as they are attempting to build their economies. Even wealthy Asian nations, such as Japan, Singapore and Taiwan also have very elderly populations and thus have to try to sustain their economies and society with small younger generations while caring for their elderly citizens. The elderly have been traditionally well-respected and well cared for in most Asian cultures; experts predict that younger generations in the future are less likely to be concerned and involved in the health care of their older relatives due to various factors such as more women joining the workforce, the separation of families because of urbanization or migration and the proliferation of Western ideals such as individualism.

### *Australia*

The health patterns found on the continent of Australia, which includes the Pacific Islands, have been very much influenced by European colonization. While indigenous medicinal beliefs are not significantly prevalent in Australia, traditional ideas are still influential in the health care problems in many of the islands of the Pacific. The rapid urbanization of Australia led to epidemics of typhoid fever and the Bubonic plague. Because of this, public health was professionalized beginning in the late 1870s in an effort to control these and other diseases. Since then, Australia's health system has evolved similarly to Western countries and the main cultural influence affecting health care are the political ideologies of the parties in control of the government.

Australia has had treatment facilities for 'drinkers' problem since the 1870s. In the 1960s and 1970s it was recognized that Australia had several hundred thousand alcoholics and prevention became a priority over cures, as there was a societal consensus that treatments are generally ineffective. The government began passing laws attempting to curb alcohol consumption but consistently met opposition from the wine making regions of southern Australia. The government has also waged a war on illegal drugs, particularly heroin, which in the 1950s became widely used as a pain reliever.

Experts believe that many of the history of the Pacific Islands health problems can be traced to European colonization and the subsequent globalization and modernization of island communities. European colonization and late independence meant modernization but also slow economic growth, which had an enormous impact on health care, particularly on nutrition in the Pacific Islands. The end of colonization meant a loss of medical resources, and the fledgling independent governments could not afford to continue the health policies put in place by the colonial governments. Nutrition was changed radically, contributing to various other health problems. While more prosperous, urban areas could afford food, they chose poor diets, causing 'over nourishment', and leading to extremely high levels of obesity, type 2 diabetes, and cardiovascular diseases. Poorer rural communities, on the other hand, continue to suffer from malnutrition and malaria.

Traditional diets in the Pacific are very low in fat, but since World War II there has been a significant increase in fat and protein in Pacific diets. Unfortunately, native attitudes towards weight contribute to the obesity problem. Tongan natives see obesity as a positive thing, especially in men. They also believe that women should do as little physical work as possible while the men provide for them, which means they get very little exercise.

### *Europe*

The largest endeavour to improve health across Europe is the World Health Organization, European Region. The goal is to improve the health of poor and disadvantaged populations by promoting healthy lifestyles including environmental, economic, social and providing health care. Overall health in Europe is very high, compared to the rest of the world. The average life expectancy is around 78 years in EU countries but there is a wide gap between Western and Eastern Europe. It is as low as 67 in Russia and 73 in the Balkan states. Europe is seeing an increase in the spread of HIV/AIDS in Eastern Europe because of a worsening socio-economic situation. Cardiovascular disease, cancer and diabetes mellitus are more prevalent is Eastern Europe. The WHO claims that poverty is the most important factor bringing on ill-health across Europe. Those at low socio-economic status levels and many young people are also at risk because of their increased tobacco, alcohol and drug abuse. Health and illness prevention in Europe is largely funded by governmental services including: regulating health care, insurance and social programmes. The role of religion and traditional medicine are harder to examine because no where in the report are the words religion or healing.

The study of hypertension within the United Kingdom has turned to examining the role that beliefs play in its diagnosis and treatment. Hypertension is an essential topic for study since it is linked to increased risk of stroke and coronary heart disease. The most common treatment for hypertension is medication, but compliance for this treatment plan is low. A study conducted in the UK examined the differences between 'white' patients and first generation immigrants from the West Indies. There were differing reasons for non-compliance that involve the patient's perception and beliefs about the diagnosis. Patients commonly believe that high levels of anxiety when first diagnosed are the major cause and think that when stress levels decline, so too will their hypertensions. Other respondents in this UK-based study had varying beliefs concerning the necessity of medication while others still argued that it was the side effects of medication that made them end their prescribed regimen. West Indian respondents whose lay culture teaches them to reject long-term drug therapy, opted instead for folk remedies in higher numbers than the 'white' respondents. What can be seen here is that some people will choose to ignore a doctor's expert advice and will employ 'lay consultation' instead.

Before people seek medical help they try to interpret the symptoms themselves and often consult people in their lives or use 'self-help' measures. A study of 'everyday illness' in Finland including: influenza, infections and musculo-skeletal problems focused on reasons for consulting medical experts and explanations of illness. These common illnesses were examined not because of their seriousness but because of their frequency. The researchers explain 5 possible triggers that people seek medical aid: (1) the occurrence of an interpersonal crisis (2) perceived interference with social and personal relations (3) perceived interference with vocational and physical activity (4) sanctioning by other people (5) sufferers ideas about how long certain complaints should last. These kinds of explanatory models are part of the process that people use to construct medical culture. They give meaning to illness and health, answer questions about personal responsibility about health and most importantly are part of the dialogue between patients' and professionals' illness explanations. It can help explore why some patients will follow a doctors instructions to the letter and others ignore them completely. A patient's explanation or understanding of their illness can be much broader than a physician's and this dynamic has become a major criticism of modern medical practice since it normally excludes the 'social, psychological and experiential dimensions of illness'.

The Finnish study examined 127 patients and the results have been different from findings in other countries where there is more 'lay consultation'. Half of the respondents did not have any lay consultation before coming to the doctor's office. One-third did not try any self-treatment and three-quarters of the sample consulted the doctor within three days of symptoms developing. Possible explanations are that in Finland there is an avid 'over-protectiveness' within their health care system. Many might conclude that the Finnish people are dependent and helpless but the researchers of this study found that people chose to consult professionals because they trusted them over some lay explanation. These results echo similar studies in Ireland that explain this phenomenon as being based in a strong work ethics. Illness in these countries will affect their work and Finnish people will quickly get treatment so they can return to work. This interesting research out of Finland also describes that this relationship between patient and doctor is based on: (1) national and municipal administrative bureaucracies that demand more output and more satisfied patients, (2) the public demanding better care, (3) nurses criticizing physicians for not taking a holistic view of patients and (4) hospital specialists wanting better/earlier screening for serious illnesses (e.g. cancer).

The conflict between medical and lay worlds is prominent. On one hand many patients believe they are the experts of their own body and view the Doctor-patient relationship as authoritarian. These people will often use knowledge outside the medical field to deal with health and illness. Others, see the doctor as the expert and are shy about describing their symptoms and, therefore, rely on the doctor for diagnosis and treatment.

### North America

North America is a fairly recent settled continent, made up of the United States, Canada, Mexico, Central America and the Caribbean. It was built by an amalgamation of wealth, ideas, culture and practices. North America is highly advanced intellectually, technologically and traditionally. This advantageous character of North American nations has caused a high average life expectancy of 75 years for males and 80 years for females. This leads to the conclusion that North America has cultivated a comparatively healthy society. As North America contains several core nations, the growing economies in those nations are able to maintain and develop medical institutions. This, subsequently provides more access to health care for American citizens but health care is not universal. North America is known for being a leading nation in regard to industrialization and modernization, but the United States still lacks federal laws regarding health care as a right. This lag of health care security causes subsequent issues with pharmaceutical competition, lack of care for the elderly and little attention to alternative medicine. Health care and education are plentiful at a price and illness still persists for many reasons. A main reason being that a lower- and middle-class population still exists in plentiful, maintaining a group that is highly vulnerable to physical ailment.

North America's primary risk factors for illness are currently alcohol abuse, malnutrition, obesity, tobacco use and water sanitation. Obesity is a recent pandemic in North America. The 1990s brought a rise in the average Body Mass Index, or BMI. From the beginning and to the end of the decade, the median percentage of adults who were obese went from 12 per cent to 20 per cent. This may be because of the materialistic and individualistic character of North America. Alcoholism is the addiction of overconsumption of alcohol and is highly prevalent in the US. There are high incidence rates in many other world regions. Roughly 61 per cent of American adults drank in 2007, and 21 per cent of current drinkers consumed 5 or more drinks at one point in the last year. There have also been 22,073 alcohol induced deaths in the United States in the past year with about 13,000 of them related to liver disease. Alcoholism has many risk factors ingrained in North American culture, such as heredity, stress from competition or availability. The ideological individualism and the competitive capitalism may play a part in increased risk of alcohol abuse as well.

The Swine Flu (also known as (H1N1) epidemic is a recent disease emerging in the early 21st century. Its origins were traced back to Mexico from where it rapidly infected the rest of North America. In April 2009, during the early days of the outbreak, a molecular biologist name Dr Henry Miller wrote in the *Wall Street Journal* about New York City's high-school students. These students apparently brought the virus back from Mexico and infected their classmates. All six cases so far reported in Canada were connected directly or indirectly with travel to Mexico as well. Flu viruses can be directly transmitted (via droplets from sneezing or coughing) from pigs to people, and vice versa. These cross-species infections occur most commonly when people are in close proximity to large numbers of pigs, such as in barns, livestock exhibits at fairs and slaughterhouses. The flu is transmissible from human to human, either directly or via contaminated surfaces.

### *South America*

There is a laundry list of diseases that affect South America, but two of the major conditions are Malaria and Hepatitis D. Malaria affects every country in South America except: Uruguay, Chile. The Falkland Islands also are not affected by malaria. Elevation has a key influence on areas where Malaria is found. The disease is spread from person to person via mosquito bites. People are typically bitten by mosquitoes in the dusk or dawn. Symptoms of this disorder are: high fever, chills, sweating, headaches, body aches, weakness, vomiting and diarrhea. New symptoms can develop if Malaria worsens; people who are infected may experience seizures, delirium and coma. Severe cases may end in death. Malaria can be cured, but the symptoms may not become noticeable until months later. There are three forms of medication that will help cure Malaria. An infected person's accessibility is dependent on if the person has the money or proper doctors to help them with the matter. Literature about Malaria treatment typically is focused towards people who are tourists. They have a more lighthearted tone because typically, tourist have access to doctors so they can get the proper care to overcome the disease, however, this does not account for the health of the natives.

The first sign of Hepatitis D was detected in 1978 when a strange and unrecognizable internuclear antigen was discovered during a liver biopsy of several Italians who suffered HBV infection. Scientists initially thought that it was an antigenic specificity of HBV, but they soon found that it was a protein from another disease altogether. They called it 'Hepatitis Delta Virus'. This new virus was found to be defective. HDV needed HBV to act as a helper function in order for it to be detected. Normally, Hepatitis B is transmitted through blood or any type of blood product. In South America Hepatitis D was found to be fatal. Scientist are still unsure in what way this disease was being transmitted throughout certain South American countries. Sexual contact and Drug use are the most common means of transmission. HDV is still considered an unusual form of hepatitis. Agents of this virus resemble that of plant viroids. It is still hard to tell how many stereotypes exist because HDV is under the umbrella of HBV. HDV causes very high titers in the blood of people whom are infected.

Incubation of Hepatitis D typically lasts for thirty five days. Most often Hepatitis D is a co-infection with Hepatitis B or a super-infection with chronic hepatitis. In terms of super infections there are high mortality rates, ranging seventy to eighty per cent; in contrast with co-infections which have a one to three per cent mortality rate. There is little information with the ecology of Hepatitis D. Epidemics have been found in Venezuela, Peru, Columbia, and Brazil. People who are treated for Hepatitis B have been able to control Hepatitis D. People whom have chronic HDB will continue to get HDV.

Another disease that affects South America is HIV along with AIDS. In 2008, roughly two million people had HIV and AIDS. By the end of 2008 one hundred and seventy thousand people were infected with AIDS and HIV. Seventy-seven thousand people died from this disease by the end of that year. Brazil has the most people that are affected with AIDS and HIV in South America. Forty-three per cent of people in Brazil have HIV. In Brazil sixty per cent of the inhabitants use drugs, are HIV positive, and are HIV positive because of their drug use. Usually, this disease is transmitted by either drug use involving needles or men having sex with other men unprotected. Unprotected sex between two men is the most common. Roughly twenty-five to thirty-three per cent of these men also have sex with women and in turn infect them also. Sharing needles and being infected with HIV and AIDS is most common in Paraguay and Uruguay. South America is trying to get treatment to the thousands of people infected by this disease. Brazil is offering generic AIDS prescriptions that are much less expensive than the name brand drugs. One hundred and eighty-one thousand of inhabitants in Brazil whom were infected are being treated. That accounts for eighty per cent of those who needed immediate help. This aid from the government has had positive results. Statistics show that there was a fifty per cent decrease in mortality rates, approximately sixty to eighty per cent decrease in morbidity rates and a seventy per cent decrease in hospitalization of infected people.

In very remote areas of South America traditional healers are the only forms of health care people have. In north Aymara and south Mapuche, where the indigenous groups have the strongest voices they still heavily use traditional medicine. The government in Chile has implemented an Indigenous Health System to help strengthen the health care system. Even with Chile's indigenous groups, Chile still has the best public health services in South America. They also have the lowest mortality rates in the area. Their health care policies are centred on family and community well-being by focusing on the strategies for prevention health strategies. Reports have shown an increase in mental health issues, diabetes and cardiovascular diseases.

South America's economy is developing rapidly and has a great deal of industries. There major industry in South America is agriculture. Other industries are fishing, handicrafts and natural resources. Its trade and import/export market is continually thriving. In the past, South American countries moved slowly in regard to economic development. South America began to build their economy ever since World War II. South America largest economies are Brazil, Chile, Argentina, and Columbia. Venezuela, Peru and Argentina's economy are growing very rapidly.

### Sociological Concepts in Health

Sociology in health is reflected in the myriad of sociological concepts that pervade the practice of health. More than any other social science, sociology has the discussion of socio-economic status at its very core. Social class variation within society is the key explanatory variable in sociology – for everything from variation in social structure to differential life experiences of health and illness. Indeed, there appears to be overwhelming evidence that Western industrialized societies that have little variation in social class experience have far better health outcomes than societies characterized by wide social class dispersion. In short, inequalities in health are directly related to social and economic inequalities. Much of later twentieth-century health is devoted to the reduction of these inequalities.

There is limited opportunity to intervene rapidly, directly, or simply because many sociological variables are at the so-called macro level, For example, the socio-economic status (SES) of a group is affected by complex components, such as education and occupation that are part of the total life course of individuals within the group. Thus, to change the SES of a group would require significant redistribution of resources of the larger social structure. A significant period of time and concerted effort is needed to change such macro variables. This is, however, not dissimilar to many other challenges in health, such as the long-term and time-consuming effort to change lifestyles and reduce behavioural risk factors related to chronic diseases.

The chief role of sociology in health remains its evaluation of those macro components of society that affect health at the population level. Such evaluations provide an understanding of why inequalities in health exist, and they help elaborate upon the mechanisms and processes that sustain these inequalities. This relates to the long-standing theoretical concern with social structure among sociologists. Further, sociology reveals the mechanisms for long-term changes that may lead to a reduction in health inequalities. The product of sociological thinking in health is not immediate or easily understood by those who seek quick and easy solutions to the suffering of humanity. Nonetheless, the long-term role of sociology in health is to change and improve the health.

### The Sick Role and Illness

The Sick Role was a concept invented by Talcott Parsons in 1951. Parsons was a functionalist sociologist, who argued that being sick means that the sufferer enters a role of 'sanctioned deviance'. This is because, from a functionalist perspective, when you are ill you are not being a productive member of society. Therefore, this deviance needs to be policed, which is the role of the medical profession.

The Sick Role is a term widely used in medical sociology concerning the social aspects of falling ill. The general idea is that the individual who has fallen ill is not only physically sick, but now adheres to the specifically patterned social role of being sick. 'Being Sick' is not simply a 'state of fact' or 'condition', it contains within itself customary rights and obligations based on the social norms that surround it. Sociologists conceptualize social roles as the expected behaviours (including rights and obligations) of someone with a given position (status) in society. Generally, people hold a status (position) and perform a role (behaviours).

Parsons (1951) utilized these concepts to construct a theoretical view of individuals who are sick, hence the 'sick role'. This theory outlines two rights and two obligations of individuals who become sick in our society

The theory outlined two rights of a sick person and two obligations:

#### *Rights*

- *The sick person is exempt from 'normal' social roles:* An individual's illness is grounds for his or her exemption from normal role performance and social responsibilities. This exemption, however, is relative to the nature and severity of the illness. The more severe the illness, the greater the exemption. Exemption requires legitimation by the physician as the authority on what constitutes sickness.

Legitimation serves the social function of protecting society against malingering (attempting to remain in the sick role longer than social expectations allow – usually done to acquire secondary gains or additional privileges afforded to ill persons).

- *The sick person is not responsible for his or her condition:* An individual's illness is usually thought to be beyond his or her own control. A morbid condition of the body needs to be changed and some curative process apart from person's will power or motivation is needed to get well.

### *Obligations*

- *The sick person should try to get well:* The first two aspects of the sick role are conditional upon the third aspect, which is recognition by the sick person that being sick is undesirable. Exemption from normal responsibilities is temporary and conditional upon the desire to regain normal health. Thus, the sick person has an obligation to get well.
- *The sick person should seek technically competent help and cooperate with the physician:* The obligation to get well involves a further obligation on the part of the sick person to seek technically competent help, usually from a physician. The sick person is also expected to cooperate with the physician in the process of trying to get well.

Although this concept presents some flaws, it is a valuable contribution to understanding illness behaviours and social perceptions of sickness. (It is perhaps best considered an ideal type – a general statement about social phenomena that highlights patterns of 'typical'.) We discussed a number of criticisms of Sick Role theory, including: a violation in the 'ability to get well' for a number of conditions (particularly chronic illnesses); individuals or groups may not possess the resources to 'seek technically competent help' or to 'cooperate with the physician' based upon health insurance, income, role conflicts to compliance, etc.; certain illnesses may reflect an element of personal 'blame' due to unhealthy lifestyle choices (i.e. smoking leads to emphysema); the potential inability to be 'exempt from normal social roles' due to issues of status (i.e. parent), income (need to work), gender, age, etc.

*Sick-Role Behaviour and Illness:* Generally, health-related behaviours of healthy people and those who try to maintain their health are considered as behaviours related to primary prevention of disease. Such behaviours are intended to reduce susceptibility to disease, as well as to reduce the effects of chronic diseases when they occur in the individual. Secondary prevention of disease is more closely related to the control of a disease that an individual has or that is incipient in the individual. This type of prevention is most closely tied to illness behaviour. Tertiary prevention is generally seen as directed towards reducing the impact and progression of symptomatic disease in the individual. This type of prevention is highly related to the concept of sick-role behaviour. In general, illness and sick-role behaviours are viewed as characteristics of individuals and as concepts derived from sociological and socio-psychological theories.

*Sick-Role Behaviour*: The 'sick-role' is a concept arising from the work of the important American sociologist Talcott Parsons (1902–1979). Parsons was a structural functionalist who argued that social practices should be seen in terms of their function in maintaining order or structure in society. Thus, Parsons was concerned with understanding how the sick person related to the whole social system, and what the person's function is in that system. Ultimately, the sick role and sick-role behaviour could be seen as the logical extension of illness behaviour to complete integration into the medical care system. Parsons' argument is that sick-role behaviour accepts the symptomatology and diagnosis of the established medical care system, and thus allows the individual to take on behaviours compliant with the expectations of the medical system. Basically, Parsons defined the 'sick role' as having four chief characteristics. First, the sick person is freed or exempt from carrying out normal social roles. The more severe the illness, the more one is freed from normal social roles. Everyone in society experiences this; for example, a minor chest cold 'allows' one to be excused from small obligations such as attending a social gathering. By contrast, a major heart attack 'allows' considerable time away from work and social obligations. Second, people in the sick role are not directly responsible for their plight. Third, the sick person needs to try to get well. The sick role is regarded as a temporary stage of deviance that should not be prolonged at all if possible. Finally, in the sick role the sick person or patient must seek competent help and cooperate with medical care to get well. This conceptual schema implies many reciprocal relations between the sick person (the patient), and the healer (the physician). Thus, the function of the physician is one of social control.

The complicated theoretical explanations of Parsons, yielded a voluminous research literature in the second half of the twentieth century, and they continue to stimulate much research today. In particular, there has been much study of the norms and values that define the behaviours of both the sick and those providing treatment. These studies form the basis for present-day research on the patient-physician relationship. They inform the various strategies undertaken by behavioural scientists to intervene in this relationship to bring about positive behavioural changes in both patient and practitioner that will lead to better health outcomes.

There are many research issues attendant to understanding this complicated relationship between patient and practitioner. One paramount issue is that of the differential power of the participants in the relationship. According to this view, the superior power of the physician, in terms of technical expertise and status, will more effectively induce the patient toward a positive medical outcome. It is this superior power that helps make possible the often painful procedures to which the patient concedes.

*Illness Behaviour:* The concept of illness behaviour was largely defined and adopted during the second half of the twentieth century. Broadly speaking, it is any behaviour undertaken by an individual who feels ill to relieve that experience or to better define the meaning of the illness experience. There are many different types of illness behaviour that have been studied. Some individuals who experience physical or mental symptoms turn to the medical care system for help; some may turn to self-help strategies; while others may decide to dismiss the symptoms. In everyday life, illness behaviour may be a mixture of behavioural decisions. For example, an individual faced with recurring symptoms of joint pain may turn to complementary or alternative medicine for relief. However, sudden, sharp and debilitating symptoms may lead one directly to a hospital emergency room. In any event, illness behaviour is usually mediated by strong subjective interpretations of the meaning of symptoms. As with any type of human behaviour, many social and psychological factors intervene and determine the type of illness behaviour expressed in the individual.

Considerable research exists showing the importance of age and gender in illness behaviour. Illness behaviour, as shown in the use of medical services, is far greater in women. Many studies have linked illness-behaviour variation to ethnicity, education, family structure and social networks. Illness behaviour is also shown to be related to health care coverage and insurance. Most importantly, illness behaviour is highly related to socio-economic status. Classic studies done in the 1950s, powerfully demonstrated that socio-economic class influenced how symptoms were acted on, with lower-class individuals (lower in socio-economic status) most likely to delay seeking professional health care even when presented with severe symptoms.

While much of the early work on illness behaviour was seen in the context of understanding patient's help-seeking behaviour, the large research literature on illness behaviour has gone well beyond this more narrow medicalized view. Many studies have considered the different perspectives of illness behaviour held by individuals and health care practitioners. The differing world-views of patients and practitioners are now seen as highly relevant to illness behaviour. The medical practitioner and the individual experiencing symptoms go through very different appraisals of the meaning of the symptoms. Increasingly in the literature, there is the recognition of the strong relationship between the physical and mental experience of symptoms and the meaning of that experience for illness behaviour. David Mechanic, a pioneer in the study of illness behaviour, best summarizes the current perspective on illness behaviour: 'Illness behaviours arise from complex causes, including biological predispositions, the nature of symptomatology, learned patterns of response, attributional predispositions, situational influences, and the organization and incentives characteristic of the health care system that affect access, responsiveness and the availability of secondary benefits' (Mechanic, 1994).

### *Concept of Sick-Role and Illness Behaviour in Public Health*

In present-day public health practice, which is based on population and community-based approaches with an emphasis on participation, the research from these concepts of behaviour has helped immensely in clarifying critical approaches to public health. The concept of diversity in populations has been greatly enhanced through the articulation of the concepts of illness behaviour and the sick role. Researchers now have a significant body of research showing the wide variation in these behaviours with respect to all the key demographic variables. For example, there has been excellent work showing how the presentation of symptoms to a physician is highly dependent on gender, ethnic background and other socio-cultural characteristics. Research on the sick-role concept has elucidated the issue of power and its many manifestations in doctors' offices, hospitals and other medical settings. It would be difficult, given this literature, for a practicing health educator not to consider the role of power in patient-physician interactions.

Present-day health education has also been heavily influenced by the research on illness and sick-role behaviour. These concepts have helped inform part of the scientific basis for the educational and environmental approach to health promotion planning elucidated by L.W. Green and M.W. Kreuter in their widely used *recedeproceed* model. At the same time, the conceptual components of illness and sick-role behaviour continue to be explored in narrative analyses of the written and spoken traditions of peoples to describe their experiences of illness and sickness.

# 2

# Health, Society and Education

Medical sociology is concerned with individual and group responses aimed at assessing well-being, maintaining health, acting upon real or perceived illness, interacting with health care systems and maximizing health in the face of physiologic or functional derangement. It also analyses the impact of the psychological conditions resulting from our environment on our health. Medical sociology includes the study of medical professional, as well as the study of and human behavioural responses to health and illness

Health care is a prevention, treatment and management of illness, and the preservation of health through services offered by the medical, dental, nursing and allied health professions. Health care embraces all the goods and services designed to promote health, including 'preventive, curative and palliative interventions, whether directed to individuals or to populations'. The organized provision of such services may constitute a health care system. This can include specific governmental organizations such as, in the UK, the National Health Service or cooperation across the National Health Service and Social Services as in Shared Care. Before the term health care became popular, English-speakers referred to medicine or to the health sector and spoke of the treatment and prevention of illness and disease.

## Emerging Relationship between Medicine and Sociology

Good health is prerequisite for the adequate functioning of any individual or society. If our health is sound we can engage in numerous types of activities. But if we are ill or injured, we may face the curtailment of our usual round of daily life and we may also become so preoccupied with our state of health that other pursuits are of secondary importance or quite meaningless. Obviously, nobody likes to feel unequal to his or her daily schedule. This natural concern with the healthy functioning of our bodies has probably been with us throughout our existence on this planet. Rene DuBos has suggested in *Man, Medicine and Environment* (1969) that primitive human beings were closer to the animals, in that they too relied upon their instincts to stay healthy. Yet some primitive humans recognized a cause and effect relationship between doing certain things and alleviating symptoms of a disease or improving the condition of a wound.

Since there was so much that primitive human did not understand about the functioning of the body, magic became an integral component of the beliefs about the causes and cures of health disorders. Actually, an uncritical acceptance of magic and the supernatural pervaded practically every aspect of primitive life. So it is not surprising that early humans thought that illness was caused by evil spirits. Primitive medicines made from vegetables or animals were invariably used in combination with some form of ritual to expel the harmful spirit from a diseased body. During the Neolithic age, some 4,000 to 5,000 years ago, people living in what is today the Eastern Mediterranean and North Africa are known to have even engaged in a surgical procedure called 'trepanation' or trephining, which consists of a hole being bored in the skull in order to liberate the evil spirit supposedly contained in a person's head. The finding by anthropologists of more than one hole in some skulls and the lack of signs of osteomyelitis (erosion of bone tissue) suggests that the operation was not always fatal. Some estimates indicate that the mortality rate from trepanation was as low as ten per cent, an amazing accomplishment considering the difficulty of the procedure and the crude conditions under which it must have been performed.

Therefore, as DuBos explains, medicine has had a dual nature from its very inception in that it included knowledge about the definite medical procedures and a belief in some magic or religious power involving forces beyond human comprehension. This dual nature of medicine is still with us today, as a patient's family and friends will attempt to supplement the modern physician's skill and experience with prayer. The prevailing structure of medical science, regardless of a society's level of medical knowledge and technology, still functions within the context of the values, attitudes, and beliefs of the people who comprises that society.

### *Medicine and Behavioural Science*

As Howard Rasmussen (1975) has made clear, medicine is now faced with two distinct alternatives. It can either redefine disease and restrict its treatment to specifically medical conditions, or it can accept a broad concept of disease and change medical education programmes to deal effectively with the wider spectrum of illness. This later alternative forecasts a close association between medicine and the behavioural sciences of sociology, anthropology, and psychology, the beginnings of which are already in evidence. In 1969 a study originated within the American Sociological Association that reviewed behavioural science programmes in nine major medical schools and found that such programmes were well accepted. Wexler characterized the findings of this study by noting that:

> The case studies are impressive documents. They describe in detail the enormous amount of effort that has been expended in trying to effect a major change in medical education and thinking. It would be necessary to have been a participant in medical education prior to 1960 to appreciate how drastically the scene has changed for the behavioural sciences. Anthropologists, psychologists, and sociologists are increasingly familiar figures in the lecture halls and seminar rooms, on ward walks, at grand rounds, on admissions committees, etc.

As for sociologists, many hold joint teaching and research appointments between departments of sociology and health institutions, or are employed full time in these institutions. Medical, nursing pharmacy and health schools are all expanding the number of faculty positions for sociologists and adding courses in the behavioural sciences at a significant rate. The growing interest of medicine human behaviour is also reflected in the much larger proportion of questions dealing with the behavioural sciences on national board examinations taken by medical students. In addition to courses in the behavioural sciences, sociologists lecture on medical sociology, social psychiatry, epidemiology, preventive medicine, community medicine, health, and the social aspects of pharmacy. They also participate in studies of the utilization and evaluation of health services and the development of health policies on local state and national levels.

Some premedical students who major in sociology are now being admitted to medical schools. And one physician, George Reader, has argued that medical schools should require a background in sociology of all students who apply for admission on the grounds that sociological principles are basic to understanding how to be a better medical student and a better practising physician.

According to Reader (1972), 'Interviewing patients can be made more of a science and less and art; obstacles to compliance with the therapeutic regime can be more easily recognized; quality of care can be measured more accurately; effects of health legislation can be made more predictable; and epidemiology gains new dimensions'.

This is not to say, however, that the growing acceptance of the behavioural sciences in medicine is proceeding without any serious problems. Not all medical educators and physicians agree about the importance of the behavioural sciences in the medical school curriculum, and the behavioural scientists themselves have yet to identify those aspects of their subject matter best suited for solving practical medical problems. Nevertheless, the indication is that inclusion of the behavioural sciences in medical education is here and will continue for some time.

### *Sociology and Medicine*

While the development of modern medicine emphasized the biological and neglected the behavioural sciences, the development of sociology, in turn, originally spurned the influence of biological elements upon human social behaviour. For that matter, a case can be made that modern sociology developed largely in opposition to biological theories that explained differences in human behaviour on the basis of innate biological characteristics. One of the most significant factors in the thought of the French sociologist Emile Durkheim (1858–1917), whose theories have dominated a large portion of sociology's approach to human behaviour, was his strong rejection of biology. Neither in the gene pool of a particular race nor in the genetic composition of an individual did Durkheim find relevant evidence for sociology. Although recognizing that biological explanations of human behaviour contribute to our understanding of human interaction, Durkheim argued that they can never be totally sufficient explanations. Instead, the basis for sound explanations of social behaviour was to be found in the social processes of culture, environment, and human thought. Thus, social behaviour must be explained from the standpoint of such social elements as norms, values and statuses that comprise the basis of human group life. The persuasiveness of Durkheim's argument and its support by other sociologists led to the nearly total disregard of biology by social theorists. Only within the past few years have the contributions of biology once again been given serious sociological consideration; today the field of social biology represents a promising but still highly underdeveloped area of study.

What prompted sociologists to organize medical sociology as an area of sociological inquiry in its own right was neither medicine nor biology, but the realization that medical practice represented a distinct segment of society with its own unique social institutions, social processes, occupations, problems, and behavioural settings. The development of the sociology of medicine was greatly influenced by the expansion of the National Institutes of Health in the United States during the late 1940s, especially the establishment of the National Institute of Mental Health, which provided the funding and encouraged the interaction researchers from both the social and the medical sciences. According to August Hollingshead (1973), one of the early participants, a major result of this interaction was the stimulus to both social and medical scientists to formulate and implement joint projects. Thereafter, the growth of medical sociology proceeded at such a rate that since 1960 it has become one of the largest and most active sections of the American Sociological Associations. The position of medical sociology was further strengthened in 1966 when the *Journal of Health and Social Behaviour* became an official American Sociological Association publication.

The preceding discussion has briefly outlined the convergence of medicine and sociology in contemporary American society. John McKinlay (1971) has ventured to suggest that the time may come when the research contributions of medical sociology will stand in the same relation to medicine as do those of physiology, endocrinology, and biology as a body of knowledge explaining human functioning in the medical sphere. It is too early to surmise whether or not McKinlay's prediction will prove true, because medical sociology is a relatively new field and a considerable amount of research still needs to be compiled and precisely formulated. However, the work to date has been most impressive and promises even more exciting contributions in the future. John Knowles (1972) is correct when he states that medicine is a social science as well as a biological science and that it needs the social sciences as never before.

## Social Perspectives of Health and Health Care

In order to understand the social perspectives of health it is important also to consider the manner in which physicians are selected and trained as medical professionals. The relationship between social conditions and factors that influence health and the development of disease has long been a major interest of human kind. Throughout history, people have generally tended to view health problems from the perspective of their own particular societies and cultures. As a result, they have usually responded to the threat of disease in predictable ways.

Knowledge about norms, values, beliefs, social structures and life-styles has provided insight not only about the social organization of human resources designed to cope with health hazards, but also about the nature and causes of illness. The recognition, therefore, of the significance of the complex relationship between social factors and the level of health characteristic of specific social groups has led to the development of medical sociology as an important substantive area within the general field of sociology.

As an academic discipline, sociology is concerned with the function, structure and the roles of social institutions along with social processes and social behaviour of persons and groups. Thus, it follows that medical sociology is concerned with the social facets of health and illness, the social functions of health institutions and organizations, the relationship of systems of health care delivery to other social systems, and the social behaviour of health personnel and those people who are consumers of health care.

In recent years we have acquired a new philosophy of health which may be stated as below:

- Health is a fundamental human right.
- Health is intersectoral.
- Health is an integral part of development.
- Health is central to the concept and quality of life.
- Health involves individual, state and international responsibility.
- Health and its maintenance is a major social investment.
- Health is a worldwide social goal.

### *Health Care Services*

There is broad agreement on the issue that health services should be comprehensive, accessible and acceptable, which should provide scope for community participation and be available at a cost that community and country can afford. The purpose of health care services is to contribute to the improvement of the health condition of the population and widen the scope of health services so that it includes ever-changing national, state and local health problems. In India, the health care services is represented by the five major sectors or agencies applying distinct health technology and having difference sources of funds for operation. A brief classification of these sectors is given in succeeding paragraphs. However, it may be noted that there could be sectoral overlapping, i.e. indigenous system can be found in public as well as private sector and so on.

### *Official and Lay Definitions of Health*

According to World Health Organization (WHO, 1946), 'Health is state of complete physical, mental and social well-being and not merely the absence of disease or infirmity. Providing conditions for achieving normal health for all is the duty of the state and society. In fact, it is the deepest urge of humanity to be healthy. Health is one of the essentials of life without which nothing can be achieved. The sick and hungry child can't learn and the sick and hungry adult can't produce. Health is a means of social development and vice versa. The success of any health care delivery system to meet health needs of a society is depending upon the extent of people's participation or utilization of services by the people. Various factors: social, economic and psychological have important significance in Health Care Service. On the basis of some of the studies by sociologists, anthropologists, social workers and medical scientists it has been advocated that health and diseases are not merely biological phenomena. The socio-cultural and economic environment, faith in supernatural powers and other related belief style, nature of medical profession and services and their utilization also affect the health and disease profile of a community. It indicates that the consideration of such factors is indispensable to planning, organizing, implementing and monitoring the medical and health care programmes in any community for far-reaching results'.

While WHO views health as an absence of disease, injury or distress, most studies suggest that lay persons tend to view health as the capacity to carry out one's daily activities (Calnan, 1987; Field, 1984; Evans and Stoddart, 1990). Many individuals consider health to be a state of functional fitness and apply this definition to their everyday lives.

Good health is a prerequisite for the adequate functioning of any individual or society; if our health is sound, we can engage in numerous types of activities. But if we are ill, distressed or injured, we may face the curtailment of our usual round of daily life and we may also become so preoccupied with our state of health that other pursuits are of secondary importance or quite meaningless. Therefore, as Rene DuBos (1981) explains, health can be defined as the ability to function. This does not mean that healthy people are free from all health problems; it means that they can function to the point that they can do what they want to do.

As Thomas McKeown (1979) observes, we know from personal experience that the feeling of well-being is more than the perceived absence of disease and disability. Many influences social, religious, economic, personal and medical contribute to such a state. The role of medicine in health promotion is the prevention of illness and premature death and care of the sick and disabled. Thus, McKeown concludes that medicine's task is not to create happiness, but to remove a major source of unhappiness – disease and disability from people's attempts to understand the relationship between social behaviour and health have their origin in history. DuBos (1969) suggested that primitive humans were closer to the animals, in that, they too relied upon their instincts to stay healthy. Yet some primitive humans recognized a cause and effect relationship between doing certain things and alleviating symptoms of a disease or improving the condition of a wound. Since there was so much that primitive humans did not understand about the functioning of the body, magic became an integral component of the beliefs about the causes and cures of health disorders. Actually, an uncritical acceptance of magic and the supernatural pervaded practically every aspect of primitive life. So it is not surprising that early humans thought the illness was caused by evil spirits. Primitive medicines made from vegetables or animals were invariably used in combination with some form of ritual to expel the harmful spirit from a diseased body. During the Neolithic age, some 4,000 to 5,000 years age, and people living in what is today the Eastern Mediterranean and North Africa are known to have even engaged in a surgical procedure called 'trepanation' or 'trephining', which consists of a hole being bored in the skull in order to liberate the evil spirit supposedly contained in a person's head. The finding by anthropologists of more than one hole in some skulls and the lack of signs of osteomyelitis (erosion of bone tissue) suggest that the operation was not always fatal. Some estimates indicate tat the mortality rate from trepanation was as low as 10 per cent, an amazing accomplishment considering the difficulty of the procedure and the crude conditions under which it must have been performed (Mora, 1985).

One of the earliest attempts in the Western world to formulate principles of health care based upon rational thought and the rejection of supernatural phenomena is found in the work of the Greek physician Hippocrates. Little is known of Hippocrates, who lived around 400 BC, not even whether he actually authored the collection of books that bears his name. Nevertheless, the writings attributed to him have provided a number of principles underlying modern medical practice. One of his most famous contributions, the Hippocratic Oath, is the foundation of contemporary medical ethics. Among other things, it requires the physician to swear that he or she will help the sick, refrain from intentional wrongdoing or harm, and keep confidential all matters pertaining to the doctor-patient relationship.

Hippocrates also argued that medical knowledge should be derived from an understanding of the natural sciences and the logic of cause and effect relationships. In his classic treatise, on Airs, Waters, and Places, Hippocrates pointed out that human well-being is influenced by the totality of environmental factors; living habits or lifestyle, climate, topography of the land, and the quality of air, water and food. Interestingly enough, concerns about our health, the quality of air, water and places are still very much with us today.

In their intellectual orientation toward disease, Hippocrates and the ancient Greeks held views that were more in line with contemporary thinking about health than was found in the middle ages and the Renaissance. Much of the medical knowledge of the ancient world was lost during the Dark Ages that descended on Europe after the fall of the Roman Empire. What knowledge remained in the West was preserved by the Catholic Church. The Church took responsibility for dealing with mental suffering and adverse social conditions like poverty, while physicians focused more or less exclusively on treating physical ailments. The human body was regarded as a machine-like entity that operated according to principles of physics and chemistry. The result was that both Western religion and medical science sponsored the idea 'of the body as a machine, of disease as a break down of the machine, and of the doctor's task as repair of the machine' (Engel, 1977).

A few physicians, such as Paracelsus, a famous Swiss doctor who lives in the early sixteenth century, did show interest in understanding more than the physical functioning of the body. Paracelsus demonstrated that specific diseases common among miners were related to their work conditions. But Paracelsus was an exception and few systematic measures were employed to either research or to cope with the effects of adverse social situations on health until the late eighteenth and early nineteenth centuries.

### *Health in a Social Context*

Health is a common theme in the elements of culture. In fact, all communities have their own concept of health as a part of culture, yet health continues to be a neglected area. However, during the past few decades there has been a reawakening that health is a fundamental human right and a worldwide social goal. It is essential to the satisfaction of basic human needs and to an improved quality of life and is to be attained by all. This unit gives an idea about the concept of health and hygiene, and it also deals with the role that can be played by social workers in promotion of health and hygiene. This unit also throws light on education and changing philosophy of health, the Mous models for community health-work and identifying the basic health and hygiene problems in India and making appropriate interventions.

## Health Disparities

Health disparities (also called health care inequality in some countries) refer to gaps in the quality of health and health care across racial, ethnic, sexual orientation and socio-economic groups. The Health Resources and Services Administration defines health disparities as 'population-specific differences in the presence of disease, health outcomes, or access to health care'.

In the United States, health disparities are well documented in minority populations such as African Americans, Native Americans, Asian Americans, and Latinos. When compared to whites, these minority groups have higher incidence of chronic diseases, higher mortality and poorer health outcomes. Among the disease-specific examples of racial and ethnic disparities in the United States is the cancer incidence rate among African Americans, which is 10 per cent higher than among whites. In addition, adult African Americans and Latinos have approximately twice the risk as whites of developing diabetes. Minorities also have higher rates of cardiovascular disease, HIV/AIDS and infant mortality than whites.

Health disparities are evident in the developing world, where the importance of equitable access to health care has been cited as crucial to achieving many of the Millennium Development Goals.

### *Ethnic and Racial Disparities*

There is debate about what causes health disparities between ethnic and racial groups. However, it is generally accepted that disparities can result from three main areas:

- From the personal, socio-economic and environmental characteristics of different ethnic and racial groups (such as how certain racial groups, on average, live in poorer areas with high incidence of lead-based paint, which can harm children). A great deal of research on social determinants of health and the socio-ecological model have also surfaced, which connect economic and social conditions in determining a community's or a population's health.

- From the barriers certain racial and ethnic groups encounter when trying to enter into the health care delivery system; and
- From the quality of health care different ethnic and racial groups receive.

Each of these dimensions has been suggested as possible causes for disparities between racial and ethnic groups. However, most attention on the issue has been given to the health outcomes that result from differences in access to medical care among groups and the quality of care different groups receive. Additionally, attention on health care disparities is largely focused on race and ethnicity; data on racial and ethnic disparities are relatively widely available. In contrast, data on socio-economic health care disparities are collected less often, often using education as the indicator of socio-economic status.

The goal of eliminating disparities in health care in the United States remains elusive. Even as quality improves on specific measures, disparities often persist. Addressing these disparities must begin with the fundamental step of bringing the nature of the disparities and the groups at risk for those disparities to light by collecting health care quality information stratified by race, ethnicity and language data. Then attention can be focused on where interventions might be best applied, and on planning and evaluating those efforts to inform the development of policy and the application of resources. A lack of standardization of categories for race, ethnicity and language data has been suggested as one obstacle to achieving more widespread collection and utilization of these data.

The Institute of Medicine report, *Race, Ethnicity, and Language Data* identifies current models for collecting and coding race, ethnicity and language data; ascertains the challenges involved in obtaining these data in health care settings; and makes recommendations for improvement.

A study of 20,000 cancer patients in the United States found that African Americans are less likely than European Americans to survive breast, prostate and ovarian cancer even when given equal care, but that other forms of cancer had equal survival chances, which suggests that biological factors may be at work.

Transplantation rates differ based on race, sex and income. A study done with patients beginning long-term dialysis showed that the socio-demographic barriers to renal transplantation present themselves even before patients are on the transplant list. For example, different groups express definite interest and complete the pretransplant workup at different rates. Previous efforts to create fair transplantation policies had focused on patients currently on the transplantation waiting list.

### *Disparities in Access to Health Care*

Reasons for disparities in access to health care are many, but can include the following:

- *Lack of insurance coverage:* Without health insurance, patients are more likely to postpone medical care, more likely to go without needed medical care, and more likely to go without prescription medicines. Minority groups in the United States lack insurance coverage at higher rates than whites.
- *Lack of a regular source of care:* Without access to a regular source of care, patients have greater difficulty obtaining care, fewer doctor visits, and more difficulty obtaining prescription drugs. Compared to whites, minority groups in the United States are less likely to have a doctor they go to on a regular basis and are more likely to use emergency rooms and clinics as their regular source of care.
- *Lack of financial resources:* Although the lack of financial resources is a barrier to health care access for many Americans, the impact on access appears to be greater for minority populations.
- *Legal barriers:* Access to medical care by low-income immigrant minorities can be hindered by legal barriers to public insurance programmes. For example, in the United States, federal law bars states from providing Medicaid coverage to immigrants who have been in the country fewer than five years.
- *Structural barriers:* These barriers include poor transportation, an inability to schedule appointments quickly or during convenient hours, and excessive time spent in the waiting room, all of which affect a person's ability and willingness to obtain needed care.
- *The health care financing system:* The Institute of Medicine in the United States says fragmentation of the US health care delivery and financing system is a barrier to accessing care. Racial and ethnic minorities are more likely to be enrolled in health insurance plans which place limits on covered services and offer a limited number of health care providers.
- *Scarcity of providers:* In inner cities, rural areas and communities with high concentrations of minority populations, access to

medical care can be limited due to the scarcity of primary care practitioners, specialists and diagnostic facilities.

- *Linguistic barriers:* Language differences restrict access to medical care for minorities in the United States who are not English-proficient.
- *Health literacy:* This is where patients have problems obtaining, processing and understanding basic health information. For example, patients with a poor understanding of good health may not know when it is necessary to seek care for certain symptoms. While problems with health literacy are not limited to minority groups, the problem can be more pronounced in these groups than in whites due to socio-economic and educational factors.
- *Lack of diversity in the health care workforce:* A major reason for disparities in access to care is the cultural differences between predominantly white health care providers and minority patients. Only four per cent of physicians in the United States are African American, and Hispanics represent just 5 per cent, even though these percentages are much less than their groups' proportion of the United States population.
- *Age:* Age can also be a factor in health disparities for a number of reasons. As many older Americans exist on fixed incomes, which may make paying for health care expenses difficult. Additionally, they may face other barriers such as impaired mobility or lack of transportation which make accessing health care services challenging for them physically. Also, they may not have the opportunity to access health information via the internet as less than 15 per cent of Americans over the age of 65 have access to the internet. This could put older individuals at a disadvantage in terms of accessing valuable information about their health and how to protect it.

### *Disparities in Quality of Health Care*

Health disparities in the quality of care different ethnic and racial groups receive can include:

- *Problems with Patient-provider Communication:* This communication is critical for the delivery of appropriate and effective treatment and care, regardless of a patient's race; miscommunication can lead to incorrect diagnosis, improper use of medications and failure to receive follow-up care. Among non-English speaking populations in the United States, the linguistic barrier is even greater. Less than half of non-English speakers who say they need an interpreter during health care visits report having one. Additional communication problems stem from a lack of cultural understanding on the part of white providers for their minority patients. For example, patient health decisions can be influenced by religious beliefs, mistrust of Western medicine, and familial and hierarchical roles, all of which a white provider may not be familiar with. Other type of communication problems are seen in LGBT health care with the spoken heterosexist (conscious or unconscious) attitude on LGBT patients, lack of understanding on issues like having no sex with men (lesbians, gynecologic examinations) and other issues.

- *Provider Discrimination:* This is where health care providers either unconsciously or consciously treat certain racial and ethnic patients differently than other patients. Some research suggests that ethnic minorities are less likely than whites to receive a kidney transplant once on dialysis or to receive pain medication for bone fractures. Critics question this research and say further studies are needed to determine how doctors and patients make their treatment decisions. Others argue that certain diseases cluster by ethnicity and that clinical decision-making does not always reflect these differences.
- *Lack of Preventive Care:* According to the 2009 National Healthcare Disparities Report, uninsured Americans are less likely to receive preventive services in health care. For example, minorities are not regularly screened for colon cancer and the death rate for colon cancer has increased among African Americans and Hispanic people.

### *Ending Health Disparities*

The Commonwealth Fund, in a report on how to eliminate health disparities, says that the following steps should be considered in developing policies to eliminate racial and ethnic disparities:

- Consistent racial and ethnic data collection by health care providers.
- Effective evaluation of disparities-reduction programmes.
- Minimum standards for culturally and linguistically competent health services.
- Greater minority representation within the health care workforce.
- Establishment or enhancement of government offices of minority health.

- Expanded access to services for all ethnic and racial groups.
- Involvement of all health system representatives in minority health improvement efforts.

Other methods for ending health disparities or reducing health disparities have been suggested based on research that observes cultural differences within health care systems. According to the Agency for Healthcare Research and Quality and the assisting authors Cindy Brach and Irene Fraserirector, in an effort to reduce disparities between racial and ethnic groups, the health care system should consider the following nine cultural competency techniques:

- *Interpreter Services:* If agencies take an active approach in hiring professional interpreters, for both foreign languages and for the speaking and hearing impaired, communication barriers will begin to decrease.
- *Recruitment and Retention:* Health care systems need to become more conscious of the staff within their facilities. It is essential to the reduction of disparities that most minority groups be represented within the various health care offices and clinics.
- *Training:* The Agency for Healthcare Research and Quality and its assisting authors emphasized the importance of health care professionals being trained to work with interpreters and minority groups.
- *Coordinating with Traditional Healers:* Health care workers should be supportive and able to adjust health care plans according to the patient's cultural beliefs and traditional health practices.
- *Use of Community Health Workers:* These individuals could be responsible for bringing in the population of people who rarely seek out health care.
- *Culturally Competent Health Promotion:* This information can be available through community health workshops, or simply by health care workers taking the necessary measures to promote early detection and treatment and outlining the good and risky health behaviours to all patients.
- *Including Family and/or Community Members:* The Agency for Healthcare Research and Quality states that this particular cultural competency may be vital to obtaining consent and adherence to treatments.
- *Immersion Into Another Culture:* Allowing yourself to step outside of your comfort zone will increase your tolerance for another culture as well as raise your awareness to new ideals and beliefs.

- *Administrative and Organizational Accommodations:* These are some aspects of the health care offices that should be considered; they include the location of the health care offices, public transportation availability, clinic hours, the physical environment of the clinic, and the rapport built with the patients.

## Towards a Social Model of Health

One of the most influential social psychological approaches designed to account for the ways in which healthy people seek to avoid illness is the Health Belief Model (see Figure 1) of Irwin Renstock (1966) and his colleagues (Becker, 1974). The health belief model is derived to a great extent from the theories of psychologists Kurt Lewin, who suggested that people exist in a life space composed of regions with both positive and negative values. An illness would be a negative value and would have the effect of pushing a person away from that region, unless doing so would cause the person to enter a region of even greater negative values (for example, risking disease might be less negative than failing at an important task). While people are pushed away from regions with negative values, they are attracted toward region of positive values. Thus, a person's behaviour might be viewed as the result of seeking regions which offer the most attractive values.

**Figure 1**

*Health Belief Model*

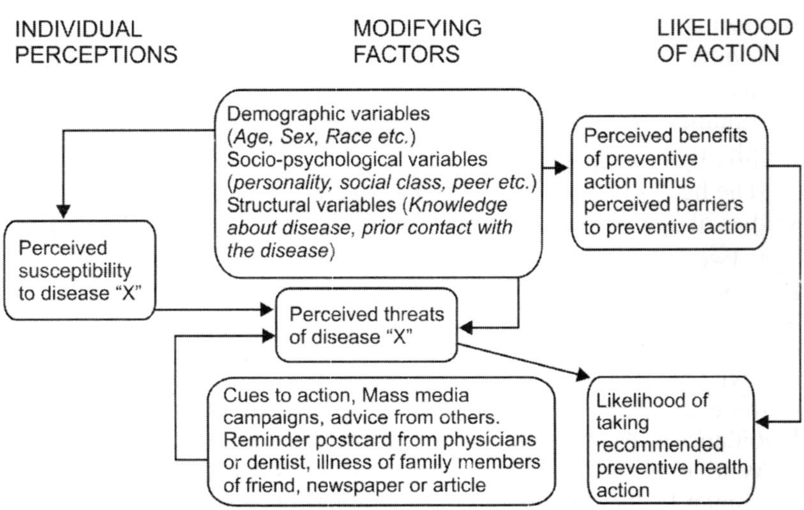

Within this framework, human behaviour is seen as being dependent upon two primary variables: (1) the value placed by a person upon a particular outcome and (2) the person's belief that a given action will result in that outcome. Accordingly, the health belief model, suggests that preventive action taken by an individual to avoid disease 'X' is due to that particular individual's perception that he or she is personally susceptible and that the occurrences of the disease would have at least some severe personal implications.

Although not directly indicated in Figure 1, the assumption in this model is that by taking a particular action, susceptibility would be reduced, or if the disease occurred, severity would be reduced. The perception of the threat posed by disease 'X', however, is affected by modifying factors. As shown in the above figure these factors are demographic, socio-psychological and structural variables that can influence both perception and the corresponding cues necessary to instigate action. Action cues are required, says Rosenstock (1988), because while and individual may perceive that a given action will be effective in reducing the threat of disease, that action may not be taken if it is further defined as too expensive, too unpleasant or painful, too inconvenient, or perhaps too traumatic.

So, despite recognition that action is necessary and the presence of energy to take that action, a person may still not be sufficiently motivated to do something. The likelihood of action also involves a weighing of the perceived benefits to action, contrasted to the perceived barriers. Therefore, Rosenstock believed that a stimulus in the form of an action cue was required to 'trigger' the appropriate behaviour. Such a stimulus could be either internal (perception of bodily states) or external (interpersonal interaction, mass media communication, or personal knowledge of someone affected by the health problem).

The health belief model has been employed successfully in several studies of (preventive) health behaviour, such as the seeking of dental care (Gochman, 1971). Dietary compliance among obese children (Becker et al., 1977) quitting cigarette smoking in Australia (Knight and Hay, 1989), engaging in self-care in the United States and Japan (Haug et al., 1989), and ethnic differences in managing hypertension (Brown and Segal, 1966). Help seeking behaviour was observed in each of these studies to be based upon the value of the perceived outcome (avoidance of personal vulnerability) and the expectation that preventive action would result in that outcome. For example, the Gochman (1971) study found that if children are motivated to have good health in general, their perception of vulnerability to tooth disease and the benefits of visiting the dentist will result in their intentions to seek future dental care. Conversely, those children with low health motivation are not as likely to have the future intention of seeing a dentist. In the Becker et al. (1977) study, 182 pairs of mothers and their obese children were divided into three groups while the children participated in a weight reduction programme. The groups consisted of (1) a high fear group (shown alarming material about the potentially unfavourable consequences of being fat in later life), (2) a low fear group (shown similar but less threatening information) and (3) a control group (shown no additional information). Children in the control group did not lose weight. Children in the low fear group lost some weight initially but also tended to put some of it back on. The high fear group lost some weight and did not put any of it back on. The intervention of a fear arousal cue in the high fear group had a marked effect on the mother's notions of the perceived susceptibility, seriousness and benefits of compliance for their children.

Unfortunately, the usefulness of the health belief model is limited, in that, it has been applied mostly to preventive situations in which the behaviour studied is voluntary. Obviously, however, many people who seek health services are motivated to take action only by the appearance of clear and definite symptoms.

Nevertheless, the health belief model has demonstrated considerable utility in the study of health behaviour (Becker, 1979; Janz and Becker, 1984; Mullen, Hersey and Iverson, 1987). The merit of the model is that even when an individual recognizes personal susceptibility, he or she may not take action unless the individual also perceives that being ill, will result in serious difficulty. Thus, the individual's subjective assessment of the health situation becomes the critical variable in the utilization of health services. In fact, a person's subjective assessment may be more important than an objective medical diagnosis. Several studies show no (sometimes even a negative) correlation between medical estimates of health and patient compliance (Becker and Maiman, 1975). David Mechanic (1972) has noted that the difficulty in preventive medicine is that common sense approaches do not necessarily match clinic approaches, and common sense often determines whether health services are sought. Furthermore, once a patient subjectively feels well, physicians may be faced with the additional problem of encouraging the patient to continue to follow medical advice.

# 3

# Preventive and Protective Hygienic Habits

Health is a common theme in the elements of culture. In fact, all communities have their own concept of health as a part of culture, yet health continues to be a neglected area. However, during the past few decades there has been a reawakening that health is a fundamental human right and a worldwide social goal. It is essential to the satisfaction of basic human needs and to an improved quality of life and is to be attained by all. This unit gives an idea about the concept of health and hygiene and it also deals with the role that can be played by social workers in promotion of health and hygiene.

## Concept of Health and Hygiene

World Health Organization (WHO, 1946) defined health as a 'state of complete physical, mental and social well-being and not merely the absence of disease or infirmity'. Thus, it is a basic human right. Providing condusive condition for achieving normal health is the duty of state and society. In fact, the deepest urge of humanity is to be healthy. Health is one of the essentials of life, without which nothing can be achieved. The sick and hungry child cannot learn and the sick and hungry adult cannot produce. In other words, we can say that health is a condition of equilibrium between physical fitness, mental balance and social adjustment of human beings.

The term 'hygiene' is derived from 'hygeia', the goddess of health in Greek mythology. Hygiene has been variously defined, such as hygiene is 'the science of health and embraces all factors which contributes to healthful living'. According to another definition, hygiene is 'the science of preventing disease and promoting health'. Thus, the aim of hygiene is not only to preserve health but also to improve it.

An individual may be called a healthy person if he/she is physically fit, mentally sound and socially well adjusted. Any change in either components, i.e. physical, mental or social may result in discomfort or disease. It may also be regarded as the disease that is an interruption in the state of equilibrium of all the three components of health. This concept may easily be understood through a triangle of sixty degrees each with the physical, mental and social arms. Any variation in either angle or contraction/elongation in any one of the arms will produce imbalance (state of illness) in any individual and on the other hand exact degrees and equal arms are the sign of totally healthy person.

The etiology of ill health lies in the malfunctioning of the social system in terms of poverty, ignorance, population explosion, unemployment, old age, unhygienic living conditions, bad housing, poor nutrition and incompatible dietary habits, poor quality of drinking water and sanitary facilities, etc. Thus, we can say that ill health is only a symptom of social disequilibrium and not a phenomenon independent of social affairs of man. Generally, health is misunderstood with treatment which is not necessarily a precondition of good health but it involves prevention, education, rehabilitation and a number of other interventions in terms of social services which ensures the vitality of human health. The main causes of health and hygiene problems in India may be enumerated as below:

*Environmental Causes*

- lack of safe drinking water
- lack of basic sanitation
- crowded, unsanitary living conditions
- pollution of water, food, soil and air

*Social Economic Causes*

- poverty
- illiteracy
- ignorance
- prejudicial customs, traditions, beliefs and cultural pattern
- inadequate nutrition
- lack of personal hygiene

- rapid population growth

*Others*

- uneven development of health care services and social care
- inadequate primary health care

### *Identifying Basic Health and Hygiene Problems*

An assessment of the health status and health problem is the first requisite for any planned effort to develop health care services. This is also known as Community Diagnosis. The analysis of data relating to health situation and health problems comprises:

- Morbidity and mortality statistics
- Demographic conditions of the population
- Environmental conditions which have a bearing on health
- Socio-economic factors which have a direct effect on health
- Cultural background, attitudes, beliefs and practices which effect health
- Medical and health services available,
- Other services available

### *Physical, Mental and Social Aspects of Health*

*Physical Health:* Crew (1965) observed that the sign of physical health in an individual constitutes a good complexion, a clean skin, bright eyes, lustrous hair with a body well clothed with firm flesh neither too thin nor too fat, a sweet breath, a good appetite, sound sleep, regular activity of bowels and bladder and smooth, easy coordinated movements. All the organs of the body are unexceptional in size and function normally. All the special senses are intact. The resting pulse rate, blood pressure and tolerance, etc. are all within the range of 'normality' in the context of the individual's age and sex. In the young and growing individual, there is a steady gain in weight and in the mature this weight remains more or less than the individual's weight at twenty-five. On the basis of above signs the basic health needs include a hygienic and balanced diet, pure water, a good habitat, neighbourhood and community with basic sanitation, suitable clothes, well regulated lifestyle, exercise and personal hygiene. A periodic health check-up is also very essential for good health.

*Mental Health:* The old saying 'healthy mind in a healthy body' confirms the interrelationship between mental and physical health.

Poor mental health affects physical health and vice versa. According to WHO Technical Report (1964), the psychological factors are considered to play a major role in disorders such as hypertension, peptic ulcer and asthma. A mentally healthy person is free from internal conflicts and external maladjustments. He is not swayed by emotions; and has good self-control.

As such, mental health primarily needs physical health. The other important needs are a good home, a good neighbourhood, a good community and job satisfaction. The psychologists are of the opinion that the dissatisfaction of instinctual and basic life needs leads to insanity.

*Social Health:* The social health of the people in a community is determined and judged on the basis of their personal and social characteristics. One who plays one's roles, according to one's status and is apt in establishing and maintaining harmonious relationship in family and community and on job is considered socially a healthy person. On the contrary, when he fails to perform these roles, neglects social relations, indulges in bad habits and gets involved in homicide, suicide, crime, gambling, drinking, etc. he is considered abnormal.

Therefore, family and social welfare services are important. Social health needs to deal with the problems connected with social existence of individuals. But these needs are seldom integrated with health services which is a great weakness of health care delivery system in most societies. Some of the determinants of health are heredity, environment, lifestyle, socio-economic conditions, health and family welfare services, together with other factors such as food, agriculture, education, industry, social development, social welfare, etc.

## Sex Education

### *Relevance of Sex Education*

Sex education is a broad term used to describe education about human sexual anatomy, sexual reproduction, sexual intercourse, reproductive health, emotional relations, reproductive rights and responsibilities, contraception, and other aspects of human sexual behaviour. Common avenues for sex education are parents or caregivers, school programmes, and public health campaigns.

Sex education may also be described as 'sexuality education,' which means that it encompasses education about all aspects of sexuality, including information about family planning, reproduction (fertilization, conception and development of the embryo and foetus, through to childbirth), plus information about all aspects of one's sexuality including: body image, sexual orientation, sexual pleasure, values, decision-making, communication, dating, relationships, sexually transmitted infections (STIs) and how to avoid them, and birth control methods.

Sex education may be taught informally, such as when someone receives information from a conversation with a parent, friend, religious leader, or through the media. It may also be delivered through sex self-help authors, magazine advice columnists, sex columnists, or through sex education websites. Formal sex education occurs when schools or health care providers offer sex education.

Sometimes, formal sex education is taught as a full course and is a part of the curriculum in junior high school or high school. Other times, it is only one unit within a more broad biology class, health class, home economics class, or physical education class. Some schools offer no sex education, since it remains a controversial issue in several countries, particularly the United States (especially with regard to the age at which children should start receiving such education, the amount of detail that is revealed, and topics dealing with human sexual behaviour, eg. safe sex practices, masturbation, premarital sex and sexual ethics).

In 1936, Wilhelm Reich commented that sex education of his time was a work of deception, focusing on biology while concealing excitement-arousal, which is what a pubescent individual is mostly interested in. Reich added that this emphasis obscures what he believed to be a basic psychological principle: that all worries and difficulties originate from unsatisfied sexual impulses.

When sex education is contentiously debated, the chief controversial points are whether covering child sexuality is valuable or detrimental; the use of birth control such as condoms and hormonal contraception; and the impact of such use on pregnancy outside marriage, teenage pregnancy and the transmission of STIs. Increasing support for abstinence-only sex education by conservative groups has been one of the primary causes of this controversy. Countries with conservative attitudes towards sex education (including the UK and the US) have a higher incidence of STIs and teenage pregnancy.

The existence of AIDS has given a new sense of urgency to the topic of sex education. In many African nations, where AIDS is at epidemic levels, sex education is seen by most scientists as a vital public health strategy. Some international organizations such as Planned Parenthood consider that broad sex education programmes have global benefits, such as controlling the risk of overpopulation and the advancement of women's rights.

According to SIECUS, the Sexuality Information and Education Council of the United States, 93 per cent of adults they surveyed support sexuality education in high school and 84 per cent support it in junior high school. In fact, 88 per cent of parents of junior high school students and 80 per cent of parents of high school students believe that sex education in school makes it easier for them to talk to their adolescents about sex. Also, 92 per cent of adolescents report that they want both to talk to their parents about sex and to have comprehensive in-school sex education.

*Sex Education in Asia*: The state of sex education programmes in Asia is at various stages of development. Indonesia, Mongolia, South Korea and Sri Lanka have a systematic policy framework for teaching about sex within schools. Malaysia, the Philippines and Thailand have assessed adolescent reproductive health needs with a view to developing adolescent-specific training, messages and materials. India has programmes that specifically aim at school children at the age group of nine to sixteen years. These are included as subjects in the curriculum and generally involve open and frank interaction with the teachers. In India, there is a huge debate on the curriculum of sex education and when should it be increased. Attempts by state governments to introduce sex education as a compulsory part of the school curriculum have often been met with harsh criticism by political parties, who claim that sex education 'is against Indian culture' and would mislead children.(Bangladesh, Myanmar, Nepal and Pakistan have no coordinated sex education programmes.) In Japan, sex education is mandatory from age ten or eleven, mainly covering biological topics such as menstruation and ejaculation.

In China, sex education traditionally consists in reading the reproduction section of biology textbooks. However, in 2000 a new five-year project was introduced by the China Family Planning Association to 'promote reproductive health education among Chinese teenagers and unmarried youth' in twelve urban districts and three counties. This includes discussion about sex within human relationships as well as pregnancy and HIV prevention.

The International Planned Parenthood Federation and the BBC World Service ran a 12-part series known as Sexwise, which discussed sex education, family life education, contraception and parenting. It was first launched in South Asia and then extended worldwide.

### *Morality of Sex Education*

One approach to sex education is to view it as necessary to reduce risk behaviours such as unprotected sex, and equip individuals to make informed decisions about their personal sexual activity. Additionally, some proponents and opponents of comprehensive sex education contend that education about homosexuality encourages tolerance and understanding that homosexuality is not wrong.

Another viewpoint on sex education, historically inspired by sexologists like Wilhelm Reich and psychologists like Sigmund Freud and James W. Prescott, holds that what is at stake in sex education is control over the body and liberation from social control. Proponents of this view tend to see the political question as whether society or the individual should teach sexual mores. Sexual education may thus be seen as providing individuals with the knowledge necessary to liberate themselves from socially organized sexual oppression and to make up their own minds. In addition, sexual oppression may be viewed as socially harmful.

To another group in the sex education debate, the question is whether the state or the family should teach sexual mores. They believe that sexual mores should be left to the family, and sex-education represents state interference. They claim that some sex education curricula break down pre-existing notions of modesty and encourage acceptance of practices that those advocating this viewpoint deem immoral, such as homosexuality and premarital sex. They cite websites such as that of the Coalition for Positive Sexuality as examples. Naturally, those that believe that homosexuality and premarital sex are a normal part of the range of human sexuality disagree with them.

Many religions teach that sexual behaviour outside of marriage is immoral, so their adherents feel that this morality should be taught as part of sex education. Other religious conservatives believe that sexual knowledge is unavoidable, hence their preference for curricula based on abstinence.

### *Scientific Study of Sex Education*

The debate over teenage pregnancy and STIs has spurred some research into the effectiveness of different approaches to sex education. In a meta-analysis, DiCenso et al. (2002), have compared comprehensive sex education programmes with abstinence-only programmes. Their review of several studies shows that abstinence-only programmes did not reduce the likelihood of pregnancy of women who participated in the programmes, but rather increased it. Four abstinence programmes and one school programme were associated with a pooled increase of 54 per cent in the partners of men and 46 per cent in women (confidence interval 95 per cent 0.95 to 2.25 and 0.98 to 2.26 respectively). The researchers conclude:

'There is some evidence that prevention programmes may need to begin much earlier than they do. In a recent systematic review of eight trials of day care for disadvantaged children under five years of age, long-term follow up showed lower pregnancy rates among adolescents. We need to investigate the social determinants of unintended pregnancy in adolescents through large longitudinal studies beginning early in life and use the results of the multivariate analyses to guide the design of prevention interventions. We should carefully examine countries with low pregnancy rates among adolescents. For example, the Netherlands has one of the lowest rates in the world (8.1 per 1,000 young women aged 15 to 19 years), and Ketting and Visser have published an analysis of associated factors. In contrast, the rates are:

- 93.0 per 1,000 in the United States (85.8/1,000 in 1996)
- 62.6 per 1,000 in England and Wales
- 42.7 per 1,000 in Canada
- 15.1 per 1,000 in Belgium (1996)

We should examine effective programmes designed to prevent other high risk behaviours in adolescents. For example, Botvin et al. (2007), found that school based programmes to prevent drug abuse during junior high school (ages 12–14 years) resulted in important and durable reductions in use of tobacco, alcohol, and cannabis if they taught a combination of social resistance skills and general life skills, were properly implemented, and included at least two years of booster sessions. Few sexual health interventions are designed with input from adolescents. Adolescents have suggested that sex education should be more positive with less emphasis on anatomy and scare tactics; it should focus on negotiation skills in sexual relationships and communication; and details of sexual health clinics should be advertised in areas that adolescents frequent (for example, school toilets, shopping centres).'

Also, a US review, 'Emerging Answers', by the National Campaign to Prevent Teenage Pregnancy examined 250 studies of sex education programmes. The conclusion of this review was that 'the overwhelming weight of evidence shows that sex education that discusses contraception does not increase sexual activity'.

## AIDS and HIV

### *Introduction*

In the past, the world has faced many pandemics like cholera and plague. At the turn of the 20th century the world faced influenza pandemic. Every fifty to sixty years, the world has faced a new disease that has been in the nature of an epidemic. These diseases have left a trail of death and morbidity. There has been widespread fear and stigma attached to the victims due to ignorance and fear. As the diseases have progressed people have studied how, what and why of those diseases. They have found the cause of most of the diseases. They have also found how these diseases spread. Many times they have found cures and vaccines to prevent the spread of the disease. A new disease appeared and affected mankind in the early 1980s. This disease is called AIDS (Acquired Immuno Deficiency Syndrome).

*AIDS:* AIDS or acquired immunodeficiency syndrome is a disabling and deadly disease caused by HIV. ('Acquired' means something not inherent in the patient's body but transmitted from others; 'immunodeficiency' refers to the weakened ability of the body's immune system that helps it ward off infections and diseases; and 'syndrome' is the group of signs and symptoms associated with the disease.) AIDS occurs as a collection of infections (called opportunistic infections) that are usually severe, such as pneumonia or tuberculosis, manifest more often during the late stages of HIV infection. An HIV – infected person may not develop AIDS until 8 to 10 years after being infected.

*HIV:* Human immunodeficiency virus (HIV) is a lentivirus (a member of the retrovirus family) that can lead to acquired immuno deficiency syndrome (AIDS), a condition in humans in which the immune system begins to fail, leading to life-threatening opportunistic infections. Previous names for the virus include human T-lymphotropic virus III (HTLV III), lymphadenopathy – associated virus (LAV), and AIDS – associated retrovirus (ARV).

Infection with HIV occurs by the transfer of blood, semen, vaginal fluid, pre-ejaculate, or breast milk. Within these bodily fluids, HIV is present as both free virus particles and virus within infected immune cells. The four major routes of transmission are unprotected sexual intercourse, contaminated needles, breast milk, and transmission from an infected mother to her baby at birth (vertical transmission). Screening of blood products for HIV has largely eliminated transmission through blood transfusions or infected blood products in the developed world.

HIV infection in humans is now pandemic. As of January 2006, the joint United Nations programme on HIV/AIDS (UNAIDS) and the World Health Organization (WHO) estimate that AIDS has killed more than twenty-five million people since it was first recognized on 1 December 1981. It is estimated that about 0.6 per cent of the world's population is infected with HIV. In 2005 alone, AIDS claimed an estimated 2.4–3.3 million lives, of which more than 5,70,000 were children. A third of these deaths are occurring in Sub-Saharan Africa, retarding economic growth and increasing poverty. According to current estimates, HIV is set to infect 90 million people in Africa, resulting in a minimum estimate of 18 million orphans, Antiretroviral treatment reduces both the mortality and the mortality of HIV infection, but routine access to antiretroviral medication is not available in all countries.

HIV primarily infects vital cells in the human immune system such as helper T cells (specifically $CD4^+$ T cells), macrophages, and dendritic cells. HIV infection leads to low levels of $CD4^+$ T cells through three main mechanisms: firstly, direct viral killing of infected cells; secondly, increased rates of apoptosis in infected cells; and thirdly, killing of infected $CD4^+$ T cells by CD8 cytoxic lymphocytes that recognize infected cells. When $CD4^+$ T cell numbers decline below a critical level, cell-mediated immunity is lost, and the body becomes progressively more susceptible to opportunistic infections.

Eventually, most HIV infected individuals develop AIDS (Acquired Immunodeficiency Syndrome). These individuals mostly die from opportunistic infection or malignancies associated with the progressive failure of the immune system. Without treatment, about nine out of every ten persons with HIV will progress to AIDS after ten–fifteen years. Treatment with anti-retrovirals increases the life expectancy of people infected with HIV. Even after HIV has progressed to diagnosable AIDS, the average survival time with antiretroviral therapy (as of 2005) is estimated to be more than five years. Without antiretroviral therapy, death normally occurs within a year. It is hoped that current and future treatments may allow HIV-infected individuals to achieve a life expectancy approaching that of the general public

HIV or human immunodeficiency virus is a virus that infects humans. A person with HIV is infected for life and can infect others. The virus attacks the immune system and slowly weakens the body's defence against diseases. An HIV-infected person can look and feel well for a long time without developing AIDS.

### *History of HIV/AIDS in India*

When the disease appeared in the West, many people in India thought that the disease would not affect the Indians. Indians have strong family ties and consider themselves as very religious people. Homosexuality is thought to be very rare in India. HIV was seen as a disease of the West. It was seen as disease due to promiscuity. People were complacent about the disease. In 1985 the Indian Council of Medical Research (ICMR), set up a sero-surveillance programme. In 1986 the presence of the virus was first detected in sex workers in Chennai. The first Indian patient to suffer from AIDS was reported from Mumbai. In 1987, the ICMR warned the country about the impending epidemic. Soon after the reporting of the first few HIV/AIDS cases in the country in 1986, Government recognized the seriousness of the problem and took a series of important measures to tackle the epidemic. By this time, AIDS had already attained epidemic proportion in the African region and was spreading rapidly in many countries of the world. Government of India without wasting any time initiated steps and started pilot screening of high-risk population. A high-powered National AIDS Committee was constituted in 1986 itself and a National AIDS Control Programme was launched in the year 1987.

#### *National AIDS Committee*

To formulate strategy and plan for implementation of prevention and control of HIV/AIDS in the country, Ministry of Health and Family Welfare constituted a National AIDS Committee in the year 1986, under the chairmanship of the Union Minister of Health and Family Welfare with representatives from various sectors. The committee was formed with a view to bringing together various ministries, non-government organizations and private institutions for effective coordination in implementing the programme. The committee acts as the highest-level deliberation body to oversee the performance of the programme and to provide overall policy directions, and to forge multi-sectoral collaborations. In the initial years the programme focused on generation of public awareness through more communication programmes, introduction of blood screening for transfusion purpose and conducting surveillance activities in the epicentres of the epidemic. Every state began testing for HIV and several cases of HIV infections started emerging.

### *Medium-Term Plan for HIV/AIDS Control*

In year 1989, with the support of WHO a medium-term plan for HIV/AIDS Control was developed with a US$ 10 million budget to be provided from external sources. Project documents for the implementation of this plan were developed and implemented in five states and UTs which were most affected, namely, Maharashtra, Tamil Nadu, West Bengal, Manipur, and Delhi. Initial activities focused on the reinforcement of programme management capacities as well as targeted IEC and surveillance activities. Actual preventive activities like implementation of education and awareness programme, blood safety measures, control of hospital infection, condom promotion to prevent HIV/AIDS and strengthening of clinical services for STD and HIV/AIDS gained momentum only in 1992.

### *National AIDS Control Organization (NACO)*

In 1991, a number of donors indicated their interest to support India and accordingly a 'Strategic Plan for Prevention and Control of AIDS in India' was prepared for the five-year period 1992–1997. The strategic Plan has, to date, received support from the World Bank, WHO and other international agencies. The aim of the NACO was to establish a comprehensive, multi-sectoral programme for the prevention and control of HIV/AIDS in India. In order to achieve their objectives and combat the onslaught of the HIV/AIDS epidemic effectively, the Government of India established the National AIDS Control Organization in 1992, as an executive body in the Ministry of Health and Family Welfare at New Delhi, to work for the prevention and control of AIDS in the country. An Additional Secretary posted as its Project Director heads national AIDS Control. Its Secretariat consists of an Additional Project Director (Technical), subject specialists and other technical and administrative staff.

### *National AIDS Control Board*

A National AIDS Control Board has been constituted at the National level under the chairmanship of Secretary (Health), Ministry of Health and Family Welfare in order to review NACO policies, to expedite sanction, approve procurement and to undertake and award contracts to private agencies. The other major functions of the board pertain to the approval of annual operation plan budget, reallocation of funds between programme components, formation of the programme managerial teams and appointment of senior programme staff. The board exercises all financial and administrative powers, which are beyond the powers of the Addl. Secretary and Project Director, NACO and which the Department of Health, Government of India can exercise with the approval of the department of expenditure, Ministry of Finance. No separate reference to Ministry of Finance for funding planned activities is required as the Ministry of Finance is represented on the board.

The National AIDS Control Board has also been entrusted with all the functions, which hitherto were being performed by the technical Advisory Committee under the Chairmanship of the Director General of Health Services (DGHS). NACO has close collaboration and effective coordination among Central and State Governments, various Government departments, local bodies, partnership with NGOs, corporate bodies, international and bilateral collaboration for implementing and monitoring various programmes. NACO has been in the forefront for the fight against HIV/AIDS. In 2002, NACO announced the national policy for fight against HIV/AIDS.

### *Transmission of HIV*

The virus is carried from an infected person to a healthy person by blood, semen, vaginal fluids and breast milk. HIV is transmitted in several ways:

- By having unprotected sexual intercourse (vaginal, anal or oral sex); in other words, by having sex without a condom with someone who is HIV infected. Although most cases of sexual transmission involve men and women, men having sex with men are equally at risk.
- By using (or being injured by) needles, razor blades or other medical/surgical equipment which have been recently contaminated by the blood of a person infected with HIV.
- By sharing needles and syringes used by an HIV infected injecting drug user or by using needles/syringes that have been used in health care settings.
- By receiving blood transfusions, blood products or organ transplants from an HIV infected person.
- By an infected mother to her baby during pregnancy, delivery or breast-feeding.

HIV does not spread through ordinary social contact. For example, shaking hands with or travelling in the same bus with an HIV infected person, or eating from the same plates that an infected person has used, or hugging and kissing an HIV-positive individual will not spread the disease. Mosquitoes and insects do not carry the virus nor is the disease water-borne or air-borne.

### *HIV Test*

Many HIV-positive people are unaware that they are infected with the virus. For example, less than 1 per cent of the sexually active urban population in Africa has been tested and this proportion is even lower in rural populations. Furthermore, only 0.5 per cent of pregnant women attending urban health facilities are counselled, tested or receive their test results. Again, this proportion is even lower in rural health facilities. Since donors may, therefore, be unaware of their infection, donor blood and blood products used in medicine and medical research are routinely screened for HIV.

HIV-1 testing consists of initial screening with an enzyme linked immunosorbent assay (ELISA) to detect antibodies to HIV-1. Specimens with a non-reactive result from the initial ELISA are considered HIV-negative unless new exposure to an infected partner or partner of unknown HIV status has occurred. Specimens with a reactive ELISA result are retested in duplicate. If the result of either duplicate test is reactive, the specimen is reported as repeatedly reactive and undergoes confirmatory testing with a more specific supplemental test (e.g. Western blot or, less commonly, an immunofluorscence assay (IFA)). Only specimens that are repeatedly reactive by ELISA and positive by IFA or reactive by Western blot are considered HIV-positive and indicative of HIV infection. Specimens that are repeatedly ELISA-reactive, occasionally provide an indeterminate Western blot result, which may be either an incomplete antibody response to HIV in an infected person or non-specific reactions in an uninfected person. Although IFA can be used to confirm infection in these ambiguous cases, this assay is not widely used. Generally, a second specimen should be collected more than a month later and retested for persons with indeterminate Western blot results. Although much less commonly available, nucleic acid testing (e.g. viral RNA or proviral DNA amplification method) can also help diagnosis in certain situations. In addition, a few tested specimens might provide inconclusive results because of a low quantity specimen. In these situations, a second specimen is collected and tested for HIV infection.

### *Presence of Other Sexually Transmitted Infections (STIs) Facilitate HIV Transmission*

Many sexually transmitted infections (STIs) increase the risk of acquiring HIV infection as well as the chances of transmitting it to others. For example, the risk of infection increases by as much as 50 to 300 times per each sexual contact with a person who has a genital ulcer.

It is important to keep in mind that HIV transmission is more likely to occur in combination with other sexually transmitted infections for many reasons:

- HIV can easily pass through breaks and lacerations in the skin and mucous membranes caused by genital ulcers.
- HIV can attach to the white blood cells usually present in genital discharges caused by STIs.
- Large amounts of HIV are found in ulcers and genital fluid (semen, secretions from the cervix) of people with infections such as gonorrhoea, genital herpes, syphilis, and chancroid.

### *Early Detection and Treatment of Sexually Transmitted Infections (STIs)*

Early and effective treatment of STIs decreases the amount of HIV in genital secretions and reduces the risk of its spread to other sexual partners. Early treatment also reduces the risk of contracting HIV from infected partners. Furthermore, early diagnosis and treatment of STIs are important because they can prevent serious complications, such as infertility, ectopic pregnancy, genital cancer, blinding eye disease and major nervous system infections in infants, which can occur as a result of an untreated STI.

#### *HIV Transmitted From a Mother to Her Child*

Transmission from an infected mother to her baby occurs in about 30 per cent of cases, in the absence of a preventive treatment during pregnancy, delivery and breast-feeding.

- *Pregnancy:* Through the mother's blood. The baby is more at risk if the mother has been recently infected or is at a later stage of AIDS.
- *Delivery:* At the time of birth when the baby is exposed to the infected mother's blood.
- *Breast-feeding:* The virus has been found in breast milk in low concentrations and studies have shown that children of HIV-infected mothers can get HIV infection through breast milk.

Children can be both infected by HIV and affected by AIDS. Over 2.5 million children worldwide are now infected with HIV. If HIV continues to spread across the world, there will be a greater increase in deaths among infants and children. It is also estimated that by the year 2010, 25 million children will be orphans because of AIDS.

### *People Can Prevent Themselves from Being Infected*

A person can avoid HIV infection by abstaining from sex; by having a mutually faithful monogamous sexual relationship with an uninfected partner or by practising safer sex. Safer sex involves the correct use of a condom during each sexual encounter; it also includes none-penetrative sex.

Both men and women share the responsibility for avoiding behaviour that might lead to HIV infection. They also share the right to refuse sex and assume responsibility for ensuring safe sex. In many societies, however, men have much more control than women do over when, with whom and how they have sex. In such cases, men need to assume greater responsibility for their actions.

Babies born to HIV-infected mothers can be protected against HIV infection if the mother receives antiretroviral drugs during pregnancy and at delivery. While avoiding breast-feeding seems logical when a mother is HIV-infected, the benefits of breast-feeding for the baby cannot be ignored. Exclusive breast-feeding, usually recommended during the first months of life, should be discontinued as soon as it is feasible. Replacement feeding is recommended only where it is acceptable, available, feasible, affordable, sustainable and safe.

### *Vaccine for HIV/AIDS*

While there is no effective vaccine to prevent HIV/AIDS yet, many scientists agree that an AIDS vaccine is possible. Vaccines are used either to protect humans from disease or infection. Most scientific efforts focus on developing an AIDS preventive vaccine for people who are not infected with HIV. The vaccine would prepare the immune system to respond in case of an exposure to the virus.

In the past few years, AIDS vaccine research has gathered momentum and today it has become a global effort. Clinical trials of different vaccines are continuing as patients, health care workers, scientists, institutions and governments eagerly wait for an AIDS vaccine. In the South-East Asia Region, candidate vaccines are presently undergoing clinical trials in India and Thailand.

### *Cure for HIV/AIDS*

There is no cure for HIV/AIDS. Since AIDS is a collection of 'opportunistic' infections, there are medicines that can prevent and control these infections in persons affected by HIV/AIDS. While opportunistic infections would be either harmless or at least easily managed in healthy people, they can kill people with damaged and impaired immune systems, as for those with HIV/AIDS. The prevention and treatment of opportunistic infections have a beneficial impact on the progression of HIV infection.

With the advent of antiretroviral drugs today, people living with HIV are receiving treatment that can slow the pace at which HIV multiplies in the body. Antiretroviral drugs, along with prevention and treatment of opportunistic infections, have helped make HIV/AIDS a manageable chronic disease. However, taking antiretroviral drugs means following a rigid schedule: they must be taken daily for the rest of the life. If a patient misses even 1 dose in a regimen of 50, the virus can become resistant to the medicines and the drugs lose their effect. A strict adherence to regimen and proper care and treatment has been shown to prolong survival and improve the quality of life of people living with HIV/AIDS. Antiretroviral therapy is only effective if a combination of three or four antiretroviral drugs is used. Single drugs are used only for the prevention of mother-to-child transmission.

### *Importance of HIV Testing and Counselling*

More than 90 per cent of people infected with HIV do not know their HIV status. Voluntary testing and counselling have proved to be an effective public health strategy as they result in reduced risk behaviours and increased condom use. Testing and counselling serve as entry points to HIV/AIDS care and support.

### *Importance of Counselling for Treatment*

Counselling is important for effective antiretroviral treatment, as it is critical that all prescribed medicines are taken regularly and at the same time of the day. Some drugs require special instructions, as they are to be taken before or after a meal and with a certain amount of fluid. The counsellor plays an important role in assessing the patient's readiness for antiretroviral treatment, treatment literacy and adherence. All antiretroviral medicines have side effects. The counsellor can refer a patient to a physician with antiretroviral treatment experience to determine if a treatment should continue or be interrupted.

### *Post-Exposure Prophylaxis for HIV*

Prophylaxis is the treatment to prevent the onset of a particular disease or the recurrence of symptoms in an existing infection. Post-exposure prophylaxis is a short-term antiretroviral treatment to reduce the likelihood of HIV infection after potential exposure, either occupationally (as in health care settings or workplaces) or through sexual intercourse. The medications used depend on the exposure to HIV, and should be taken ideally within 2–24 hours and no later than 48–72 hours following the possible HIV exposure.

### *HIV/AIDS Prevention, Care, Support and Treatment Continuum*

The HIV/AIDS prevention, care, support and treatment continuum regards HIV/AIDS as a chronic disease requiring treatment throughout life. Experiences from several countries have demonstrated that a continuum of prevention, care and treatment from hospital to home is the optimum for those affected. WHO South-East Asia Regional Office (SEARO) is promoting a patient-centred approach through a continuum of prevention, care, support and treatment by decentralization of services, which includes an adequate referral and collaborative care network from hospital to the community and home.

Management of opportunistic infections and antiretroviral treatment cannot be seen in isolation. HIV-infected patients, including those with active tuberculosis, should benefit from additional care needs, including clinical and nursing care, in particular, for the prevention and treatment of opportunistic infections, ongoing psychosocial support and counselling, financial and employment support, assistance for housing and living in enabling environment, legal assistance, and care and support for orphans as promoted by WHO SEARO.

### *Patient-Centred Approach to HIV/AIDS Care*

The public health approach to HIV/AIDS chronic care is patient – centric. As with other chronic illnesses, such as diabetes and hypertension, patients manage their care. Patients need to be educated about the disease so that they can make informed decisions on adherence and management and be prepared to deal with the challenges of living with a chronic disease. They need to know when and how to interact with the health services available in the community. For example, a person on treatment who may experience diarrhoea should know when to rush to the health facility for medical attention, that is if blood is present or there is associated fever, or when to relieve the symptom with a locally available remedy.

### *Treatment Preparedness*

Treatment preparedness stems from the concept of a patient-centric approach and applies to building up of adequate resources and actions at the level of the individual as well as the community. It involves preparation of the community to the disease by effective messaging using mass media, effective use of community resources, ensuring inputs of people living with HIV/AIDS. At the level of the individual, it involves building of skills to enable people on treatment and their supporters to contribute to the patient-centric approach to prevention, care and treatment and to support their peers. Treatment preparedness provides a platform for enhancing the ability of civil society to deal with the disease.

### *Role of the Community/Civil Society in HIV/AIDS Control*

Community participation is required for every aspect of HIV prevention and control, and includes advocacy, delivery of services and support to patients. A strong community leadership or an effective civil society involvement in policy/decision-making will lead to better and more sustainable health outcomes. This is because HIV/AIDS is not only a medical issue. People with HIV/AIDS face other psycho-social challenges, such as stigma and discrimination, which are best addressed through strong community support. In partnership with the health sector, civil society groups (including faith-based groups) can offer a wide range of support services, education, home-based care, training in income-generating activities and treatment adherence counselling.

### *Role of Non-Governmental Organizations (NGOs) in HIV/AIDS Control*

The close interpersonal interaction that nongovernmental organizations (NGOs) have with people in the communities they work in, is extremely useful for implementing the behavioural interventions necessary for HIV/AIDS prevention and care. NGOs are also not under the same political constraints, as government programmes are. They, therefore, have greater flexibility and the capacity to accommodate changing programmes and public needs, and can innovate and implement new initiatives more easily.

# 4

# Sociology of Ageing

Ageing is the accumulation of changes in an organism or object over time. Ageing in humans refers to a multidimensional process of physical, psychological and social change. Some dimensions of ageing grow and expand over time, while others decline. Reaction time, for example, may slow with age, while knowledge of world events and wisdom may expand. Research shows that even late in life potential exists for physical, mental, and social growth and development. Aging is an important part of all human societies reflecting the biological changes that occur, but also reflecting cultural and societal conventions. Age is usually measured in full years and months for young children. A person's birthday is often an important event.

The term 'ageing' is somewhat ambiguous. Distinctions may be made between 'universal ageing' (age changes that all people share) and 'probabilistic ageing' (age changes that may happen to some, but not to all people as they grow older, such as the onset of Type Two diabetes). Chronological ageing, referring to how old a person is, is arguably the most straightforward definition of ageing and may be distinguished from 'social ageing' (society's expectations of how people should act as they grow older) and 'biological ageing' (an organism's physical state as it ages). There is also a distinction between 'proximal ageing' (age-based effects that come about because of factors in the recent past) and 'distal ageing' (age-based differences that can be traced back to a cause early in person's life, such as childhood poliomyelitis).

Differences are sometimes made between populations of children; divisions are sometimes made between the young old (65–74), the middle old (75–84) and the oldest old (those aged 85 and above). However, problematic in this is that chronological age does not correlate perfectly with functional age, i.e. two people may be of the same age, but differ in their mental and physical capacities.

Population ageing is the increase in the number and proportion of older people in society. Population ageing has three possible causes: migration, longer life expectancy (decreased death rate), and decreased birth rate. Ageing has a significant impact on society. Young people tend to commit most crimes; they are more likely to push for political and social change, to develop and adopt new technologies, and to need education. Older people have different requirements from society and government as opposed to young people, and frequently differing values as well. Older people are also far more likely to vote, and in many countries the young are forbidden from voting. Thus, the aged have comparatively more political influence.

## Senescence

In biology, 'Senescence' is the state or process of ageing. Cellular senescence is a phenomenon where isolated cells demonstrate a limited ability to divide in culture (the Hayflick Limit, discovered by Leonard Hayflick in 1965), while *Organismal senescence* is the ageing of organisms. After a period of near perfect renewal (in humans, between 20 and 35 years of age), organismal senescence is characterized by the declining ability to respond to Stress, increasing homoestatic imbalance and increased risk of disease. This irreversible series of changes inevitably ends in death. Some researchers (specifically biogerontologist) are treating ageing as a disease. As genes that have an effect on ageing are discovered, ageing is increasingly being regarded in a similar fashion to other genetic conditions, potentially 'treatable.'

Indeed, ageing is not an unavoidable property of life. Instead, it is the result of a genetic programme. Numerous species show very low signs of ageing ('negligible senescence'), the best known being trees like the bristlecone pine (however, Dr Hayflick states that the bristlecone pine has no cells older than thirty years), fish like the sturgeon and the rockfish, invertebrates like the quahog or sea anemone.

In humans and other animals, cellular senescence has been attributed to the shortening of telomeres with each cell cycle; when telomeres become too short, the cells die. The length of telomeres is therefore the 'molecular clock,' predicted by Hayflick. Telomere length is maintained in immortal cells (e.g. germ cells and keratinocyte stem cells, but not other skin cell types) by the enzyme telomerase. In the laboratory, mortal cell lines can be immortalized by the activation of their telomerase gene, present in all cells but active in few cell types. Cancerous cells must become immortal to multiply without limit. This important step towards carcinogenesis implies, in 85 per cent of cancers, the reactivation of their telomerase gene by mutation. Since this mutation is rare, the telomere 'clock' can be seen as a protective mechanism against cancer. Research has shown that the clock must be located in the nucleus of each cell and there have been reports that the longevity clock might be located in genes on either the first or fourth chromosome of the twenty–three pairs of human chromosomes.

Other genes are known to affect the ageing process; the sirtuin family of genes has been shown to have a significant effect on the lifespan of yeast and nematodes. Over-expression of the RAS2 gene increases lifespan in yeast substantially.

In addition to genetic ties to lifespan, diet has been shown to substantially affect lifespan in many animals. Specifically, caloric restriction (that is, restricting calories to 30–50 per cent less than an ad libitum animal would consume, while still maintaining proper nutrient intake), has been shown to increase lifespan in mice up to 50 per cent. Caloric restriction works on many other species beyond mice (including species as diverse as yeast and Drosophila), and appears (though the data is not conclusive) to increase lifespan in primates according to a study done on Rhesus monkeys at the National Institute of Health (US), although the increase in lifespan is only notable if the caloric restriction is started early in life. Since, at the molecular level, age is counted not as time but as the number of cell doublings, this effect of calorie reduction could be mediated by the slowing of cellular growth and, therefore, the lengthening of the time between cell divisions.

## Dividing the Lifespan

A human life is often divided into various ages. Historically, the lifespan of people are divided into seven ages; because biological changes are slow moving and vary from person to person, arbitrary dates are usually set to mark periods of human life. In some cultures the divisions given below are quite varied.

Ages can also be divided by decade:

- *Denarian:* someone between 10 and 19 years old
- *Vicenarian:* someone between 20 and 29 years old
- *Tricenarian:* someone between 30 and 39 years old
- *Quadragenarian:* someone between 40 and 49 years old

- *Quinquagenarian:* someone between 50 and 59 years old
- *Sexagenarian:* someone between 60 and 69 years old
- *Septuagenarian:* someone between 70 and 79 years old
- *Octogenarian:* someone between 80 and 89 years old
- *Nonagenarian:* someone between 90 and 99 years old
- *Centenarian:* someone between 100 and 109 years old
- *Super centenarian:* someone 110 years old and over

People from thirteen to nineteen years of age are also known as teens and the casual terms 'twentysomething' and 'thirtysomething', etc. are also in use to describe people by decade.

### Cultural Variations

In some cultures (for example Serbian and Russian) there are two ways to express age: by counting years with or without including current year. For example, it could be said about the same person that he is twenty years old or that he is in the twenty-first year of his life. In Russian the former expression is generally used, the latter one has restricted usage: it is used for age of a deceased person in obituaries and for the age of a child when it is desired to show him/her older than he/she is. (Psychologically, a boy in his 4th year seems older than one who is three years old.)

Considerable numbers of cultures have less of a problem with age compared with what has been described above, and it is seen as an important status to reach stages in life, rather than defined numerical ages. Advanced age is given more respect and status.

## Social Aspects of Ageing

### *Legal*

There are variations in many countries as to what age a person legally becomes an adult. Most legal systems define a specific age for when an individual is allowed or obliged to do something. These ages include voting age, drinking age, age of consent, age of majority, age of criminal responsibility, marriageable age, age where one can hold public office, and mandatory retirement age. Admission to a movie for instance, may depend on age according to a motion picture rating system. A bus fare might be discounted for the young or old.

Similarly in many countries in jurisprudence, the defence of infancy is a form of defence by which a defendant argues that, at the time a law was broken, they were not liable for their actions, and thus should not be held liable for a crime. Many courts recognize that defendants who are considered to be juveniles may avoid criminal prosecution on account of their age, and in borderline cases the age of the offender is often held to be a mitigating circumstance.

### Economics and Marketing

The economics of ageing are also of great importance. Children and teenagers have little money of their own, but most of it is available for buying consumer goods. They also have considerable impact on how their parents spend money.

Young adults are an even more valuable cohort. They often have jobs with few responsibilities such as a mortgage or children. They do not yet have set buying habits and are more open to new products.

The young are thus the central target of marketers. Television is programmed to attract the range of 15 to 35 year olds. Mainstream movies are also built around appealing to the young.

### Health Care Demand

Many societies in the rich world, e.g. Western Europe and Japan, have ageing populations. While the effects on society are complex, there is a concern about the impact on health care demand. The large number of suggestions in the literature for specific interventions to cope with the expected increase in demand for long-term care in ageing societies can be organized under four headings: improve system performance; redesign service delivery; support informal caregivers; and shift demographic parameters.

However, the annual growth in national health spending is not mainly due to increasing demand from ageing populations, but rather has been driven by rising incomes, costly new medical technology, a shortage of health care workers and informational asymmetries between providers and patients.

Even so, it has been estimated that population ageing only explains 0.2 percentage points of the annual growth rate in medical spending of 4.3 per cent since 1970. In addition, certain reforms to Medicare decreased elderly spending on home health care by 12.5 per cent per year between 1996 and 2000. This would suggest that the impact of ageing populations on health care costs is not inevitable.

### Cognitive Effects

Steady decline in many cognitive processes are seen across the lifespan, starting in one's thirties. Research has focused in particular on memory and ageing, and has found decline in many types of memory with ageing, but not in semantic memory or general knowledge such as vocabulary definitions, which typically increases or remains steady. Early studies on changes in cognition with age generally found declines in intelligence in the elderly, but studies were cross sectional rather than longitudinal and thus results may be an artifact of cohort rather than a true example of decline. Intelligence may decline with age, though the rate may vary depending on the type, and may in fact remain steady throughout most of the lifespan, dropping suddenly only as people near the end of their lives. Individual variations in rate of cognitive decline may, therefore, be explained in terms of people having different lengths of life.

### *Coping and Well-being*

Psychologists have examined coping skills in the elderly. Various factors, such as social support, religion and spirituality, active engagement with life and having an internal locus of control have been proposed as being beneficial in helping people to cope with stressful life events in later life. Social support and personal control are possibly the two most important factors that predict well-being, morbidity and mortality in adults. Other factors that may link to well-being and quality of life in the elderly include social relationships (possibly relationships with pets as well as humans), and health.

Individuals in different wings in the same retirement home have demonstrated a lower risk of mortality and higher alertness and self-rated health in the wing where residents had greater control over their environment, though personal control may have less impact on specific measures of health. Social control, perceptions of how much influence one has over one's social relationships, shows support as a modern variable for the relationship between social support and perceived health in the elderly, and may positively influence coping in the elderly.

### *Religion*

Religion has been an important factor used by the elderly in coping with the demands of later life, and appears more often than other forms of coping later in life. Religious commitment may also be associated with reduced mortality, though religiosity is a multidimensional variable; while participation in religious activities in the sense of participation in formal and organized rituals may decline, it may become a more informal, but still important aspect of life such as through personal or private prayer.

### *Self-rated Health*

Self-ratings of health, the beliefs in one's own health as excellent, fair or poor, has been correlated with well-being and mortality in the elderly; positive ratings are linked to high well-being and reduced mortality. Various reasons have been proposed for this association; people who are objectively healthy may naturally rate their health better than that of their ill counterparts, though this link has been observed even in studies which have controlled for socio-economic status, psychological functioning and health status. This finding is generally stronger for men than women, though the pattern between genders is not universal across all studies, and some results suggest sex-based differences only appear in certain age groups, for certain causes of mortality and within a specific sub-set of self-ratings of health.

### *Retirement*

Retirement, a common transition faced by the elderly, may have both positive and negative consequences.

### *Societal Impact*

Societal ageing refers to the demographic aging of populations and societies. Cultural differences in attitudes to aging have been studied.

### *Emotional Improvement*

Given the physical and cognitive declines seen in ageing, a surprising finding is that emotional experience improves with age. Older adults are better at regulating their emotions and experience negative effect less frequently than younger adults and show a positive effect in their attention and memory. The emotional improvements show up in longitudinal studies as well as in cross-sectional studies and so cannot be entirely due to only the happier individuals surviving.

## Successful Ageing

The concept of *successful ageing* can be traced back to the 1950s, and popularized in the 1980s. Previous research into aging exaggerated the extent to which health disabilities, such as diabetes or osteoporosis, could be attributed exclusively to age, and research in gerontology exaggerated the homogeneity of samples of elderly people.

Successful aging consists of three components:

1. Low probability of disease or disability;
2. High cognitive and physical function capacity;
3. Active engagement with life.

A greater number of people self-report successful ageing than those that strictly meet these criteria. Successful aging may be viewed an interdisciplinary concept, spanning both psychology and sociology, where it is seen as the transaction between society and individuals across the life span with specific focus on the later years of life. The terms 'healthy aging' 'optimal aging' have been proposed as alternatives to successful ageing.

Six suggested dimensions of successful ageing include:

1. No physical disability over the age of 75 as rated by a physician;
2. Good subjective health assessment (i.e. good self-ratings of one's health);
3. Length of undisabled life;
4. Good mental health;
5. Objective social support;
6. Self-rated life satisfaction in eight domains, namely marriage, income-related work, children, friendship and social contacts, hobbies, community service activities, religion and recreation/sports

## Theories of Ageing

### *Biological Theories*

At present, the biological basis of aging is unknown. Most scientists agree that substantial variability exists in the rates of aging across different species, and that this to a large extent is genetically based. In model organisms and laboratory settings, researchers have been able to demonstrate that selected alterations in specific genes can extend lifespan (quite substantially in nematodes, less so in fruit flies, and even less in mice). Nevertheless, even in the relatively simple organisms, the mechanism of aging remained to be elucidated. Because the lifespan of even the simple lab mouse is around 3 years, very few experiments directly test specific aging theories (most of the evidence for the ones listed below is correlative).

The National Institute of Aging currently funds an intervention testing programme, whereby investigators nominate compounds (based on specific molecular aging theories) to have evaluated with respect to their effects on lifespan and age-related biomarkers in outbred mice. Previous age-related testing in mammals has proved largely irreproducible, because of small numbers of animals, and lax mouse husbandry conditions. The intervention testing programme aims to address this by conducting parallel experiments at three internationally recognized mouse ageing-centres, the Barshop Institute at UTHSCSA, the University of Michigan at Ann Arbor and the Jackson Lab. While the hypotheses below reflect some of the current direction in biological aging research, none of them is accepted as a 'theory' in the sense of the 'theory of gravity' or 'theory of relativity'.

*Telomere Theory*

Telomeres (structures at the ends of chromosomes) have experimentally been shown to shorten with each successive cell division. Shortened telomeres activate a mechanism that prevents further cell multiplication. This may be an important mechanism of aging in tissues like bone marrow and the arterial lining where active cell division is necessary. Importantly though, mice lacking telomerase do not show a dramatically reduced lifespan, as the simplest version of this theory would predict.

*Reproductive-Cell Cycle Theory*

The idea that aging is regulated by reproductive hormones that act in an antagonistic pleiotropic manner via cell cycle signalling, promoting growth and development early in life in order to achieve reproduction, but later in life, in a futile attempt to maintain reproduction, become dysregulated and drive senescence (dyosis). At the same time, castrated animals, although living somewhat longer, still experience senescence, even in the absence of reproductive hormones.

*Wear-and-Tear Theory*

The very general idea that changes associated with ageing are the result of chance damage that accumulates over time.

*Somatic Mutation Theory*

The biological theory that holds that aging results from damage to the genetic integrity of the body's cells.

*Error Accumulation Theory*

This theory hold that aging results from chance events that escaped proof reading mechanisms, which gradually damages the genetic code.

***Evolutionary Theories***

These are by far the most theoretical; however, their usefulness is somewhat limited as they do not provide readily testable biochemically-based interventions.

### *Accumulative-Waste Theory*

The biological theory of aging that points to a build-up of cells of waste products that presumably interferes with metabolism.

### *Autoimmune Theory*

This theory holds the idea that ageing results from an increase in auto-antibodies that attack the body's tissues. A number of diseases associated with ageing, such as atrophic gastritis and Hashimoto's thyroiditis, are probably autoimmune in this way. While inflammation is very much evident in old mammals, even SCID mice in SPF colonies still senescence.

### *Ageing-Clock Theory*

The theory that aging results from a pre-programmed sequence, as in a clock, built into the operation of the nervous or endocrine system of the body. In rapidly dividing cells the shortening of the telomeres would provide just such a clock. This idea is indirect contradiction with the Evolutionary-Based Theory of Ageing.

### *Cross-Linkage Theory*

This theory holds the idea that aging results from accumulation of cross-linked compounds that interfere with normal cell function.

### *Free-Radical Theory*

The idea that free radicals (unstable and highly reactive organic molecules, also named reactive oxygen species or oxidative stress) create damage that gives rise to symptoms we recognize as aging.

### *Mitohormesis*

It has been known since the 1930s that restricting calories while maintaining adequate amounts of other nutrients prevents aging across a broad range of organism. Recently, Michael Ristow has shown that this delay of ageing is due to increased formation of free radicals within the mitochondria causing a secondary induction of increased antioxidant defence capacity.

## Social Gerontology

Gerontology is the study of the social, psychological and biological aspects of ageing. It is distinguished from geriatrics, which is the branch of medicine that studies the disease of the elderly.

Gerontology includes these and other endeavours:

- Studying physical, mental, and social changes in people as they age;
- Investigating the aging process itself (biogerontology);
- Investigating the interface of normal aging and age-related disease (geroscience);
- Investigating the effects of our ageing population on society, including the fiscal effects of pensions, entitlements, life and health insurance, and retirement planning;
- Applying this knowledge to policies and programmes, including a macroscopic (i.e. government planning) and microscopic (i.e. running a nursing home) perspective.

The multidisciplinary focus of gerontology means that there are a number of sub-fields, as well as associated fields such as psychology and sociology that also cross over into gerontology. However, that there is an overlap should not be taken as to construe that they are the same. For example, a psychologist may specialize in early adults (and not be a gerontologist) or specialize in older adults (and be a gerontologist).

The field of gerontology was developed relatively late, and as such often lacks the structural and institutional support needed (for example, relatively few universities offer a PhD in gerontology). Yet the huge increase in the elderly population in the post-industrial Western nations has led to this becoming one of the most rapidly growing fields. As such, gerontology is currently a well-paying field for many in the West.

Social gerontology is a multidisciplinary sub-field that specializes in studying or working with older adults. Social gerontologists may have degrees or training in social work, nursing, psychology, sociology, demography, gerontology, or other social science professions. Gerontologists are responsible for educating, researching, and advancing the broader causes of older people by giving informative presentations, publishing books and articles that pertain to the ageing population, producing relevant films and television programmes, and producing new graduates of these various disciplines in college and university settings.

Because issues of life span and life extension need numbers to quantify them, there is an overlap with demography. Those that study the demography of the human life span are different than those that study the social demographics of ageing.

### *Theories of Ageing in Social Gerontology*

There are several theories of ageing in social gerontology, but four of these Disengagement Theory, Activity Theory, Continuity Theory that have generally been accepted as the most influential to date will be considered here.

### *Disengagement Theory*

This is the idea that separation of older people from active roles in society is normal and appropriate, and benefits both society and older individuals. Disengagement theory, first proposed by Cumming and Henry, has received considerable attention in gerontology, but has been much criticized. The original data on which Cumming and Henry based the theory were from a rather small sample of older adults in Kansas City and from this select sample Cumming and Henry then took disengagement to be a universal theory. There are research data suggesting that the elderly who do become detached from society as those were initially reclusive individuals, and such disengagement is not purely a response to ageing.

### *Activity Theory*

In contrast to disengagement theory, this theory implies that the more active elderly people are, the more likely they are to be satisfied with life. The view that elderly adults should maintain well-being by keeping active has had a considerable history, and since 1972, this has become to be known as activity theory. However, this theory may be just as inappropriate as disengagement for some people as the current paradigm on the psychology of ageing is that both disengagement theory and activity theory may be optimal for certain people in old age, depending on both circumstances and personality traits of the individual concerned. There are also data which query whether, as activity theory implies, greater social activity is linked with well-being in adulthood.

Selectivity Theory mediates between Activity and Disengagement Theory, which suggests that it may benefit older people to become more active in some aspects of their lives, more disengaged in others.

### *Continuity Theory*

The view that in ageing people are inclined to maintain, as much as they can, the same habits, personalities, and styles of life that they have developed in earlier years. Continuity theory is Atchley's theory that individuals, in later life, make adaptations to enable them to gain a sense of continuity between the past and the present, and the theory implies that this sense of continuity helps to contribute to well-being in later life. Disengagement theory, activity theory and continuity theory are social theories about ageing, though all may be products of their era rather than a valid, universal theory.

# 5

# Infectious and Physical Deficient Diseases

As long as medicine has been practised as a special occupation, anyone interested in studying symptoms, causes and consequences of diseases has been faced with the problem of classification. It is a process of sorting information into categories or 'families' of data which will be useful to the investigator or practitioner. From a sociological frame of reference, one would be more interested in the impact of diseases on group life than in a particular disease entity. Diseases like some other human enemies constitute a threat to group unity and survival, whether the size of the group is a family or a society.

The present state of medical knowledge indicates that most communicable diseases are caused by a wide variety of microorganisms which become parasites on the human host e.g. bacteria, viruses, fungi, worms, rickettsiae. In fact, much of the success story of medicine stems from the identification of specific causes of disease, beginning with the contributions made by the early pioneers in the late nineteenth and early twentieth centuries.

### Tuberculosis

Tuberculosis (TB) is a potentially fatal contagious disease that can affect almost any part of the body but is mainly an infection of the lungs. It is caused by a bacterial microorganism, the tubercle bacillus or Mycobacterium tuberculosis. Although TB can be treated, cured and can be prevented if persons at risk take certain drugs, scientists have never come close to wiping it out. Few diseases have caused so much distressing illness for centuries and claimed so many lives.

Tuberculosis (TB), an infectious disease, has been present throughout ancient and modern history. TB rates in the United States are on the decline after resurgence from 1985 to 1992. However, TB continues to be a major killer in much of the world. The implications of this epidemic are global, as travel and migration are now part of everyday life.

Although the cause, diagnosis, treatment and prevention of TB are known, paradoxically, the disease continues to increase as a public health challenge. Caused by a bacterium called *Mycobacterium tuberculosis*, TB spreads via an airborne route from an infectious person coughing, sneezing, laughing or singing. The bacteria infect mainly other individuals who have frequent and prolonged contact with a contagious TB case.

### *Overview of Tuberculosis*

Tuberculosis was popularly known as consumption for a long time. Scientists know it as an infection caused by M. tuberculosis. In 1882, the microbiologist Robert Koch discovered the tubercle bacillus, at a time when one of every seven deaths in Europe was caused by TB. Because antibiotics were unknown, the only means of controlling the spread of infection was to isolate patients in private sanitoria or hospitals limited to patients with TB – a practice that continues to this day in many countries. The net effect of this pattern of treatment was to separate the study of tuberculosis from mainstream medicine. Entire organizations were set up to study not only the disease as it affected individual patients, but its impact on the society as a whole. At the turn of the twentieth century more than 80 per cent of the population in the United States were infected before age 20, and tuberculosis was the single most common cause of death. By 1938, there were more than 700 TB hospitals in this country.

Tuberculosis spread much more widely in Europe when the industrial revolution began in the late nineteenth century. The disease became widespread, somewhat later, in the United States, because the movement of the population to large cities made overcrowded housing so common. When streptomycin, the first antibiotic effective against M. tuberculosis, was discovered in the early 1940s, the infection began to come under control. Although other more effective anti-tuberculosis drugs were developed in the following decades, the number of cases of TB in the United States began to rise again in the mid-1980s. This upsurge was in part again a result of overcrowding and unsanitary conditions in the poor areas of large cities, prisons and homeless shelters. Infected visitors and immigrants to the United States also contributed to the resurgence of TB. An additional factor is the AIDS epidemic. AIDS patients are much more likely to develop tuberculosis because of their weakened immune systems. There still are an estimated 8 to 10 million new cases of TB each year worldwide, causing roughly 3 million deaths.

### *History of Tuberculosis*

TB's existence dates back many centuries. There are references to TB in third-century BCE Chinese and second-century BCE Indian texts; Plato and Hippocrates wrote about it around 400 BCE. TB was commonly known as consumption in Europe, a cause of death for hundreds of thousands in the late eighteenth and nineteenth centuries. This is when TB in close groups was first observed and assumed to have a genetic cause, since it was commonly seen in families.

In 1882, Robert Koch's discovery of *Mycobacterium tuberculosis* led to the recognition of TB as an infectious disease. This discovery also led to interventions for interrupting transmission from person-to-person.

Beginning in the late 1880s, TB patients were treated in sanitoria with various modalities, including exposure to fresh air, exercise and nourishment. About 50 per cent of patients recovered or had long-term remission. However, as is known today, their 'cure' was not due to the treatments administered but perhaps to self-healing mechanisms.

In the early twentieth-century, public health interventions became key in controlling the spread of TB in the cities, where TB was most prevalent. For example, Herman M. Biggs, General Medical Officer of New York City, actively catalogued lists of TB patients and enforced isolation and environmental mechanisms to control TB, including the opening of a TB hospital to quarantine patients. Between 1914 and 1923, the Metropolitan Life Insurance Company conducted the 'Framingham Tuberculosis Project' using community nurses to visit the homes of its clients to do assessments, teach health practices and collect data for research and policy-making purposes. The project was in response to a high rate of TB – related mortality among Metropolitan customers. As a result, mortality rates for TB in the Metropolitan pool declined by 68 per cent.

Beginning in 1921, the Bacille Calmette Guerin (BCG) vaccine was used to prevent TB. Still used in many parts of the world but not in the United States, the vaccine is not effective, except perhaps in infants. The discovery of streptomycin in 1943 brought drug treatment for TB. Between 1943 and 1952, two more TB drugs, para-amino-salicylic acid (PAS) and isoniazid (INH), were discovered. Sanitoria began to close in the early 1970s, as TB could be now be treated on an outpatient basis, as evidenced by success in the decrease in TB rates with combined drug treatment and infection-control mechanisms.

### *Predisposing Factors*

- *Age:* All ages but highly susceptible below 3 years
- Devitalized conditions such as chronic malnutrition, diabetes.
- *Economic status:* Common in poor communities due to poor sanitation, housing, state, nutrition, etc.
- *Genetic factors:* Host resistance may be lowered by genetic factors.
- Addiction to tobacco, alcohol, etc.
- Occupational diseases like silicosis, asbestosis.
- *Causative organisms:* Two species, M. tuberculosis and M. bovis affect the human race. Avian bacilli have little invasiveness. Several other species of Mycobacteria and atypical mycobacteria may produce chronic pulmonary lesion but are rare.

### *Types of Tuberculosis*

- Primary
- Post Primary

#### *Primary Tuberculosis*

Tubercle bacilli get entry into the human body through various routes; but of these respiratory, gastrointestinal and cutaneous routes are common. When the child is exposed to a diseased individual via droplet infection, the organism enters the respiratory tract. Because of adequate ventilation, lower two-thirds of the lungs are the common sites for lodgement. They multiply at the local site and ultimately are carried to the regional lymph nodes and then to other organs of the body through blood stream before specific immunity develops. During this period, as they produce no toxin and no tissue reaction so no symptom develops. Therefore, the characteristic tissue reaction develops anywhere according to the site of lodgement of the organism. This consists of central necrotic area undergoing caseation, epitheloid cells, Langhans type of giant cells and a lymphocytic barrier at the periphery. This is the characteristic lesion of tuberculosis. When caseation develops this is associated with liberation of various cytotoxic materials from T lymphocytes giving rise to marked reduction in the population of the organism. At the same time these toxic materials destroy the parenchymal tissue of the host. After this, the process of primary infection is gradually closed up by a process of healing by fibrosis, calcification, etc. During initial lesion in the toulung there will be (1) sub-pleural caseous focus anywhere in the lung about 2 cm. in diameter, (2) inflammation of lymphatics, draining the affected area and (3) hilar lymphadenopathy affecting the lymph nodes draining that particular area. These three together are called primary complex and these three components together may be seen in X-ray, though commonly (1) and sometimes (1) and (3) are seen when healing takes place by calcification; pulmonary component can be seen as an opaque spot on X-ray and it is called Ghon's focus.

*Clinical Features*

- Asymptomatic type – This is the commonest type and constitutes about 75–80 per cent of all cases. Ghon's focus in the X-rays and positive Mantoux test are evidences of past infection.
- Febrile type – In some cases the only manifestation is fever, ranging from 37.8–39.5°C (100°–103°F) lasting for 1–2 weeks. WBC count is normal but ESR remains high.
- Allergic type – In this type, patient may show erythema nodosum or phlyctenular keratitis, conjunctivitis or both.
- Progressive type – Here the patient may develop tuberculous pneumonia, broncho-pneumonia, pleurisy, pleural effusion, military tuberculosis, tuberculous meningitis, lobar or segmental collapse or even post primary tuberculosis. This is the gravest type.

*Investigation*

- *Mantoux test:* shows a positive reaction.
- Sputum examination for AFB is usually negative.
- X-Ray of chest may show enlarged hilar nodes with sub-pleural lesion.
- ESR is raised.

*Acute Miliary Tuberculosis*

*Pathogenesis*

Hilar lymphadenopathy occurs in cases of primary tuberculosis. In course of time these lymph nodes become caseous and softened and ultimately these softened materials are poured into a nearly pulmonary venule or arteriole, commonly in the former as its wall is thin. If these are poured into a venule, the tubercle bacilli are disseminated throughout the body and this is called generalized military tuberculosis; when these materials entered in arteriole only pulmonary dissemination occurred. This is called pulmonary military tuberculosis. Because lymphadenopathy occurs in primary tuberculosis and as primary tuberculosis occurs in children, military tuberculosis is also common in children. Each localized lesion resembles millet seed in appearance and therefore the disease is called military tuberculosis. Because of the marked host resistance, the lesions are not limited only to those organs with elevated PO2 but are also found in liver, spleen, lymph node, bone marrow and meninges.

*Clinical Features*

The onset is usually sudden, rarely insidious which is seen in middle aged and elderly individuals.

*Symptoms*

- Fever – high remittent or intermittent type
- Headache
- Severe sweating
- Cough – less prominent
- Dyspnoea
- Anorexia, weakness and emaciation
- Convulsive seizure
- Gradually, unconsciousness sets in.

*Special Investigation*

Blood – shows slightly leucocytosis, at times leucocyte count may be normal or low. ESR is high. There may a leukaemoid reaction and sometimes monocytosis. Mantoux test – may sometimes be negative. X-ray of chest – may show bilateral snowstorm appearance with remarkable absence of vascular markings. Hilar lymphadenopathy may be present. Sputum is usually negative for AFB. CSF may reveal features of tuberculous meningitis in late stages. Biopsy of liver, bone marrow or lymph node may show tuberculous granuloma.

*Post Primary Tuberculosis (Adult Phthisis)*

Post primary tuberculosis occurs: (1) directly from a primary lesion, (2) from reactivation of primary lesion, or (3) reinfection when the primary lesion has been completely healed up. Characteristics lesion of this is a cavity in the lungs.

*Pathogenesis*

It begins as a small caseopneumonic focus in posterior portion of upper lobe or apical portion of lower lobe, the focus is called early infiltration. Why this site is selected is still unsolved; but tubercle bacilli are strict aerobic organism and they grow at plasma oxygen tension of about 140 mm of Hg. In the apices of the lung the PO2 varies from 120–130 mm of Hg in the upright position. Possibly, that is why this is the common site of lesion. Caseation in the centre is followed by liquefaction. The liquefied central mass is discharged into a bronchus and thus a cavity is formed. There is great tendency to localize the cavity by fibrosis. Sometimes, the early infiltrate is arrested at an early stage by fibrosis and calcification.

### *Clinical Features*

*Constitutional symptoms due to tuberculous activity:* Weakness, lassitude, malaise, loss of weight, loss of appetite, sweating at night, evening temperature, palpitation, menstrual disturbances.

*Symptoms due to local infection of the lung:* Cough, pain chest, sputum, sometimes there may be haemoptysis which may be due to (1) ulceration of the bronchial mucosa, (2) erosion of a vessel wall by tubercle (3) rupture of congested vessel, (4) rupture of a mycotic aneurysm (Rasmussen's aneurysm), (5) cavitary lesion, or (6) coagulation defect.

### *Special Investigation*

- *Bacteriological examination:* Demonstration of tubercle bacilli is the sheet anchor of the diagnosis.
  - *Sputum:* Smear and staining with acid fast stain to demonstrate AFB to be confirmed by culture followed by animal inoculation test can be done.
  - Tracheal washings can also be treated in the same way as above.
  - Gastric washings particularly in children and aged can be examined in the same way.
  - Mere presence of acid fast bacilli will not indicate tuberculosis; as there are other non-tuberculous acid fast organisms. Culture and animal inoculation test are also mandatory to differentiate Mycobacterium tuberculosis from typical saprophytic and other mycobacteria.
- X-Ray of the chest usually discloses the disease to the clinician. There may be apical and subapcial infiltration (called nodular or satellite lesion), pneumonic shadow, cavitation with or without fibrotic lesions and military lesions in the X-ray. In post primary lesion, apical and subapical involvements are very common though only lower lobe involvement may occur in 3 per cent of the cases.

- *Biopsy:* If enlarged cervical lymph nodes are present biopsy should be done. Similarly in a patient with continued type of temperature when no obvious cause is found, one must try liver biopsy or sterna puncture in addition. Pleural and pulmonary biopsy may also add materials to investigation. Search should be made for typical tuberculous granuloma in the biopsied material. Apart from histological study, biopsied specimen may be cultured.
- *Study of pleural fluid:* In cases of pulmonary tuberculosis associated with pleural effusion, pleural fluid will show all features of exudates together with AFB in some cases.
- *Skin testing:* Skin test is based on hypersensitivity of skin to specific protein antigen of the mycobacteria. Skin test may be done by intracutaneous injection (Manotoux test) or by multiple puncture method (Time test, Heaf test). The intracutaneous method is best and the most reliable practice currently. Purified protein derivative (PPD-S) 0.1 c.c containing 5 tuberculin units is commonly used but much more stable standardized liquid PPD containing Tween 80 (5 TU of PPD-T) should be used. If the test is negative then 250 TU should be used.

Mantoux test is usually positive in all adult city dwellers. Therefore, mere positive Montoux test will not indicate recent infection. Conversion reaction in any age or very strongly positive reaction in children below 10 years or just positive reaction near about 3 years, usually indicate recent infection dormant or clinically pronounced. It has got no value in the diagnosis of adult tuberculosis. After BCG vaccination Mantoux test will naturally become positive. Mere erythema never indicates a positive test. Inuration is the basic criterion of a positive test.

*Blood:* Blood examination shows normal, low or high leucocyte count. Leukaemoid reaction, lymphocytosi and monocytosis are sometimes seen; ESR is usually high. These changes are never helpful in diagnosis but gradual reduction in ESR has some prognostic value during treatment.

### *Management of Tuberculosis*

- *Bed rest:* It is to be advised till symptoms like fever, haemoptysis, etc. persists. Otherwise, rest is not absolutely required. Sputum positive cases should be isolated till they become negative.
- High calorie, high protein diet supplemented with vitamins is ideal.
- Drugs:

| Drugs | Dose | Side Effects |
|---|---|---|
| Isoniazid (INH) | 5 mg/kg/day in adults. 10–15 mg/kg/day in children | Peripheral neuropathy, hepatitis, jaundice, allergic reactions including fever and skin rash, psychic upset, fits, blood dyscrasia. |
| Stereptomycin | 1 gram IM daily or twice weekly | Headache, vomiting, giddiness, circumoral parasthesia, vestibular and cochlear dysfunction, fever, rash, jaundice. |
| Ethambutol | 15 mg/kg/day | Diminished visual acuity, colour blindness usually green, skin rash, neuropathy. |
| Rifampin | 10 mg/kg/day | Cytopenia, orange colouration of different body fluids including sweat, altered liver function tests, jaundice, rash, hypersensitivity reaction. |

Therapy should be started usually with three drugs: Streptomycin, Isoniazid and Ethambutol. Streptomycin should be continued up to 1 gm in an average case of which first 30–40 injections should be given daily and the remaining 30–40 injections should preferably be given on alternate days and sometimes twice a week. Before giving Streptomycin, sensitivity test should be performed. Instead of 1 Gram dose now a days 0.75 Gram daily dose is said to be quite adequate. During the whole period of Streptomycin therapy Isoniazid 300 mg daily should be given as a single dose or in divided doses along with Ethambutol 1,000–1,200 mgm a day as a single dose. This initial three drug regime is chosen to prevent drug resistance. After 70–80 grams of Streptomycin, Isoniazid and Ethmbutol are to be continued for a period of 15–18 months of pulmonary tuberculosis but the total duration varies. In cases of bone and joint tuberculosis, tuberculosis of kidney, intestinal tuberculosis, etc. the total duration of therapy may be prolonged even to 2 years or more than that. If patient develops resistance to any one of these drugs Ethionamide, Pyrazinamide, Rifampin or others are to be substituted. In military tuberculosis, pleural, pericardial tuberculosis, tuberculuos meningitis, for drug desensitization and as substitution therapy in cases of Addison's disease steroids is given in addition to the antituberculous drugs. Without adequate antituberculous coverage steroid should never be given.

- *Surgical:* For localized chronic tuberculosis with or without cavitary lesion, surgical resection is to be considered.

**Malaria**

Malaria is caused by a parasite called Plasmodium, which is transmitted via the bites of infected mosquitoes. In the human body, the parasites multiply in the liver, and then infect red blood cells. Malaria is a vector-borne infectious disease caused by protozoan parasites. It is widespread in tropical and subtropical regions, including parts of the Americas, Asia, and Africa. Each year, there are approximately 515 million cases of malaria, killing between one and three million people, the majority of whom are young children in Sub-Saharan Africa. Ninety per cent of malaria-related deaths occur in Sub-Saharan Africa. Malaria is commonly associated with poverty, but is also a cause of poverty and a major hindrance to economic development.

Malaria is one of the most common infectious diseases and an enormous public health problem. The disease is caused by protozoan parasites of the genus Plasmodium. Only four types of the plasmodium parasite can infect humans; the most serious forms of the disease are caused by Plasmodium falciparum and Plasmodium Vivax, but other related species (Plasmodium ovale, Plasmodium malariae) can also affect humans. This group of human-pathogenic Plasmodium species is usually referred to as malaria parasites.

Usually, people get malaria when bitten by an infective female Anopheles mosquito. Only Anopheles mosquitoes can transmit malaria, and they must have been infected through a previous blood meal taken on an infected person. When a mosquito bites an infected person, a small amount of blood is taken, which contains microscopic malaria parasites. About one week later, when the mosquito takes its next blood meal, these parasites mix with the mosquito's saliva and are injected into the person being bitten. The parasites multiply within red blood cells, causing symptoms that include symptoms of anaemia (light-headedness, shortness of breath, tachycardia, etc.), as well as other general symptoms such as fever, chills, nausea, flu-like illness, and, in severe cases, coma, and death. Malaria transmission can be reduced by preventing mosquito bites with mosquito nets and insect repellents, or by mosquito control measures such as spraying insecticides inside houses and draining standing water where mosquitoes lay their eggs.

Although some are under development, no vaccine is currently available for malaria; preventive drugs must be taken continuously to reduce the risk of infection. These prophylactic drug treatments are often too expensive for most people living in endemic areas. Most adults from endemic areas have a degree of long-term infection, which tends to recur, and also possess partial immunity (resistance); the resistance reduces with time, and such adults may become susceptible to severe malaria if they have spent a significant amount of time in non-endemic areas. They are strongly recommended to take full precautions if they return to an endemic area. Malaria infections are treated through the use of antimalarial drug, such as quinine or artemisinin derivatives. However, parasites have evolved to be resistant to many of these drugs. Therefore, in some areas of the world, only a few drugs remain as effective treatments for malaria.

### *History of Malaria*

Malaria has infected humans for over 50,000 years, and may have been a human pathogen for the entire history of the species. Close relatives of the human malaria parasites remain common in chimpanzees. References to the unique periodic fevers of malaria are found throughout recorded history, beginning in 2700 BC in China. The term malaria originates from Medieval Italian: *mala aria* – 'bad air'; and the disease was formerly called ague or marsh fever due to its association with swamps and marshland.

Scientific studies on malaria made their first significant advance in 1880, when a French army doctor working in the military hospital of Constantine in Algeria named Charles Louis observed parasites for the first time, inside the red blood cells of people suffering from malaria. He, therefore, proposed that malaria is caused by this protozoan, the first time protozoa were identified as causing disease. For this and later discoveries, he was awarded the 1907 Nobel Prize for Physiology or Medicine. The protozoan was called Plasmodium by the Italian scientists Ettore Marchiafava and Angelo Celli. A year later, Carlos Finlay, a Cuban doctor treating patients with yellow fever in Havana, provided strong evidence that mosquitoes were transmitting disease to and from humans. This work followed earlier suggestions by Josiah C. Nott and work by Patrick Manson on the transmission of filariasis.

However, it was Britain's Sir Ronald Ross working in the Presidency General Hospital in Calcutta who finally proved in 1898 that malaria is transmitted by mosquitoes. He did this by showing that certain mosquito species transmit malaria to birds and isolating malaria parasites from the salivary glands of mosquitoes that had fed on infected birds. For this work Ross received the 1902 Nobel Prize in Medicine. After resigning from the Indian Medical Service, Ross worked at the newly-established Liverpool School of Tropical Medicine and directed malaria-control efforts in Egypt, Panama, Greece and Mauritius. The findings of Finlay and Ross were later confirmed by a medical board headed by Walter Reed in 1900 and its recommendations implemented by William C. Gorgas in the health measures undertaken during construction of the Panama Canal. This public-health work saved the lives of thousands of workers and helped develop the methods used in future public-health campaigns against this disease.

The first effective treatment for malaria came from the bark of cinchona tree, which contains quinine. This tree grows on the slopes of the Andes, mainly in Peru. A tincture made of this natural product was used by the inhabitants of Peru to control malaria, and the Jesuits introduced this practice to Europe during the 1640s, where it was rapidly accepted. However, it was not until 1820 that the active ingredient, quinine, was extracted from the bark, isolated and named by the French chemists Pierre Joseph Pelletier and Joseph Bienaimé Caventou.

In the early twentieth century, before antibiotics, patients with syphilis were intentionally infected with malaria to create a fever, following the work of Julius Wagner-Jauregg. By accurately controlling the fever with quinine, the effects of both syphilis and malaria could be minimized. Although some patients died from malaria, this was preferable to the almost-certain death from syphilis.

Although the blood stage and mosquito stages of the malaria life cycle were identified in the 19th and early 20th centuries, it was not until the 1980s that the latent liver form of the parasite was observed. The discovery of this latent form of the parasite finally explained why people could appear to be cured of malaria but still relapse years after the parasite had disappeared from their bloodstreams.

### *Distribution and Impact*

Malaria causes about 250 million cases of fever and approximately one million deaths annually. The vast majority of cases occur in children under 5 years old; pregnant women are also especially vulnerable. Despite efforts to reduce transmission and increase treatment, there has been little change in which areas are at risk of this disease since 1992. Indeed, if the prevalence of malaria stays on its present upwards course, the death rate could double in the next twenty years. Precise statistics are unknown because many cases occur in rural areas where people do not have access to hospitals or the means to afford health care. As a consequence, the majority of cases are undocumented.

Although co-infection with HIV and malaria does cause increased mortality, this is less of a problem than with HIV/tuberculosis co-infection, due to the two diseases usually attacking different age-ranges, with malaria being most common in the young and active tuberculosis most common in the old. Although HIV/malaria co-infection produces less severe symptoms than the interaction between HIV and TB, HIV and malaria do contribute to each other's spread. This effect comes from malaria increasing viral load and HIV infection increasing a person's susceptibility to malaria infection.

Malaria is presently endemic in a broad band around the equator, in areas of the Americas, many parts of Asia and much of Africa; however, it is in Sub-Saharan Africa where 85–90 per cent of malaria fatalities occur. The geographic distribution of malaria within large regions is complex, and malaria-afflicted and malaria-free areas are often found close to each other. In drier areas, outbreaks of malaria can be predicted with reasonable accuracy by mapping rainfall. Malaria is more common in rural areas than in cities; this is in contrast to dengue fever where urban areas present the greater risk. For example, the cities of Vietnam, Laos and Cambodia are essentially malaria-free, but the disease is present in many rural regions. By contrast, in Africa malaria is present in both rural and urban areas, though the risk is lower in the larger cities. The global endemic levels of malaria have not been mapped since the 1960s. However, the Wellcome Trust, UK, has funded the Malaria Atlas Project to rectify this, providing a more contemporary and robust means with which to assess current and future malaria disease burden.

### *Socio-economic Effects*

Malaria is not just a disease commonly associated with poverty but also a cause of poverty and a major hindrance to economic development. Tropical regions are affected most; however, malaria's furthest extent reaches into some temperate zones with extreme seasonal changes. The disease has been associated with major negative economic effects on regions where it is widespread. During the late 19th and early 20th centuries, it was a major factor in the slow economic development of the American southern states. A comparison of average per capita GDP in 1995, adjusted for parity of purchasing power, between countries with malaria and countries without malaria gives a fivefold difference ($1,526 USD versus $8,268 USD). In countries where malaria is common, average per capita GDP has risen (between 1965 and 1990) only 0.4 per cent per year, compared to 2.4 per cent per year in other countries. However, poverty is both a cause and effect, since the poor do not have the financial capacity to prevent or treat the disease. The lowest income group in Malawi carries the burden of having 32 per cent of their annual income used on this disease, compared with the 4 per cent of household incomes from low-to-high groups. In its entirety, the economic impact of malaria has been estimated to cost Africa $12 billion USD every year. The economic impact includes costs of health care, working days lost due to sickness, days lost in education, decreased productivity due to brain damage from cerebral malaria, and loss of investment and tourism. In some countries with a heavy malaria burden, the disease may account for as much as 40 per cent of public health expenditure, 30–50 per cent of inpatient admissions and up to 50 per cent of outpatient visits. The extensive use of anti-malaria campaigns in recent decades seeks to address the correlation between the disease and poverty. Government subsidies and public health care providers made available in closer proximity to all of the people in a town are efficient methods to reduce the cost of treatment for the poor and the rest of the social classes as that would allow equal accessibility and utilization of treatment.

### *Symptoms of Malaria*

Symptoms of malaria include fever, shivering, arthralgia (joint pain), vomiting, anaemia (caused by hemolysis), hemoglobinuria, retinal damage and convulsions. The classic symptom of malaria is cyclical occurrence of sudden coldness followed by rigour and then fever and sweating lasting four to six hours, occurring every two days in P. vivax and P. ovale infections, while every three for P. malariae. P. falciparum can have recurrent fever every 36–48 hours or a less pronounced and almost continuous fever. For reasons that are poorly understood, but that may be related to high intracranial pressure, children with malaria frequently exhibit abnormal posturing, a sign indicating severe brain damage. Malaria has been found to cause cognitive impairments, especially in children. It causes widespread anaemia during a period of rapid brain development and also direct brain damage. This neurologic damage results from cerebral malaria to which children are more vulnerable.

| Species | Appearance | Periodicity | Persistent in Liver? |
|---|---|---|---|
| Plasmodium vivax | | Tertian | Yes |
| Plasmodium ovale | 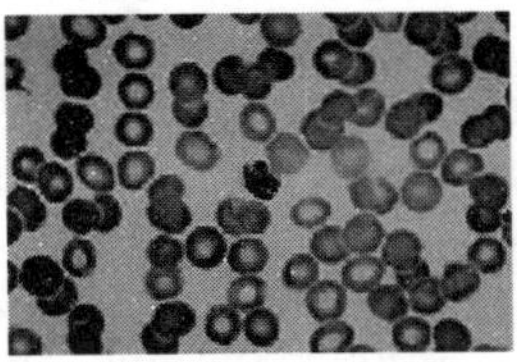 | Tertian | Yes |
| Plasmodium falciparum | | Tertian | No |
| Plasmodium malariae | | Quartan | No |

Severe malaria is almost exclusively caused by P. falciparum infection and usually arises 6–14 days after infection. Consequences of severe malaria include coma and death if untreated – young children and pregnant women are especially vulnerable. Splenomegaly (enlarged spleen), severe headache, cerebral ischemia, hepatomegaly (enlarged liver), hypoglycemia, and hemoglobinuria with renal failure may occur. Renal failure may cause blackwater fever, where hemoglobin from lysed red blood cells leaks into the urine. Severe malaria can progress extremely rapidly and cause death within hours or days. In the most severe cases of the disease fatality rates can exceed 20 per cent, even with intensive care and treatment. In endemic areas, treatment is often less satisfactory and the overall fatality rate for all cases of malaria can be as high as one in ten. Over the longer term, developmental impairments have been documented in children who have suffered episodes of severe malaria.

Chronic malaria is seen in both P. vivax and P. ovale, but not in P. falciparum. Here, the disease can relapse months or years after exposure, due to the presence of latent parasites in the liver. Describing a case of malaria as cured by observing the disappearance of parasites from the bloodstream can, therefore, be deceptive. The longest incubation period reported for a P. vivax infection is 30 years. Approximately one in five of P. vivax malaria cases in temperate areas involve overwintering by hypnozoites (i.e. relapses begin the year after the mosquito bite).

### *Causes of Malaria*

*Malaria parasites:* Malaria is caused by protozoan parasites of the genus Plasmodium (phylum Apicomplexa). In humans, malaria is caused by P. Falciparum, P. malariae, P. ovale, P. vivax and P. knowlesi. P.

falciparum is the most common cause of infection and is responsible for about 80 per cent of all malaria cases and is also responsible for about 90 per cent of the deaths from malaria. Parasitic Plasmodium species also infect birds, reptiles, monkeys, chimpanzees and rodents. There have been documented human infections with several simian species of malaria, namely P. knowlesi, P. inui, P. cynomolgi, P. simiovale, P. brazilianum, P. schwetzi and P. simium; however, with the exception of P. knowlesi, these are mostly of limited public health importance. Although avian malaria can kill chickens and turkeys, this disease does not cause serious economic losses to poultry farmers. However, since being accidentally introduced by humans it has decimated the endemic birds of Hawaii, which evolved in its absence and lacks any resistance to it.

### *Mosquito Vectors and the Plasmodium Life Cycle*

The parasite's primary (definitive) hosts and transmission vectors are female mosquitoes of the Anopheles genus. Young mosquitoes first ingest the malaria parasite by feeding on an infected human carrier and the infected Anopheles mosquitoes carry Plasmodium sporozoites in their salivary glands. A mosquito becomes infected when it takes a blood meal from an infected human. Once ingested, the parasite gametocytes taken up in the blood will further differentiate into male or female gametes and then fuse in the mosquito gut. This produces an ookinete that penetrates the gut lining and produces an oocyst in the gut wall. When the oocyst ruptures, it releases sporozoites that migrate through the mosquito's body to the salivary glands, where they are then ready to infect a new human host. This type of transmission is occasionally referred to as anterior station transfer. The sporozoites are injected into the skin, alongside saliva, when the mosquito takes a subsequent blood meal.

Only female mosquitoes feed on blood, thus males do not transmit the disease. The females of the Anopheles genus of mosquito prefer to feed at night. They usually start searching for a meal at dusk, and will continue throughout the night until taking a meal. Malaria parasites can also be transmitted by blood transfusions, although this is rare.

### *Pathogenesis*

A mosquito infects a person, by taking a blood meal. First, sporozoites enter the bloodstream, and migrate to the liver. They infect liver cells (hepatocytes), where they multiply into merozoites, rupture the liver cells, and escape back into the bloodstream. Then, the merozoites infect red blood cells, where they develop into ring forms, then trophozoites (a feeding stage), then schizonts (a reproduction stage), then back into merozoites. Sexual forms called gametocytes are also produced which, if taken up by a mosquito, will infect the insect and continue the life cycle.

*Malaria in humans develops via two phases:* an exoerythrocytic and an erythrocytic phase. The exoerythrocytic phase involves infection of the hepatic system, or liver, whereas the erythrocytic phase involves infection of the erythrocytes, or red blood cells. When an infected mosquito pierces a person's skin to take a blood meal, sporozoites in the mosquito's saliva enter the bloodstream and migrate to the liver. Within 30 minutes of being introduced into the human host, the sporozoites infect hepatocytes, multiplying asexually and asymptomatically for a period of 6–15 days. Once in the liver, these organisms differentiate to yield thousands of merozoites, which, following rupture of their host cells, escape into the blood and infect red blood cells, thus beginning the erythrocytic stage of the life cycle. The parasite escapes from the liver undetected by wrapping itself in the cell membrane of the infected host liver cell.

Within the red blood cells, the parasites multiply further, again asexually, periodically breaking out of their hosts to invade fresh red blood cells. Several such amplification cycles occur. Thus, classical descriptions of waves of fever arise from simultaneous waves of merozoites escaping and infecting red blood cells.

Some P. vivax and P. ovale sporozoites do not immediately develop into exoerythrocytic – phase merozoites, but instead produce hypnozoites that remain dormant for periods ranging from several months (6–12 months is typical) to as long as three years. After a period of dormancy, they reactivate and produce merozoites. Hypnozoites are responsible for long incubation and late relapses in these two species of malaria.

The parasite is relatively protected from attack by the body's immune system because for most of its human life cycle, it resides within the liver and blood cells and is relatively invisible to immune surveillance. However, circulating infected blood cells are destroyed in the spleen. To avoid this fate, the P. falciparum parasite displays adhesive proteins on the surface of the infected blood cells, causing the blood cells to stick to the walls of small blood vessels, thereby sequestering the parasite from passage through the general circulation and the spleen. This 'stickiness' is the main factor giving rise to hemorrhagic complications of malaria. High endothelial venules (the smallest branches of the circulatory system) can be blocked by the attachment of masses of these infected red blood cells. The blockage of these vessels causes symptoms such as in placental and cerebral malaria. In cerebral malaria the sequestrated red blood cells can breach the blood brain barrier possibly leading to coma.

Although the red blood cell surface adhesive proteins (called PfEMP1, for Plasmodium falciparum erythrocyte membrane protein 1) are exposed to the immune system, they do not serve as good immune targets because of their extreme diversity; there are at least 60 variations of the protein within a single parasite and perhaps limitless versions within parasite populations. Like a thief changing disguises or a spy with multiple passports, the parasite switches between broad repertoires of PfEMP1 surface proteins, thus staying one step ahead of the pursuing immune system.

Some merozoites turn into male and female gametocytes. If a mosquito pierces the skin of an infected person, it potentially picks up gametocytes within the blood. Fertilization and sexual recombination of the parasite occurs in the mosquito's gut, thereby defining the mosquito as the definitive host of the disease. New sporozoites develop and travel to the mosquito's salivary gland, completing the cycle. Pregnant women are especially attractive to the mosquitoes, and malaria in pregnant women is an important cause of stillbirths, infant mortality and low birth weight, particularly in P. falciparum infection, but also in other species infection, such as P. vivax.

### *Diagnosis*

Blood smear from a P. falciparum culture (K1 strain). Several red blood cells have ring stages inside them. Close to the centre there is a schizont and on the left a trophozoite. Severe malaria is commonly misdiagnosed in Africa, leading to a failure to treat other life-threatening illnesses. In malaria-endemic areas, parasitemia does not ensure a diagnosis of severe malaria because parasitemia can be incidental to other concurrent diseases. Recent investigations suggest that malarial retinopathy is better (collective sensitivity of 95 per cent and specificity of 90%) than any other clinical or laboratory feature in distinguishing malarial from non-malarial coma.

#### *Symptomatic Diagnosis*

Areas that cannot afford even simple laboratory diagnostic tests often use only a history of subjective fever as the indication to treat for malaria. Using Giemsa-stained blood smears from children in Malawi, one study showed that unnecessary treatment for malaria was significantly decreased when clinical predictors (rectal temperature, nailbed pallor, and splenomegaly) were used as treatment indications, rather than the current national policy of using only a history of subjective fevers (sensitivity increased from 21% to 41%).

### *Microscopic Examination of Blood Films*

The most economic, preferred and reliable diagnosis of malaria is microscopic examination of blood films because each of the four major parasite species has distinguishing characteristics. Two sorts of blood films are traditionally used. Thin films are similar to usual blood films and allow species identification because the parasite's appearance is best preserved in this preparation. Thick films allow the microscopist to screen a larger volume of blood and are about eleven times more sensitive than the thin film, so picking up low levels of infection is easier on the thick film, but the appearance of the parasite is much more distorted and therefore distinguishing between the different species can be much more difficult. With the pros and cons of both thick and thin smears taken into consideration, it is imperative to utilize both smears while attempting to make a definitive diagnosis.

From the thick film, an experienced microscopist can detect parasite levels (or parasitemia) down to as low as 0.0000001 per cent of red blood cells. Diagnosis of species can be difficult because the early trophozoites ('ring form') of all four species look identical and it is never possible to diagnose species on the basis of a single ring form; species identification is always based on several trophozoites.

### *Field Tests*

In areas where microscopy is not available, or where laboratory staff are not experienced at malaria diagnosis, there are antigen detection tests that require only a drop of blood. Immunochromatographic tests (also called: Malaria Rapid Diagnostic Tests, Antigen-Capture Assay or 'Dipsticks') have been developed, distributed and field-tested. These tests use finger-stick or venous blood, the completed test takes a total of 15–20 minutes and a laboratory is not needed. The threshold of detection by these rapid diagnostic tests is in the range of 100 parasites/Fl of blood compared to 5 by thick film microscopy. The first rapid diagnostic tests were using P. falciparum glutamate dehydrogenase as antigen. PGluDH was soon replaced by P. falciparum lactate dehydrogenase, a 33 kDa oxidoreductase [EC 1.1.1.27]. It is the last enzyme of the glycolytic pathway, essential for

ATP generation and one of the most abundant enzymes expressed by P. falciparum. PLDH does not persist in the blood but clears about the same time as the parasites following successful treatment. The lack of antigen persistence after treatment makes the pLDH test useful in predicting treatment failure. In this respect, pLDH is similar to pGluDH. The OptiMAL-IT assay can distinguish between P. falciparum and P. vivax because of antigenic differences between their pLDH isoenzymes. OptiMAL-IT will reliably detect falciparum down to 0.01 per cent parasitemia and non-falciparum down to 0.1 per cent. Paracheck-Pf will detect parasitemias down to 0.002 per cent but will not distinguish between falciparum and non-falciparum malaria. Parasite nucleic acids are detected using polymerase chain reaction. This technique is more accurate than microscopy. However, it is expensive, and requires a specialized laboratory. Moreover, levels of parasitemia are not necessarily correlative with the progression of disease, particularly when the parasite is able to adhere to blood vessel walls. Therefore, more sensitive low-tech diagnosis tools need to be developed in order to detect low levels of parasitaemia in the field.

### *Molecular Methods*

Molecular methods are available in some clinical laboratories and rapid real-time assays (for example, QT-NASBA based on the polymerase chain reaction) are being developed with the hope of being able to deploy them in endemic areas.

### *Laboratory Tests*

OptiMAL – IT will reliably detect falciparum down to 0.01 per cent parasitemia and non-falciparum down to 0.1 per cent. Paracheck-Pf will detect parasitemias down to 0.002 per cent but will not distinguish between falciparum and non-falciparum malaria. Parasite nucleic acids are detected using polymerase chain reaction. This technique is more accurate than microscopy. However, it is expensive and requires a specialized laboratory. Moreover, levels of parasitemia are not necessarily correlative with the progression of disease, particularly when the parasite is able to adhere to blood vessel walls. Therefore, more sensitive, low-tech diagnosis tools need to be developed in order to detect low levels of parasitaemia in the field.

### *Treatment*

Active malaria infection with P. falciparum is a medical emergency requiring hospitalization. Infection with P. vivax, P. ovale or P. malariae can often be treated on an outpatient basis. Treatment of malaria involves supportive measures as well as specific antimalarial drugs. When properly treated, someone with malaria can expect a complete recovery.

#### *Antimalarial Drugs*

There are several families of drugs used to treat malaria. Chloroquine is very cheap and, until recently, was very effective, which made it the antimalarial drug of choice for many years in most parts of the world. However, resistance of Plasmodium falciparum to chloroquine has spread recently from Asia to Africa, making the drug ineffective against the most dangerous Plasmodium strain in many affected regions of the world. In those areas where chloroquine is still effective it remains the first choice. Unfortunately, chloroquine-resistance is associated with reduced sensitivity to other drugs such as quinine and amodiaquine.

There are several other substances which are used for treatment and, partially, for prevention. Many drugs may be used for both purposes; larger doses are used to treat cases of malaria. Their deployment depends mainly on the frequency of resistant parasites in the area where the drug is used. One drug currently being investigated for possible use as an anti-malarial, especially for treatment of drug-resistant strains, is the beta blocker propranolol. Propranolol has been shown to block both Plasmodium's ability to enter red blood cell and establish an infection, as well as parasite replication. A December 2006 study by Northwestern University researchers suggested that propranolol may reduce the dosages required for existing drugs to be effective against P. falciparum by 5 to 10-fold, suggesting a role in combination therapies.

Currently available anti-malarial drugs include:

- Artemether – lumefantrine (Therapy only, commercial names Coartem and Riamet)
- Artesunate – amodiaquine (Therapy only)
- Artesunate – mefloquine (Therapy only)
- Artesunate – Sulfadoxine/pyrimethamine (Therapy only)

- Atovaquone – proguanil, trade name Malarone (Therapy and prophylaxis)
- Quinine (Therapy only)
- Chloroquine (Therapy and prophylaxis; usefulness now reduced due to resistance)
- Cotrifazid (Therapy and prophylaxis)
- Doxycycline (Therapy and prophylaxis)
- Mefloquine, trade name Lariam (Therapy and prophylaxis)
- Primaquine (Therapy in P. vivax and P. ovale only; not for prophylaxis)
- Proguanil (Prophylaxis only)
- Sulfadoxine – pyrimethamine (Therapy; prophylaxis for semi-immune pregnant women in endemic countries as 'Intermittent Preventive Treatment' – IPT)
- Hydroxychloroquine, trade name Plaquenil (Therapy and prophylaxis)

The development of drugs was facilitated when Plasmodium falciparum was successfully cultured. This allowed in vitro testing of new drug candidates.

Extracts of the plant Artemisia annua, containing the compound artemisinin or semi-synthetic derivatives (a substance unrelated to quinine), offer over 90 per cent efficacy rates, but their supply is not meeting demand. In 2007, the Bill and Melinda Gates Foundation contributed $13.6 million to support research at the University of York to develop fast and high-yield strains of artemisia, with researchers predicting an increase in yield of up to 1,000 per cent compared to current varieties. One study in Rwanda showed that children with uncomplicated P. falciparum malaria demonstrated fewer clinical and parasitological failures on post-treatment day 28 when amodiaquine was combined with artesunate, rather than administered alone (OR = 0.34). However, increased resistance to amodiaquine during this study period was also noted. Since 2001, the World Health Organization has recommended using artemisinin-based combination therapy (ACT) as first-line treatment for uncomplicated malaria in areas experiencing resistance to older medications. The most recent WHO treatment guidelines for malaria recommend four different ACTs. While numerous countries, including most African nations, have adopted the change in their official malaria treatment policies, cost remains a major barrier to ACT implementation. Because ACTs cost up to twenty times as much as older medications, they remain unaffordable in many malaria-endemic countries. The molecular target of artemisinin is controversial, although recent studies suggest that SERCA, a calcium pump in the endoplasmic reticulum may be associated with artemisinin resistance. Malaria parasites can develop resistance to artemisinin and resistance can be produced by mutation of SERCA. However, other studies suggest the mitochondrion is the major target for artemisinin and its analogs.

In February 2002, the journal *Science* and other press outlets announced progress on a new treatment for infected individuals. A team of French and South African researchers had identified a new drug they were calling 'G25'. It cured malaria in test primates by blocking the ability of the parasite to copy itself within the red blood cells of its victims. In 2005, the same team of researchers published their research on achieving an oral form, which they refer to as 'TE3' or 'te3'. As of early 2006, there is no information in the mainstream press as to when this family of drugs will become commercially available.

In 1996, Professor Geoff McFadden stumbled upon the work of British biologist Ian Wilson, who had discovered that the plasmodia responsible for causing malaria retained parts of chloroplasts, an organelle usually found in plants, complete with their own functioning genomes. This led Professor McFadden to the realization that any number of herbicides may, in fact, be successful in the fight against malaria, and so he set about trialing large numbers of them, and enjoyed a 75 per cent success rate.

These 'apicoplasts' are thought to have originated through the endosymbiosis of algae and play a crucial role in fatty acid bio-synthesis in plasmodia. To date, 466 proteins have been found to be produced by apicoplasts and these are now being looked at as possible targets for novel anti-malarial drugs.

*Counterfeit Drugs*

Sophisticated counterfeits have been found in several Asian countries such as Cambodia, China, Indonesia, Laos, Thailand, Vietnam and are an important cause of avoidable death in these countries. WHO have said that studies indicate that up to 40 per cent of artesunate-based malaria medications are counterfeit, especially in the Greater Mekong region and have established a rapid alert system to enable information about counterfeit drugs to be rapidly reported to the relevant authorities in participating countries. There is no reliable way for doctors or lay people to detect counterfeit drugs without help from a laboratory. Companies are attempting to combat the persistence of counterfeit drugs by using new technology to provide security from source to distribution.

### *Prevention and Disease Control*

Anopheles albimanus mosquito is a vector of malaria and mosquito control is a very effective way of reducing the incidence of malaria. Methods used to prevent the spread of disease, or to protect individuals in areas where malaria is endemic, include prophylactic drugs, mosquito eradication and the prevention of mosquito bites. The continued existence of malaria in an area requires a combination of high human population density, high mosquito population density, and high rates of transmission from humans to mosquitoes and from mosquitoes to humans. If any of these is lowered sufficiently, the parasite will sooner or later disappear from that area, as happened in North America, Europe and much of Middle East. However, unless the parasite is eliminated from the whole world, it could become re-established if conditions revert to a combination that favours the parasite's reproduction. Many countries are seeing an increasing number of imported malaria cases due to extensive travel and migration.

There is currently no vaccine that will prevent malaria, but this is an active field of research. Many researchers argue that prevention of malaria may be more cost-effective than treatment of the disease in the long run, but the capital costs required are out of reach of many of the world's poorest people. Economic adviser, Jeffrey Sachs estimates that malaria can be controlled for US$3 billion in aid per year. It has been argued that, in order to meet the Millennium Development Goals, money should be redirected from HIV/AIDS treatment to malaria prevention, which for the same amount of money would provide greater benefit to African economies.

The distribution of funding varies among countries. Countries with large populations do not receive the same amount of support. The 34 countries that received a per capita annual support of less than $1 included some of the poorest countries in Africa, Brazil, Eritrea, India, and Vietnam have, unlike many other developing nations, successfully reduced the malaria burden. Common success factors included conducive country conditions, a targeted technical approach using a package of effective tools, data-driven decision-making, active leadership at all levels of government, involvement of communities, decentralized implementation and control of finances, skilled technical and managerial capacity at national and sub-national levels, hands-on technical and programmatic support from partner agencies, and sufficient and flexible financing.

### *Vector Control*

Before DDT, malaria was successfully eradicated or controlled also in several tropical areas by removing or poisoning the breeding grounds of the mosquitoes or the aquatic habitats of the larva stages, for example by filling or applying oil to places with standing water. These methods have seen little application in Africa for more than half a century.

Efforts to eradicate malaria by eliminating mosquitoes have been successful in some areas. Malaria was once common in the United States and southern Europe, but the draining of wetland breeding grounds and better sanitation, in conjunction with the monitoring and treatment of infected humans eliminated it from affluent regions. In 2002, there were 1,059 cases of malaria reported in the US, including eight deaths. In five of those cases, the disease was contracted in the United States. Malaria was eliminated from the northern parts of the USA in the early twentieth century, and the use of the pesticide DDT eliminated it from the South by 1951. In the 1950s and 1960s, there was a major public health effort to eradicate malaria worldwide by selectively targeting mosquitoes in areas where malaria was rampant. However, these efforts have so far failed to eradicate malaria in many parts of the developing world – the problem is most prevalent in Africa.

Sterile insect technique is emerging as a potential mosquito control method. Progress towards transgenic, or genetically modified, insects suggest that wild mosquito populations could be made malaria-resistant. Researchers at Imperial College London created the world's first transgenic malaria mosquito, with the first plasmodium-resistant species announced by a team at Case Western Reserve University in Ohio in 2002. Successful replacement of existent populations with genetically modified populations relies upon a drive mechanism, such as transposable elements to allow for non-Mendelian inheritance of the gene of interest. However, this approach contains many difficulties and 34 per cent of the malaria research and control community say that such an approach 'will never fly'. Furthermore, such an approach is at least 5 to 10 years away from introduction and the progress which has been made in developing a vaccine could influence further research in genetic modification of malaria mosquitoes negatively.

### *Prophylactic Drugs*

Several drugs, most of which are also used for treatment of malaria, can be taken preventively. Generally, these drugs are taken daily or weekly, at a lower dose than would be used for treatment of a person who had actually contracted the disease. Use of prophylactic drugs is seldom practical for full-time residents of malaria-endemic areas, and their use is usually restricted to short-term visitors and travellers to malarial regions. This is due to the cost of purchasing the drugs, negative side effects from long-term use and because some effective anti-malarial drugs are difficult to obtain outside of wealthy nations.

Quinine was used starting in the seventeenth century as a prophylactic against malaria. The development of more effective alternatives such as quinacrine, chloroquine, and primaquine in the twentieth century reduced the reliance on quinine. Today, quinine is still used to treat chloroquine resistant Plasmodium falciparum, as well as severe and cerebral stages of malaria, but is not generally used for prophylaxis. Of interesting historical note is the observation by Samuel Hahnemann in the late 18th century that overdosing of quinine leads to a symptomatic state very similar to that of malaria itself. This leads Hahnemann to develop the Law of Similars, and the subsequent pseudo-medical system of Homeopathy.

Modern drugs used preventively include mefloquine (Lariam), doxycycline (available generically), and the combination of atovaquone and proguanil hydrochloride (Malarone). The choice of which drug to use depends on which drugs the parasites in the area are resistant to, as well as side effects and other considerations. The prophylactic effect does not begin immediately upon starting taking the drugs, so people temporarily visiting malaria-endemic areas usually begin taking the drugs one to two weeks before arriving and must continue taking them for 4 weeks after leaving (with the exception of atovaquone proguanil that only needs to be started 2 days prior and continued for 7 days afterwards).

### *Indoor Residual Spraying*

Indoor residual spraying (IRS) is the practice of spraying insecticides on the interior walls of homes in malaria affected areas. After feeding, many mosquito species rest on a nearby surface while digesting the bloodmeal, so if the walls of dwellings have been coated with insecticides, the resting mosquitos will be killed before they can bite another victim, transferring the malaria parasite.

The first and historically the most popular insecticide used for IRS is DDT. While it was initially used exclusively to combat malaria, its use quickly spread to agriculture. In time, pest-control, rather than disease-control came to dominate DDT use and this large-scale agricultural use led to the evolution of resistant mosquitoes in many regions. If the use of DDT was limited agriculturally, DDT may be more effective now as a method of disease-control. The DDT resistance shown by Anopheles mosquitoes can be compared to antibiotic resistance shown by bacteria. The overuse of anti-bacterial soaps and antibiotics have led to antibiotic resistance in bacteria, similar to how overspraying of DDT on crops have led to DDT resistance in Anopheles mosquitoes. During the 1960s, awareness of the negative consequences of its indiscriminate use increased ultimately leading to bans on agricultural applications of DDT in many countries in the 1970s.

Though DDT has never been banned for use in malaria control and there are several other insecticides suitable for IRS, some advocates have claimed that bans are responsible for tens of millions of deaths in tropical countries where DDT had once been effective in controlling malaria. Furthermore, most of the problems associated with DDT use stem specifically from its industrial-scale application in agriculture, rather than its use in public health.

The World Health Organization (WHO) currently advises the use of twelve different insecticides in IRS operations. These include DDT and a series of alternative insecticides (such as the pyrethroids permethrin and deltamethrin) to combat malaria in areas where mosquitoes are DDT-resistant, and to slow down the evolution of resistance. This public health use of small amounts of DDT is permitted under the Stockholm Convention on Persistent Organic Pollutants (POPs), which prohibits the agricultural use of DDT. However, because of its legacy, many developed countries discourage DDT use even in small quantities.

One problem with all forms of Indoor Residual Spraying is insecticide resistance via evolution of mosquitos. According to a study published on Mosquito Behaviour and Vector Control, mosquito breeds that are affected by IRS are endophilic species (Species which tend to rest and live indoors) and due to the irritation caused by spraying, their evolutionary descendants are trending towards becoming exophilic (Species which tend to rest and live out of doors), meaning that they are not as affected – if affected at all – by the IRS, rendering it somewhat useless as a defence mechanism.

*Mosquito Nets and Bedclothes*

Mosquito nets help keep mosquitoes away from people and thus greatly reduce the infection and transmission of malaria. The nets are not a perfect barrier, so they are often treated with an insecticide designed to kill the mosquito before it has time to search for a way past the net. Insecticide-treated nets (ITN) are estimated to be twice as effective as untreated nets and offer greater than 70 per cent protection compared with no net. Although ITN are proven to be very effective against malaria, less than 2 per cent of children in urban areas in Sub-Saharan Africa are protected by ITNs. Since the Anopheles mosquitoes feed at night, the preferred method is to hang a large 'bed net' above the centre of a bed such that it drapes down and covers the bed completely.

The distribution of mosquito nets impregnated with insecticide (often permethrin or deltamethrin) has been shown to be an extremely effective method of malaria prevention and it is also one of the most cost-effective methods of prevention. ITNs have been shown to be the most cost-effective prevention method against malaria and are actively part of WHO's Millennium Development Goals (MDGs).

For maximum effectiveness, the nets should be re-impregnated with insecticide every six months. This process poses a significant logistical problem in rural areas. New technologies like Olyset or DawaPlus allow for production of long-lasting insecticidal mosquito nets (LLINs), which release insecticide for approximately 5 years. ITNs have the advantage of protecting people sleeping under the net and simultaneously killing mosquitoes that contact the net. This has the effect of killing the most dangerous mosquitoes. Some protection is also provided to others, including people sleeping in the same room but not under the net.

Unfortunately, the cost of treating malaria is high relative to income, and the illness results in lost wages. Consequently, the financial burden means that the cost of a mosquito net is often unaffordable to people in developing countries, especially for those most at risk. Only one out of 20 people in Africa own a bed net. Although shipped into Africa mainly from Europe as free development help, the nets quickly become expensive trade goods. They are mainly used for fishing, and by combining hundreds of donated mosquito nets, the whole river sections can be completely shut off, catching even the smallest fish. Nets are also often distributed though vaccine campaigns using vouchers subsidies, such as the measles campaign for children. Vouchers subsidies are an effective way of getting protective nets to those who cannot afford them off the market.

A study among Afghan refugees in Pakistan found that treating top-sheets and chaddars (head coverings) with permethrin has similar effectiveness to using a treated net, but is much cheaper.

A new approach, announced in *Science* on 10 June 2005, uses spores of the fungus Beauveria bassiana, sprayed on walls and bed nets, to kill mosquitoes. While some mosquitoes have developed resistance to chemicals, they have not been found to develop a resistance to fungal infections.

### *Vaccination*

Vaccines for malaria are under development, with no completely effective vaccine yet available. The first promising studies demonstrating the potential for a malaria vaccine were performed in 1967 by immunizing mice with live, radiation-attenuated sporozoites, providing protection to about 60 per cent of the mice upon subsequent injection with normal, viable sporozoites. Since the 1970s, there has been a considerable effort to develop similar vaccination strategies within humans. It was determined that an individual can be protected from a P. falciparum infection if they receive over 1,000 bites from infected, irradiated mosquitoes.

It has been generally accepted that it is impractical to provide at-risk individuals with this vaccination strategy, but that has been recently challenged with work being done by Dr Stephen Hoffman of Sanaria, one of the key researchers who originally sequenced the genome of Plasmodium falciparum. His work most recently has revolved around solving the logistical problem of isolating and preparing the parasites equivalent to 1,000 irradiated mosquitoes for mass storage and inoculation of human beings. The company has recently received several multimillion dollar grants from the Bill and Melinda Gates Foundation and the US government to begin early clinical studies in 2007 and 2008. The Seattle Biomedical Research Institute (SBRI), funded by the Malaria Vaccine Initiative, assures potential volunteers that 'the [2009] clinical trials won't be a life-threatening experience. While many volunteers [in Seattle] will actually contract malaria, the cloned strain used in the experiments can be quickly cured, and does not cause a recurring form of the disease'. 'Some participants will get experimental drugs or vaccines, while others will get placebo'.

Instead, much work has been performed to try and understand the immunological processes that provide protection after immunization with irradiated sporozoites. After the mouse vaccination study in 1967, it was hypothesized that the injected sporozoites themselves were being recognized by the immune system, which was in turn creating antibodies against the parasite. It was determined that the immune system was creating antibodies against the circumsporozoite protein (CSP) which coated the sporozoite. Moreover, antibodies against CSP prevented the sporozoite from invading hepatocytes. CSP was, therefore, chosen as the most promising protein on which to develop a vaccine against the malaria sporozoite. It is for these historical reasons that vaccines based on CSP are the most numerous of all malaria vaccines.

Presently, there is a huge variety of vaccine candidates on the table. Pre-erythrocytic vaccines (vaccines that target the parasite before it reaches the blood), in particular, vaccines based on CSP make up the largest group of research for the malaria vaccine. Other vaccine candidates include: those that seek to induce immunity to the blood stages of the infection; those that seek to avoid more severe pathologies of malaria by preventing adherence of the parasite to blood venules and placenta; and transmission-blocking vaccines that would stop the development of the parasite in the mosquito, right after the mosquito has taken a bloodmeal from an infected person. It is hoped that the sequencing of the P. falciparum genome will provide targets for new drugs or vaccines.

The first vaccine developed that has undergone field trials, is the SPf66, developed by Manuel Elkin Patarroyo in 1987. It presents a combination of antigens from the sporozoite (using CS repeats) and merozoite parasites. During phase I trials, a 75 per cent efficacy rate was demonstrated and the vaccine appeared to be well tolerated by subjects and immunogenic. The phase IIb and III trials were less promising, with the efficacy falling to between 38.8 per cent and 60.2 per cent. A trial was carried out in Tanzania in 1993, demonstrating the efficacy to be 31 per cent after a year's follow up, however, the most recent (though controversial) study in The Gambia did not show any effect. Despite the relatively long trial periods and the number of studies carried out, it is still not known how the SPf66 vaccine confers immunity; it therefore, remains an unlikely solution to malaria. The CSP was the next vaccine developed that initially appeared promising enough to undergo trials. It is also based on the circumsporoziote protein, but additionally has the recombinant (Asn-Ala-Pro15Asn-Val-Asp-Pro) 2-Leu-Arg (R32LR) protein covalently bound to a purified Pseudomonas aeruginosa toxin (A9). However, at an early stage a complete lack of protective immunity was demonstrated in those inoculated. The study group used in Kenya had an 82 per cent incidence of parasitaemia whilst the control group only had an 89 per cent incidence. The vaccine intended to cause an increased T-lymphocyte response in those exposed, this was also not observed.

The efficacy of Patarroyo's vaccine has been disputed with some US scientists concluding in *The Lancet* (1997) that 'the vaccine was not effective and should be dropped' while the Colombian accused them of 'arrogance' putting down their assertions to the fact that he came from a developing country.

The RTS, S/AS02A vaccine is the candidate furthest along in vaccine trials. It is being developed by a partnership between the PATH Malaria Vaccine Initiative (a grantee of the Gates Foundation), the pharmaceutical company, GlaxoSmithKline and the Walter Reed Army Institute of Research. In the vaccine, a portion of CSP has been fused to the immunogenic 'S antigen' of the hepatitis B virus; this recombinant protein is injected alongside the potent AS02A adjuvant. In October 2004, the RTS, S/AS02A researchers announced results of a Phase IIb trial, indicating the vaccine reduced infection risk by approximately 30 per cent and severity of infection by over 50 per cent. The study looked at over 2,000 Mozambican children. More recent testing of the RTS, S/AS02A vaccine has focused on the safety and efficacy of administering it earlier in infancy: In October 2007, the researchers announced results of a phase I/IIb trial conducted on 214 Mozambican infants between the ages of 10 and 18 months in which the full three-dose course of the vaccine led to a 62 per cent reduction of infection with no serious side-effects save some pain at the point of injection. Further research will delay this vaccine from commercial release until around 2011.

### *Other Methods*

Education in recognizing the symptoms of malaria has reduced the number of cases in some areas of the developing world by as much as 20 per cent. Recognizing the disease in the early stages can also stop the disease from becoming a killer. Education can also inform people to cover over areas of stagnant, still water e.g. water tanks which are ideal breeding grounds for the parasite and mosquito, thus cutting down the risk of the transmission between people. This is mostly put in practice in urban areas where there are large centres of population in a confined space and transmission would be most likely in these areas.

The Malaria Control Project is currently using downtime computing power donated by individual volunteers around the world to simulate models of the health effects and transmission dynamics in order to find the best method or combination of methods for malaria control. This modelling is extremely computer intensive due to the simulations of large human populations with a vast range of parameters related to biological and social factors that influence the spread of the disease. It is expected to take a few months using volunteered computing power compared to the 40 years it would have taken with the current resources available to the scientists who developed the programme.

An example of the importance of computer modelling in planning malaria eradication programmes is shown in the paper by Águas and others. They showed that eradication of malaria is crucially dependent on finding and treating the large number of people in endemic areas with asymptomatic malaria, who act as a reservoir for infection. The malaria parasites do not affect animal species and, therefore, eradication of the disease from the human population would be expected to be effective.

## Physical Deficient Diseases

Physical deficient or deficiency diseases can be caused by insufficient intake of iron or protein and there are other diseases that occur when a person's diet lacks or is too low in a certain vitamins. Among the most well-known of these are beriberi, pellagra, pernicious anemia, scurvy, rickets and osteomalacia. Generally, such diseases can be treated successfully and even cured by ensuring that the nutritional needs of the body are met on a daily basis unless a person is fasting. Iron deficiency can result if a person suffers significant blood loss, if a person has a diet which is poor in this mineral or if a person's body has a decreased ability to absorb iron. A common form of anemia can usually be prevented by ingesting foods that are naturally high in iron, like legumes, molasses, whole heirloom grains such as spelt and leafy green vegetables, preferably those that have been organically grown. Certain groups of people, such as women of childbearing age, have a higher risk of suffering iron deficiency. Among the symptoms of this condition are fatigue, pain in chest and shortness of breath.

The nutrients that serve functions other than energy production can be classified into four different groups: vitamins, fats, proteins and minerals. All are necessary for proper body function and survival. Protein deficiency diseases could be caused by a person's failure to consume sufficient amounts of high-quality protein, resulting in abnormal growth and maintenance of tissues. Wounds generally do not heal as quickly as they should in these individuals. Most people are aware that scurvy can develop if the diet lacks ascorbic acid or vitamin C. Eating fresh citrus fruits and a variety of fresh, organically grown vegetables is all that is required to prevent, treat or cure scurvy, which rarely is seen in industrialized nations. Pernicious anemia is a condition that can develop if a person's diet is lacking in vitamin B12, also known as cobalamin. Vegans run a considerably higher risk of developing pernicious anemia than do individuals who consume meat and dairy products. Those who have insufficient amounts of the protein known as the intrinsic factor also can develop pernicious anemia.

# 6

# Heart Diseases

As we probably know, the heart is a muscle in the chest that pumps blood through the body by way of the blood vessels that make up the circulatory system. The heart has four chambers:

- Left atrium
- Left ventricle
- Right atrium
- Right ventricle

After blood travels throughout the circulatory system it runs out of oxygen and must return to the heart through the right atrium. Then the blood moves to the right ventricle, where it is pumped to the lungs so it can be re-oxygenated. Once the blood is oxygenated, it goes to the left ventricle. The left ventricle then gives the blood a forceful push into the arteries. That powerful push stems from a high-pressure contraction of the heart.

The heart's powerful contraction raises your blood pressure so that the blood has the force behind it that it needs to make its way through the entire circulatory system. It takes a strong and healthy heart to achieve this goal. Furthermore, the heart's strength is dependent on the blood that it is supplied through the coronary arteries – flexible tubes with a smooth inner lining that enables blood to flow easily without clotting.

## Heart Disease

Heart disease is not a single disease, but a complex of diseases of varied etiology. Some of the recognized causes of heart disease include damage to the heart muscle or valves due to a congenital defect; or to inflammation and damage associated with various viral, bacterial, fungal, rickettsial or parasitic diseases. Rheumatic fever or syphilis can lead to heart disease, as can genetic or autoimmune disorders in which cellular proteins in the heart muscle are deranged or which disrupt enzymes affecting cardiac function.

These factors probably contributed to most cases of heart disease recorded in the early part of the century, when rates of infectious diseases were much higher and antibiotics were not in use. But by 1950, heart disease was the leading cause of mortality, causing more than 30 per cent of all deaths, and the figure has been climbing ever since. Today, coronary heart disease accounts for about 45 per cent of all deaths. The incidence rose most precipitously between 1920 and 1960. Since that time, mortality rates from coronary heart disease have declined somewhat. This means that victims of heart disease are living longer, due most likely to improved surgical techniques, the advent of angioplasty and the use of anti-clotting drugs given to heart attack victims. But the morbidity rates – the incidence of heart disease – continue to rise, although at a lower rate than before. Of greatest concern is the high rate of heart disease in American men between the ages of 45 to 65 – during the period of greatest family and career responsibilities.

The interesting thing is that most cases of heart disease in the twentieth century are of a form that is new, namely heart attack or myocardial infarction – a massive blood clot leading to obstruction of a coronary artery and consequent death to the heart muscle. Myocardial infarction (MI) was almost nonexistent in 1910 and caused no more than 3,000 deaths per year in 1930. Dr Paul Dudley White, who introduced the electrocardiograph machine to America, stated the following during a 1956 American Heart Association televised fund – raiser: 'I began my practice as a cardiologist in 1921 and I never saw an MI patient until 1928'. By 1960, there were at least 5,00,000 MI deaths per year in the US. Rates of stroke have also increased and the cause is similar – blockage in the large arteries supplying the brain with blood.

### Factors for Heart Attack

The factors that initiate a heart attack (or a stroke) are twofold. One is the pathological build-up of abnormal plaque, or atheromas, in the arteries, plaque that gradually hardens through calcification. Blockage most often occurs in the large arteries feeding the heart or the brain. This abnormal plaque or atherosclerosis should not be confused with the fatty streaks and thickening that is found in the arteries of both primitive and industrialized peoples throughout the world. This thickening is a protective mechanism that occurs in areas where the arteries branch or make a turn and, therefore, incur the greatest levels of pressure from the blood. Without this natural thickening, our arteries would weaken in these areas as we age, leading to aneurysms and ruptures. With normal thickening, the blood vessel usually widens to accommodate the change. But with atherosclerosis the vessel ultimately becomes narrower so that even small blood clots may cause an obstruction.

The other half of the MI equation is the blood clot or thrombus that blocks blood flow to the heart or brain. Thus, any search for the causes of heart disease must consider complex factors in the blood that promote clotting at inappropriate times, that is, other than in response to bleeding from a rupture or wound. In fact, while a great deal of attention has been focused on the cause and solution to atherosclerosis, the role played by clotting factors in the blood has been relatively neglected. Yet a heart attack due to a clot can occur even in the absence of arterial blockages.

Inflammation may also cause blockages. In fact, a new view of coronary artery disease is that it is an inflammatory process, characterized by cycles of irritation, injury, healing and reinjury inside the blood vessels. The inflammatory response is actually a defense mechanism that helps the body heal but when the inflammatory process goes awry, plaques may rupture, provoking clots that lead to heart attacks.

The health and integrity of the blood vessel walls is another factor that must be considered. Aneurysms, the dilation and rupture of blood vessels due to weakness in the vessel walls, will naturally provoke a clotting response, not to mention the more immediate danger of rapid blood loss. In addition, biochemical imbalances in the smooth muscle cells may result in spasms that can be just as effective as a blood clot in cutting off blood flow to the heart.

Finally, arrhythmias – abnormalities in the rhythm of the heart's pumping mechanism – can lead to interrupted blood flow, oxygen starvation of the heart muscle or complete shut down of the heart – the so-called cardiac arrest. Regulation of the nervous impulses that govern the heart depends on a large number of factors – from mineral status to the integrity of the myelin sheath.

## Types of Heart Disease

### *Coronary Heart Disease*

Coronary artery disease is a disease of the artery caused by the accumulation of atheromatous plaques within the walls of the arteries that supply the myocardium. Angina pectoris (chest pain) and myocardial infarction (heart attack) are symptoms of and conditions caused by coronary heart disease. Over 4,59,000 Americans die of coronary heart disease every year. In the UK, 1,01,000 deaths annually are due to coronary heart disease.

#### *Cardiomyopathy*

Cardiomyopathy literally means 'heart muscle disease' (Myo= muscle, pathy= disease) It is the deterioration of the function of the mycardium (i.e. the actual heart muscle) for any reason. People with cardiomyopathy are often at risk of arrhythmia and/or sudden cardiac death.

- *Extrinsic cardiomyopathies:* cardiomyopathies where the primary pathology is outside the myocardium itself. Most cardiomyopathies are extrinsic, because by far the most common cause of a cardiomyopathy is ischemia. The World Health Organisation calls these specific cardiomyopathie:
  - Alcoholic cardiomyopathy
  - Coronary artery disease
  - Congenital heart disease
  - Nutritional diseases affecting the heart
  - Ischemic cardiomyopathy
  - Hypertensive cardiomyopathy
  - Valvular cardiomyopathy
  - Inflammatory cardiomyopathy
  - Cardiomyopathy secondary to a systematic metabolic disease
- *Intrinsic cardiomyopathies:* weakness in the muscle of the heart that is not due to an identifiable external cause.
  - *Dilated cardiomyopathy (DCM):* most common form and one of the leading indications for heart transplantation. In DCM the heart (especially the left ventricle) is enlarged and the pumping function is diminished.
  - *Hypertrophic cardiomyopathy (HCM or HOCM):* genetic disorder caused by various mutations in genes encoding sarcomeric proteins. In HCM the heart muscle is thickened, which can obstruct blood flow and prevent the heart from functioning properly.
  - *Arrhythmogenic right ventricular cardiomyopathy (ARVC):* arises from an electrical disturbance of the heart in which heart muscle is replaced by fibrous scar tissue. The right ventricle is generally most affected.

— *Restrictive cardiomyopathy (RCM):* least common cardiomyopathy. The walls of the ventricles are stiff, but may not be thickened, and resist the normal filling of the heart with blood.

— *Noncompaction Cardiomyopathy:* the left ventricle wall has failed to properly grow from birth and such has a spongy appearance when viewed during an echocardiogram.

### Cardiovascular Disease

Cardiovascular disease is any of a number of specific diseases that affect the heart itself and/or the blood vessel system, especially the veins and arteries leading to and from the heart. Research on disease dimorphism suggests that women who suffer with cardiovascular disease usually suffer from forms that affect the blood vessels while men usually suffer from forms that affect the heart muscle itself. Known or associated causes of cardiovascular disease include diabetes mellitus, hypertension, and hyperhomocystinemia.

### Ischaemic Heart Disease

Ischaemic heart disease – another disease of the heart itself, characterized by reduced blood supply to the organs.

Coronary heart disease is when the arteries that supply the oxygen and the nutrients gets stopped and the heart will not get enough of the oxygen and the nutrients and will eventually stop beating.

### Heart Failure

Heart failure, also called congestive heart failure (or CHF), and congestive cardiac failure (CCF), is a condition that can result from any structural or functional cardiac disorder that impairs the ability of the heart to fill with or pump a sufficient amount of blood throughout the body.

### Hypertensive Heart Disease

Hypertensive heart disease is heart disease caused by high blood pressure, especially localized high blood pressure. Conditions that can be caused by hypertensive heart disease include:

- Left ventricular hypertrophy
- Coronary heart disease
- (Congestive) heart failure
- Hypertensive cardiomyopathy
- Cardiac arrhythmias

### *Inflammatory Heart Disease*

Inflammatory heart disease involves inflammation of the heart muscle and/or the tissue surrounding it.

- *Endocarditis:* inflammation of the inner layer of the heart, the endocardium. The most common structures involved are the heart valves.
- Inflammatory cardiomegaly.
- *Mycocarditis:* inflammation of the mycocardium, the muscular part of the heart.

### *Valvular Heart Disease*

Valvular heart disease is a disease process that affects one or more valves of the heart. The valves in the right side of the heart are the tricuspid valve and the pulmonic valve. The valves in the left side of the heart are the mital valve and the aortic valve.

- Aortiv valve stenosis
- Mitral valve prolapse
- Valvular cardiomyopathy

## Symptoms

### *Chest Pain or Chest Discomfort*

Few symptoms are more alarming than chest pain. In the minds of many people, chest pain equals heart pain. And while many other conditions can cause chest pain, cardiac disease is so common and so dangerous that the symptom of chest pain should never be dismissed out of hand as being insignificant.

'Chest pain' is an imprecise term. It is often used to describe any pain, pressure, squeezing, choking, numbness or any other discomfort in the chest, neck, or upper abdomen and is often associated with pain in the jaw, head or arms. It can last from less than a second to days or weeks, can occur frequently or rarely and can occur sporadically or predictably. This description of chest pain is obviously very vague, and as you might expect, many medical conditions aside from heart disease can produce symptoms like this.

### *Palpitations*

Palpitation, an unusual awareness of the heartbeat, is an extremely common symptom. Most people who complain of palpitations describe them either as 'skips' in the heartbeat (that is, a pause, often followed by a particularly strong beat,) or as periods of rapid and/or irregular heartbeats.

Most people with palpitations have some type of cardiac arrhythmia. Virtually any arrhythmia can cause palpitations, but the most common causes of palpitations are premature atrial complexes (PACs), premature ventricular complexes (PVCs), episodes of atrial fibrillation, and episodes of supraventricular tachycardia (SVT). Unfortunately, on occasion palpitations can be a manifestation of a more dangerous heart arrhythmia, such as ventricular tachycardia.

### *Lightheadedness or Dizziness*

Episodes of lightheadedness or dizziness can have many causes, including anaemia (low blood count) and other blood disorders, dehydration, viral illnesses, deconditioning (such as prolonged bed rest), diabetes, thyroid disease, gastrointestinal disturbances, liver disease, kidney disease, vascular disease, neurological disorders, the dysautonomias, vasovagal episodes, heart failure and cardiac arrhythmias. Because so many different conditions can produce these symptoms, anybody experiencing episodes of lightheadedness or dizziness ought to have a thorough and complete examination by a physician. And since disorders of so many organ systems can cause these symptoms, a good general internist or family doctor may be the best place to start.

### *Syncope (Loss of Consciousness)*

Syncope is a sudden and temporary loss of consciousness, or fainting. It is a common symptom – most people pass out at least once in their lives – and often does not indicate a serious medical problem. However, sometimes syncope indicates a dangerous or even life-threatening condition, so when syncope occurs it is important to figure out the cause. The causes of syncope can be grouped into four major categories, neurologic, metabolic, vasomotor and cardiac. Of these, only cardiac syncope commonly leads to sudden death. Fortunately, most syncope is not cardiac in nature, and thus is not life-threatening.

### *Fatigue, Lethargy or Somnolence*

Fatigue, lethargy or somnolence (daytime sleepiness) is very common symptoms. Fatigue or lethargy can be thought of as an inability to continue functioning at one's normal levels. Somnolence implies, in addition, that one either craves sleep – or worse, finds oneself suddenly asleep, a condition known as narcolepsy – during the daytime.

While fatigue and lethargy can be symptoms of heart disease (particularly, of heart failure), these common and non-specific symptoms can also be due to disorders of virtually any other organ system in the body. Similar to lightheadedness and dizziness, individuals with fatigue and lethargy need a good general medical evaluation in order to begin pinning down a specific cause. Somnolence is often caused by nocturnal sleep disorders such as sleep apnea, restless leg syndrome or insomnia. All these sleep disturbances, however, are more common in patients with heart disease.

### *Shortness of Breath*

Shortness of breath is most often a symptom of cardiac or pulmonary (lung) disorders. Heart failure and coronary artery disease frequently produce shortness of breath. Patients with heart failure commonly experience shortness of breath with exertion, or when lying flat on their backs. They also can suddenly wake up at night gasping for breath, a condition known as paroxysmal nocturnal dyspnea. Coronary artery disease can manifest as shortness of breath on exertion. Other cardiac conditions such as valvular heart disease or pericardial disease can produce this symptom, as can cardiac arrhythmias. Numerous lung conditions can produce shortness of breath including asthma, emphysema, bronchitis, pneumonia, or pleural effusion (a fluid accumulation between the lung and chest wall). Shortness of breath is almost always a sign of a significant medical problem, and should always be evaluated by a doctor.

### *Miscellaneous Symptoms*

- Abdominal pain
- Abnormal pulsation
- Anxiety
- Appetite loss
- Balance problems
- Breathing problem
- Chest pain
- Cough
- Depression
- Edema
- Fainting
- Fast heart beat

- Fever
- Headache
- Hemoptysis (couging blood)
- Jaw pain
- Irregular heart beat
- Memory problem
- Muscle cramps
- Palpitation
- Skipped beats
- Syncope
- Tachycardia
- Vertigo
- Weight gain
- Weight loss

## Treatment

### *Medical Treatment*

Medical treatment may be started immediately, before a definite diagnosis of a heart problem is made. General treatment measures include the following:

- Oxygen through a tube in the nose or face mask
- Nitroglycerin under the tongue
- Pain medicines (morphine or meperidine)
- *Aspirin:* Those with allergy to aspirin may be given clopidogrel (Plavix).

*Clot-dissolving medicines:* The tissue plasminogen activators (tPAs) can actually dissolve clots in some circumstances.

- The earlier these drugs are given, the better the chance of opening the blocked artery and of protecting the cardiac muscle from further injury.
- If more than 6 hours has passed since the onset of chest pain, these drugs are less helpful.
- Potential risks of this therapy include bleeding.
- The most serious risk is a stroke (bleeding into the brain).

*Angioplasty*: Emergency coronary angiography and coronary balloon angioplasty (percutaneous transluminal coronary angioplasty, or PTCA) are available in hospitals equipped with a full-service cardiac catheterization laboratory. This is the most direct method of relieving blockage in a coronary artery.

- Coronary balloon angioplasty is an extension of coronary angiography.
- A long, thin tube (catheter) is inserted in an artery in the groin or arm.
- At the tip of the catheter is a tiny, elongated balloon, which is threaded over a hair-thin guidewire into the narrowed coronary artery.
- Once the balloon is positioned at the blockage in the coronary artery, it is inflated.
- The balloon pushes aside the plaque and clot that are blocking the artery, allowing blood to flow more freely.
- The balloon is then deflated and removed with the catheter.

*Stenting*: A stent is a small, springlike device that may be inserted into a coronary artery after balloon angioplasty. After the catheter and balloon are removed, the stent stays in place, holding the artery open. A stent is better than angioplasty alone at keeping the artery from narrowing again.

*Atherectomy*: Sometimes the plaques are too rigid, bulky, or calcified to be treated by balloon angioplasty. In these cases, the plaque often can be removed by cutting it out with a drill-like rotary blade or a laser or other tool.

### *Medications*

- Intravenous (IV) nitroglycerin has been shown to improve blood flow to the heart muscle by relaxing (dilating) the coronary arteries and increasing blood flow. It is usually given for 24–48 hours continuously.
- Heparin is a 'blood thinner,' or anticoagulant, which may be given after a heart attack. Heparin does not remove an existing clot, but it reduces the tendency of blood to clot in the coronary arteries. Some newer forms of heparin have recently been introduced that can be given as a shot instead of through an IV line.
- Beta-blockers are medications that decrease the heart rate and blood pressure. This reduces the heart's workload and thus the amount of oxygen it needs. Beta-blockers may provide immediate as well as long-term benefit for people who have a heart attack.

- Angiotensin-converting enzyme (ACE) inhibitors may prevent repeat heart attacks and other problems when started early during a heart attack. They are especially useful in people with diabetes and those with a weakened heart muscle congestive heart failure.

### *Surgery*

Sometimes cardiac catheterization reveals extensive coronary artery disease. In such cases, it is needed to undergo coronary bypass surgery.

- Standard coronary artery bypass grafting (CABG) is performed if many coronary arteries are narrowed or blocked. This is especially recommended when the left main coronary artery shows significant blockage. This is 'open heart surgery', meaning that the chest wall is opened. When performing a bypass, heart surgeons use sections of the mammary artery from the chest or veins from the legs to create detours around the blocked arteries. For this surgery, you will be connected to a bypass pump, which does the work of the heart during the operation. Although this sounds dangerous, this surgery is considered very safe and has a very low rate of complications.
- *Off-pump bypass surgery:* Sometimes the surgeon can perform open heart surgery without using a bypass pump. The heart continues to beat during surgery. This type of surgery has even fewer complications than the standard procedure but is not always feasible.
- *Minimally invasive coronary bypass:* If just the front or the right coronary artery needs bypass, the bypass may be performed via a small keyhole-type incision without a large incision in the chest. The internal mammary artery is used for the bypass.

# 7

# Diabetes

Diabetes mellitus often referred to simply as diabetes (Ancient Greek: 'to pass through'), is a syndrome of disordered metabolism, usually due to a combination of hereditary and environmental causes, resulting in abnormally high blood sugar levels (hyperglycemia). Blood glucose levels are controlled by a complex interaction of multiple chemicals and hormones in the body, including the hormone insulin made in the beta cells of the pancreas. Diabetes mellitus refers to the group of diseases that lead to high blood glucose levels due to defects in either insulin secretion or insulin action.

Diabetes develops due to a diminished production of insulin (in type 1) or resistance to its effects (in type 2 and gestational). Both lead to hyperglycaemia, which largely causes the acute signs of diabetes: excessive urine production, resulting compensatory thirst and increased fluid intake, blurred vision, unexplained weight loss, lethargy, and changes in energy metabolism. Monogenic forms, e.g. maturity onset diabetes of the young (MODY), constitute 1–5 per cent of all cases.

All forms of diabetes have been treatable since insulin became medically available in 1921, but there is no cure. The injections by a syringe, insulin pump, or insulin pen deliver insulin, which is a basic treatment of type 1 diabetes. Type 2 is managed with a combination of dietary treatment, exercise, medications and insulin supplementation.

Diabetes and its treatments can cause many complications. Acute complications (hypoglycemia, ketoacidosis, or nonketotic hyperosmolar coma) may occur if the disease is not adequately controlled. Serious long-term complications include cardiovascular disease (doubled risk), chronic renal failure, retinal damage (which can lead to blindness), nerve damage (of several kinds), and microvascular damage, which may cause erectile dysfunction and poor wound healing. Poor healing of wounds, particularly of the feet, can lead to gangrene, and possibly to amputation. Adequate treatment of diabetes, as well as increased emphasis on blood pressure control and lifestyle factors (such as not smoking and maintaining a healthy body weight) may improve the risk profile of most of the chronic complications. In the developed world, diabetes is the most significant cause of adult blindness in the non-elderly and the leading cause of non-traumatic amputation in adults, and diabetic nephropathy is the main illness requiring renal dialysis in the United States.

According to the World Health Organization (2006), at least 171 million people worldwide suffer from diabetes, or 2.8 per cent of the population. Its incidence is increasing rapidly, and it is estimated that by the year 2030, this number will almost double. Diabetes mellitus occurs throughout the world, but is more common (especially type 2) in the more developed countries. The greatest increase in prevalence is, however, expected to occur in Asia and Africa, where most patients will likely be found by 2030. The increase in incidence of diabetes in developing countries follows the trend of urbanization and lifestyle changes, perhaps most importantly a 'Western-style' diet. This has suggested an environmental (i.e. dietary) effect, but there is little understanding of the mechanism(s) at present, though there is much speculation, some of it most compellingly presented.

For at least 20 years, diabetes rates in North America have been increasing substantially. In 2008 there were about 24 million people with diabetes in the United States alone, from those 5.7 million people remain undiagnosed. Other 57 million people are estimated to have pre-diabetes.

The Centers for Disease Control and Prevention (CDC) has termed the change an epidemic. The National Diabetes Information Clearinghouse estimates that diabetes costs $132 billion in the United States alone every year. About 5 per cent to 10 per cent of diabetes cases in North America is type 1, with the rest being type 2. The fraction of type 1 in other parts of the world differs; this is likely due to both differences in the rate of type 1 and differences in the rate of other types, most prominently type 2. Most of this difference is not currently understood. The American Diabetes Association points out the 2003 assessment of the National Center for Chronic Disease Prevention and Health

Promotion (Centers for Disease Control and Prevention) that 1 in 3 Americans born after 2000 will develop diabetes in their lifetime.

According to the American Diabetes Association (2005), approximately 18.3 per cent (8.6 million) of Americans aged 60 and older has diabetes. Diabetes mellitus prevalence increases with age, and the numbers of older persons with diabetes are expected to grow as the elderly population increases in number. The National Health and Nutrition Examination Survey (NHANES III) demonstrated that, in the population over 65 years old, 18 per cent to 20 per cent have diabetes, with 40 per cent having either diabetes or its precursor form of impaired glucose tolerance.

Indigenous populations in First World countries have a higher prevalence and increasing incidence of diabetes than their corresponding non-indigenous populations. In Australia the age-standardized prevalence of self-reported diabetes in Indigenous Australians is almost 4 times that of non-indigenous Australians. Preventative community health programmes such as Sugar Man (diabetes education) are showing some success in tackling this problem.

### History of Diabetes

Diabetes is not a newly born disease, it has been with the human race from long back but, we came to knew about it in 1552 BC. Since this period, many of Greek as well French physicians had worked on it and made us aware of the nature of disease, organs responsible for it, etc. In 1870s, a French physician had discovered a link between diabetes and diet intake, and an idea to formulate individual diet plan came into picture.

The term *diabetes* was coined by Aretaeus of Cappadocia. It was derived from the Greek verb *diabaínein*, itself formed from the prefix *dia* –, 'across, apart,' and the verb *bainein*, 'to walk, stand.' The verb *diabeinein* meant 'to stride, walk, or stand with legs asunder'; hence, its derivative *diabçtçs* meant 'one that straddles,' or specifically 'a compass, siphon'. The sense 'siphon' gave rise to the use of *diabçtçs* as the name for a disease involving the discharge of excessive amounts of urine. Diabetes is first recorded in English, in the form diabete, in a medical text written around 1,425. In 1675, Thomas Willis added the word *mellitus*, from the Latin meaning 'honey', a reference to the sweet taste of the urine. This sweet taste had been noticed in urine by the ancient Greeks, Chinese, Egyptians, Indians and Persians. In 1776, Matthew Dobson confirmed that the sweet taste was because of an excess of a kind of sugar in the urine and blood of people with diabetes.

Sushruta (6th century BCE) identified diabetes and classified it as *Medhumeha*. He further identified it with obesity and sedentary lifestyle, advising exercises to help cure it. The ancient Indians tested for diabetes by observing whether ants were attracted to a person's urine, and called the ailment 'sweet urine disease' (Madhumeha). The Korean, Chinese and Japanese words for diabetes are based on the same ideographs which mean 'sugar urine disease'. In medieval Persia, Avicenna (980–1037) provided a detailed account on diabetes mellitus in *The Canon of Medicine*, 'describing the abnormal appetite and the collapse of sexual functions and he documented the sweet taste of diabetic urine'. Like Aretaeus before him, Avicenna recognized primary and secondary diabetes. He also described diabetic gangrene, and treated diabetes using a mixture of lupine, trigonella (fenugreek), and zedoary seed, which produces a considerable reduction in the excretion of sugar, a treatment which is still prescribed in modern times. Avicenna also 'described diabetes insipidus very precisely for the first time', though it was later Johann Peter Frank (1745–1821) who first differentiated between diabetes mellitus and diabetes insipidus.

Although diabetes has been recognized since antiquity, and treatments of various efficacy have been known in various regions since the Middle Ages, and in legend for much longer, pathogenesis of diabetes has only been understood experimentally since about 1900. The discovery of a role for the pancreas in diabetes is generally ascribed to Joseph von Mering and Oskar Minkowski, who in 1889 found that dogs whose pancreas was removed developed all the signs and symptoms of diabetes and died shortly afterwards. In 1910, Sir Edward Albert Sharpey-Schafer suggested that people with diabetes were deficient in a single chemical that was normally produced by the pancreas – he proposed calling this substance *insulin*, from the Latin *insula*, meaning island, in reference to the insulin-producing islets of Langerhans in the pancreas.

The endocrine role of the pancreas in metabolism, and indeed the existence of insulin, was not further clarified until 1921, when Sir Frederick Grant Banting and Charles Herbert Best repeated the work of Von Mering and Minkowski, and went further to demonstrate they could reverse induced diabetes in dogs by giving them an extract from the pancreatic islets of Langerhans of healthy dogs. Banting, Best and colleagues (especially the chemist Collip) went on to purify the hormone insulin from bovine pancreases at the University of Toronto. This led to the availability of an effective treatment – insulin injections

– and the first patients were treated in 1922. For this, Banting and laboratory director MacLeod received the Nobel Prize in Physiology or Medicine in 1923; both shared their Prize money with others in the team who were not recognized, in particular Best and Collip. Banting and Best made the patent available without charge and did not attempt to control commercial production. Insulin production and therapy rapidly spread around the world, largely as a result of this decision. Banting is honoured by World Diabetes Day which is held on his birthday, 14 November.

Diabetic diet was formulated with inclusion of milk, oats and other fibre containing foods in 1900–1915. Function of insulin, its nature, along with its use started from 1920–1923, discovered by Dr Banting, Prof. Macleod and Dr Collip, who were awarded a Noble prize. In the decade of 1940, it has been discovered that different organs like kidney and skin are also affected if diabetes is creeping from a long term. A major turn in this research was in the year 1955, when the oral hypogycemic drugs had been manufactured.

Diabetes was recognized with complete details and its types (Type 1 and Type 2 diabetes – that is insulin dependent and non-insulin dependent) in the year, 1959. As we know this is one of the old diseases, existing in many individuals and still on rising charts. Hence, scientists are continuously working to relieve us from it, by discovering the relevant drugs and making new researches.

According to WHO estimates, by 2025 total 300 million of the worldwide population will be affected by diabetes. For every 21 seconds, someone is diagnosed with diabetes, an estimation given by American Diabetes Association. And, there are 20.8 million diabetics in US at present, which is roughly estimated as 7 per cent of US population; out of this figure about 6.2 millions are unaware of the diabetes existence in there life.

## Classification of Diabetes

The term *diabetes*, without qualification, usually refers to diabetes mellitus, which is associated with excessive sweet urine (known as 'glycosuria') but there are several rarer conditions also named diabetes. The most common of these is diabetes insipidus in which the urine is not sweet (insipidus meaning 'without taste' in Latin); it can be caused by either kidney (nephrogenic DI) or pituitary gland (central DI) damage.

The term 'type1 diabetes' has universally replaced several former terms, including childhood-onset diabetes, juvenile diabetes and insulin-dependent diabetes (IDDM). Likewise, the term 'type 2 diabetes' has replaced several former terms, including adult-onset diabetes, obesity-related diabetes and non-insulin-dependent diabetes (NIDDM). Beyond these two types, there is no agreed upon standard nomenclature. Various sources have defined 'type 3 diabetes' as, among others, gestational diabetes, insulin-resistant type 1 diabetes (or 'double diabetes'), type 2 diabetes which has progressed to require injected insulin and latent autoimmune diabetes of adults (or LADA or 'type 1.5' diabetes.) There is also maturity onset diabetes of the young (MODY) which is a group of several single gene (monogenic) disorders with strong family histories that present as type 2 diabetes before 30 years of age.

### *Type I Diabetes Mellitus*

Type 1 diabetes mellitus is characterized by loss of the insulin-producing beta cells of the islets of Langerhans in the pancreas, leading to a deficiency of insulin. This type of diabetes can be further classified as immune-mediated or idiopathic. The majority of type 1 diabetes is of the immune-mediated variety, where beta cell loss is a T-cell mediated autoimmune attack. There is no known preventive measure which can be taken against type 1 diabetes; it is about 10 per cent of diabetes mellitus cases in North America and Europe (though this varies by geographical location), and is a higher percentage in some other areas. Most affected people are otherwise healthy and of a healthy weight when onset occurs. Sensitivity and responsiveness to insulin are usually normal, especially in the early stages. Type 1 diabetes can affect children or adults but was traditionally termed 'juvenile diabetes' because it represents a majority of the diabetes cases in children.

The principal treatment of type 1diabetes, even in its earliest stages, is the delivery of artificial insulin via injection combined with careful monitoring of blood glucose levels using blood testing monitors. Without insulin, diabetic ketoacidosis often develops which may result in coma or death. Treatment emphasis is now also placed on lifestyle adjustments (diet and exercise) though these cannot reverse the progress of the disease. Apart from the common subcutaneous injections, it is also possible to deliver insulin by a pump, which allows continuous infusion of insulin 24 hours a day at preset levels, and the ability to programme doses (a bolus) of insulin as needed at meal times. An inhaled form of insulin was approved by the FDA in January 2006, although it was discontinued for business reasons in October 2007. Non-insulin treatments, such as monoclonal antibodies and stem-cell based therapies, are effective in animal models but have not yet completed clinical trials in humans.

Type 1 treatment must be continued indefinitely in essentially all cases. Treatment need not significantly impair normal activities, if sufficient patient training, awareness, appropriate care, discipline in testing and dosing of insulin is taken. However, treatment is burdensome for patients; insulin is replaced in a non-physiological manner and this approach is, therefore, far from ideal. The average glucose level for the type 1 patient should be as close to normal (80–120 mg/dl, 4–6 mmol/l) as is *safely* possible. Some physicians suggest up to 140–150 mg/dl (7–7.5 mmol/l) for those having trouble with lower values, such as frequent hypoglycemic events. Values above 400 mg/dl (20 mmol/l) are sometimes accompanied by discomfort and frequent urination leading to dehydration. Values above 600 mg/dl (30 mmol/l) usually require medical treatment and may lead to ketoacidosis, although they are not immediately life-threatening. However, low levels of blood glucose, called hypoglycemia, may lead to seizures or episodes of unconsciousness and absolutely must be treated immediately, via emergency high-glucose gel placed in the patient's mouth or an injection of glucagon.

### *Type 2 Diabetes Mellitus*

Type 2 diabetes mellitus is characterized differently and is due to insulin resistance or reduced insulin sensitivity, combined with relatively reduced insulin secretion which in some cases becomes absolute. The defective responsiveness of body tissues to insulin almost certainly involves the insulin receptor in cell membranes. However, the specific defects are not known. Diabetes mellitus due to a known specific defect are classified separately.

In the early stage of type 2 diabetes, the predominant abnormality is reduced insulin sensitivity, characterized by elevated levels of insulin in the blood. At this stage hyperglycemia can be reversed by a variety of measures and medications that improve insulin sensitivity or reduce glucose production by the liver. As the disease progresses, the impairment of insulin secretion worsens, and therapeutic replacement of insulin often becomes necessary.

There are numerous theories as to the exact cause and mechanism in type 2 diabetes. Central obesity (fat concentrated around the waist in relation to abdominal organs, but not subcutaneous fat) is known to predispose individuals to insulin resistance. Abdominal fat is especially active hormonally, secreting a group of hormones called adipokines that may possibly impair glucose tolerance. Obesity is found in approximately 55 per cent of patients diagnosed with type 2 diabetes. Other factors include ageing (about 20 per cent of elderly patients in North America have diabetes) and family history (type 2 is much more common in those with close relatives who have had it). In the last decade, type 2 diabetes has increasingly begun to affect children and adolescents, likely in connection with the increased prevalence of childhood obesity seen in recent decades in some places. Environmental exposures may contribute to recent increases in the rate of type 2 diabetes. A positive correlation has been found between the concentration in the urine of bisphenol A, a constituent of polycarbonate plastic, and the incidence of type 2 diabetes.

Type 2 diabetes may go unnoticed for years because visible symptoms are typically mild, non-existent or sporadic, and usually there are no ketoacidotic episodes. However, severe long-term complications can result from unnoticed type 2 diabetes, including renal failure due to diabetic nephropathy, vascular disease (including coronary artery disease), vision damage due to diabetic retinopathy, loss of sensation or pain due to diabetic neuropathy, liver damage from non-alcoholic steatohepatitis and heart failure from diabetic cardiomyopathy.

Type 2 diabetes is usually first treated by increasing physical activity, decreasing carbohydrate intake, and losing weight. These can restore insulin sensitivity even when the weight loss is modest, for example around 5 kg (10 to 15 lb), most especially when it is in abdominal fat deposits. It is sometimes possible to achieve long-term, satisfactory glucose control with these measures alone. However, the underlying tendency to insulin resistance is not lost, and so, attention to diet, exercise and weight loss must continue. The usual next step, if necessary, is treatment with oral antidiabetic drugs. Insulin production is initially only moderately impaired in type 2 diabetes, so oral medication (often used in various combinations) can be used to improve insulin production (e.g. sulfonylureas), to regulate inappropriate release of glucose by the liver and attenuate insulin resistance to some extent (e.g. metformin), and to substantially attenuate insulin resistance (e.g. thiazolidinediones). According to one study, overweight patients treated with metformin compared with diet alone, had relative risk reductions of 32 per cent for any diabetes endpoint, 42 per cent for diabetes related death and 36 per cent for all cause mortality and stroke. Oral medication may eventually fail due to further impairment of beta cell insulin secretion. At this point, insulin therapy is necessary to maintain normal or near normal glucose levels.

### Gestational Diabetes Mellitus (GDM)

Gestational diabetes mellitus (GDM) resembles type 2 diabetes in several respects, involving a combination of relatively inadequate insulin secretion and responsiveness. It occurs in about 2 per cent to 5 per cent of all pregnancies and may improve or disappear after delivery. Gestational diabetes is fully treatable but requires careful medical supervision throughout the pregnancy. About 20 per cent to 50 per cent of affected women develop type 2 diabetes later in life.

Even though it may be transient, untreated gestational diabetes can damage the health of the foetus or mother. Risks to the baby include macrosomia (high birth weight), congenital cardiac and central nervous system anomalies and skeletal muscle malformations. Increased foetal insulin may inhibit foetal surfactant production and cause respiratory distress syndrome. Hyperbilirubinemia may result from red blood cell destruction. In severe cases, perinatal death may occur, most commonly as a result of poor placental perfusion due to vascular impairment. Induction may be indicated with decreased placental function. A cesarean section may be performed if there is marked foetal distress or an increased risk of injury associated with macrosomia, such as shoulder dystocia.

A 2008 study, completed in the US found that more American women are entering pregnancy with pre-existing diabetes. In fact, the rate of diabetes in expectant mothers has more than doubled in the past 6 years. This is particularly problematic as diabetes raises the risk of complications during pregnancy, as well as increasing the potential that the children of diabetic mothers will also become diabetic in the future.

### Other Types

Most cases of diabetes mellitus fall into the two broad etiologic categories of type 1 or type 2 diabetes. However, many types of diabetes mellitus have known specific causes, and thus fall into separate categories, as diabetes due to a specific cause. As more research is done into diabetes, many patients who were previously diagnosed as type 1 or type 2 diabetes will be reclassified as diabetes due to their known specific cause.

Some cases of diabetes are caused by the body's tissue receptors not responding to insulin (even when insulin levels are normal, which is what separates it from type 2 diabetes); this form is very uncommon. Genetic mutations (autosomal or mitochondrial) can lead to defects in beta cell function. Abnormal insulin action may also have been genetically determined in some cases. Any disease that causes extensive damage to the pancreas may lead to diabetes (for example, chronic pancreatitis and cystic fibrosis). Diseases associated with excessive secretion of insulin – antagonistic hormones can cause diabetes (which is typically resolved once the hormone excess is removed). Many drugs impair insulin secretion and some toxins damage pancreatic beta cells. The ICD–10 (1992) diagnostic entity, *malnutrition-related diabetes mellitus* (MRDM or MMDM, ICD–10 code E12), was deprecated by the World Health Organization when the current taxonomy was introduced in 1999.

## Symptoms of Diabetes

In both types of diabetes, signs and symptoms are more likely to be similar as the blood sugar is high, either due to less or no production of insulin, or insulin resistance. In any case, if there is inadequate glucose in the cells, it is identifiable through certain signs and symptoms. These symptoms are quickly relieved once the diabetes is treated and also reduce the chances of developing serious health problems.

### *Diabetes Type 1*

In type 1, the pancreas stops producing insulin due to autoimmune response or possibly viral attack on pancreas. In absence of insulin, body cells do not get the required glucose for producing ATP (Adenosin Triphosphate) units which results into primary symptom in the form of nausea and vomiting. In later stage, which leads to ketoacidosis, the body starts breaking down the muscle tissue and fat for producing energy hence, causing fast weight loss. Dehydration is also usually observed due to electrolyte disturbance. In advanced stages, coma and death is witnessed.

### *Diabetes Type 2*

- *Increased fatigue:* Due to inefficiency of the cell to metabolize glucose, reserve fat of body is metabolized to gain energy. When fat is broken down in the body, it uses more energy as compared to glucose; hence body goes in negative calorie effect, which results in fatigue.
- *Polydipsia:* As the concentration of glucose increases in the blood, brain receives signal for diluting it and, in its counteraction we feel thirsty.

- *Polyuria:* Increase in urine production is due to excess glucose present in body. Body gets rid of the extra sugar in the blood by excreting it through urine. This leads to dehydration because along with the sugar, a large amount of water is excreted out of the body.
- *Polyphegia:* The hormone insulin is also responsible for stimulating hunger. In order to cope up with high sugar levels in blood, body produces insulin which leads to increased hunger.
- *Weight fluctuation:* Factors like loss of water (polyuria), glucosuria, metabolism of body fat and protein may lead to weight loss. Few cases may show weight gain due to increased appetite.
- *Blurry vision:* Hyperosmolar hyperglycemia nonketotic syndrome is the condition when body fluid is pulled out of tissues including lenses of the eye, which affects its ability to focus, resulting blurry vision.
- *Irritability:* It is a sign of high blood sugar because of the inefficient glucose supply to the brain and other body organs, which make us feel tired and uneasy.
- *Infections:* The body gives few signals whenever there is fluctuation in blood sugar (due to suppression of immune system) by frequent skin infections like fungal or bacterial or UTI (urinary tract infection).
- *Poor wound healing:* High blood sugar resists the flourishing of WBC, (white blood cell) which is responsible for body immune system. When these cells do not function accordingly, wound healing is not at good pace. Secondly, long standing diabetes leads to thickening of blood vessels which affect proper circulation of blood in different body parts.

### Symptoms of Diabetes and How It Can Affect Our Health

Symptoms are the complaints of disease which are felt by the patient themselves. Diabetes is of two types which exhibit delicate primary symptoms. Both type 1 and type 2 diabetes have similar symptoms owing to their high blood sugar levels and defective insulin metabolism. If diabetes is treated at the earliest then these symptoms can be annihilated without any complications.

### Symptoms of Diabetes Type I

The primary symptoms exhibited in type 1 diabetes are nausea and vomiting. These symptoms are ketoacidosis which leads to breaking down of energy giving muscles and tissues, thus resulting in loss of weight. This leads to severe electrolyte disturbances and dehydration which may have a poor prognosis leading to coma and death.

### *Symptoms of Diabetes Type 2*

The major symptoms exhibited by a type 2 diabetes patient are polydipsia, polyuria, polyphegia, blurry vision, fatigue, irritability, etc. Polydipsia is a condition of increased thirst resulting from dilution of blood caused by hormonal imbalance. In order to remove the excess blood sugar which is excreted through urine, large amount of water is also excreted along with the excess sugar which is known as polyuria. Excess of insulin is secreted by the body for metabolism of excess blood sugar which results in extreme hunger known as polyphegia. The combination of the effects of polyphegia, polyuria and polydipsia result in severe weight fluctuation. Similar to type 1 diabetes, muscle and fat tissues are broken down for production of energy. This results in improper overall body metabolism and causes fatigue.

### *Effect of Diabetes on Blood and Circulatory System*

Diabetes patients also exhibit a defective blood metabolism which is a result of excessive blood sugar. This results in severe hormonal imbalance and also leads to defective formation of various blood components. Diabetes also results in poor blood circulation to various parts which may result in blurred vision, aching pain, etc.

### *Diabetes Symptoms as Autoimmune Disorders*

Various skins, genito-urinary tract and respiratory complaints occur as a result of autoimmune infections. Defective formation of various blood components like WBCs and platelets result in poor blood composition. This may result in complications like poor wound healing and easy susceptibility to injuries.

Few complications may arise if not annihilated at the earliest. They may result in blindness, cataract, gangrene, diabetic nephropathy, diabetic neuropathy, diabetic foot, etc.

## Prediabetes

Prediabetes is a stage between normal and diabetes stage. It is an alarming sign for upcoming diabetes or a chance to change future. Universally, numerous terms are given like, Borderline Diabetes, Chemical Diabetes, Touch of Diabetes, etc. The term Prediabetic was given by the US Department of Health and Human Services and American Diabetes Association (ADA) on 27 March 2002, with an intention to create awareness and convey seriousness of the condition. Also, they motivated people to opt for appropriate treatment and lifestyle modification. According to the ADA statistics 17 million US citizens are diabetic and 16 million are prediabetic. ADA defines it as a stage before the development of diabetes, with normal glucose tolerance, but with an increased risk of developing diabetes in near future.

Prediabetes is a condition when blood sugar level triggers higher than normal, but not so high that we can justify it as type 2 diabetes. According to the Centers for Disease Control and Prevention, 41 million US adults aged 40 to 74 have prediabetes. And the same reports from The American Academy of Pediatrics show that one of every 10 males and one of every 25 females aged from 12 to 19 years have prediabetes.

### *Screening and Diagnosis of Prediabetes*

Prediabetics will never know on their own about their high blood sugar. If they are suffering from the mentioned factors which indicates risk zone, they should periodically go for routine check-up and should be cautious enough about the given signs and symptoms. Once they have crossed the age of 45, they must routinely visit a doctor and ask for its diagnosis.

There are two types of blood tests to determine whether a person is suffering from prediabetes or not, they are as follows:

- *Fasting Blood Glucose Test:* A fasting blood sugar level less than 100 milligrams of glucose per decilitre of blood (mg/dl) is considered normal. If blood sugar level is 100 to 125mg/dl, have prediabetes also called impaired fasting glucose (IFG). If a person is suffering from prediabetes then the fasting blood sugar as well as postprandial blood sugar will fluctuate easily.
- *Oral Glucose Tolerance Test (OGTT):* After fasting for at least eight hours, FBS (fasting blood sugar) is checked and then an oral dose of 8 ounce sugary syrup is administered. The blood glucose level is checked after an hour and if it reaches 144–199 mg/dl after two hours, the person has impaired glucose tolerance.

## Causes of Diabetes

The precise etiology of most cases of diabetes is uncertain, although certain contributing factors are as follows:

*Type 1 Diabetes:* Type 1 diabetes is autoimmune disease that affects 0.3 per cent on average. It is result of destruction of beta cells due to aggressive nature of cells present in the body. Researchers believe that some of the etiology and risk factors which may trigger type 1 diabetes may be genetic, poor diet (malnutrition) and environment (virus affecting pancreas). Secondly, in most of the cases, diabetes occurs because there is abnormal secretion of some hormones in the blood which act as antagonists to insulin, example – Adrenocortical hormone, Adrenaline hormone and Thyroid hormone.

*Type 2 Diabetes:* Type 2 diabetes is also called non-insulin dependent diabetes mellitus (NIDDM) or adult-onset diabetes. It occurs when the body produces enough insulin but cannot utilize it effectively. This type of diabetes usually develops in middle age. A general observation says that about 90–95 per cent of people suffering with diabetes are type 2; about 80 per cent are overweight. It is more common among people who are older; obese; have a family history of diabetes; have had gestational diabetes. There are number of risk factors found to be responsible for type 2 diabetes like, the more the etiology and risk factors carried by an individual, the higher the risk for developing diabetes.

### Major Causes of Diabetes

- *Hereditary or Inherited Traits:* It is strongly believed that due to some genes which passes from one generation to another, a person can inherit diabetes. It depends upon closeness of blood relationship as mother is diabetic, the risk is 2 to 3 per cent, father is diabetic, the risk is more than the previous case and if both the parents are diabetic, the child has much greater risk for diabetes.
- *Age:* Increased age is a factor which gives more possibility than in younger age. This disease may occur at any age, but 80 per cent of cases occur after 50 year, incidences increase with the age factor.
- *Poor Diet (Malnutrition Related Diabetes):* Improper nutrition, low protein and fiber intake, high intake of refined products are the expected reasons for developing diabetes.
- *Obesity and Fat Distribution:* Being overweight means increased insulin resistance that is if body fat is more than 30 per cent, BMI 25+, waist grith 35 inches in women or 40 inches in males.
- *Sedentary Lifestyle:* People with sedentary lifestyle are more prone to diabetes, when compared to those who exercise thrice a week, are at low risk of falling prey to diabetes.
- *Stress:* Either physical injury or emotional disturbance is frequently blamed as the initial cause of the disease. Any disturbance in corticosteroid or ACTH therapy may lead to clinical signs of the disease.
- *Drug Induced:* Clozapine (Clozaril), olanzapine (Zyprexa), risperidone (Risperdal), quetiapine (Seroquel) and ziprasidone (Geodon) are known to induce this lethal disease.

- *Infection:* Some of the strephylococci is supposed to be responsible factor for infection in pancreas.
- *Sex:* Diabetes is commonly seen in elderly especially males but, strongly in women and those females with multiple pregnancy or suffering from (PCOS) Polycystic Ovarian Syndrome.
- *Hypertension:* It had been reported in many studies that there is direct relation between high systolic pressure and diabetes.
- *Serum Lipids and Lipoproteins:* High triglyceride and cholesterol level in the blood is related to high blood sugars, in some cases it has been studied that risk is involved even with low HDL levels in circulating blood.

**Prevention**

- Type 1 diabetes risk is known to depend upon a genetic predisposition based on HLA types (particularly types DR3 and DR4), an unknown environmental trigger (suspected to be an infection, although none has proven definitive in all cases), and an uncontrolled autoimmune response that attacks the insulin producing beta cells. Some research has suggested that breastfeeding decreased the risk in later life; various other nutritional risk factors are being studied, but no firm evidence has been found. Giving children 2000 IU of Vitamin D during their first year of life is associated with reduced risk of type 1 diabetes, though the causal relationship is obscure.
- Children with antibodies to beta cell proteins (i.e. at early stages of an immune reaction to them) but no overt diabetes, and treated with vitamin B-3 (niacin), had less than half the diabetes onset incidence in a 7-year time span as did the general population, and an even lower incidence relative to those with antibodies as above, but who received no vitamin B3.
- Type 2 diabetes risks can be reduced in many cases by making changes in diet and increasing physical activity. The American Diabetes Association (ADA) recommends maintaining a healthy weight, getting at least 2½ hours of exercise per week (several brisk sustained walks appear sufficient), having a modest fat intake, and eating sufficient fiber (e.g. from whole grains). The ADA does not recommend alcohol consumption as a preventive, but it is interesting to note that moderate alcohol intake may reduce the risk (though heavy consumption absolutely and clearly increases damage to bodily systems significantly); a similarly confused

connection between low dose alcohol consumption and heart disease is termed the French Paradox.

- There is inadequate evidence that eating foods of low glycemic index is clinically helpful despite recommendations and suggested diets emphasizing this approach.
- There are numerous studies which suggest connections between some aspects of type 2 diabetes with ingestion of certain foods or with some drugs. Some studies have shown delayed progression to diabetes in predisposed patients through prophylactic use of metformin, rosiglitazone, or valsartan. In patients on hydroxychloroquine for rheumatoid arthritis, incidence of diabetes was reduced by 77 per cent though causal mechanisms are unclear. Breastfeeding may also be associated with the prevention of type 2 of the disease in mothers. Clear evidence for these and any of many other connections between foods and supplements and diabetes is sparse to date; none, despite secondary claims for (or against), is sufficiently well established to justify as a standard clinical approach.

### Treatment and Management

Diabetes mellitus is currently a chronic disease, without a cure, and medical emphasis must necessarily be on managing/avoiding possible short-term as well as long-term diabetes-related problems. There is an exceptionally important role for patient education, dietetic support, sensible exercise, self-monitoring of blood glucose, with the goal of keeping both short-term blood glucose levels, and long-term levels as well, within acceptable bounds. Careful control is needed to reduce the risk of long-term complications. This is theoretically achievable with combinations of diet, exercise and weight loss (type 2), various oral diabetic drugs (type 2 only), and insulin use (type 1 and for type 2 not responding to oral medications, mostly those with extended duration diabetes). In addition, given the associated higher risks of cardiovascular disease, lifestyle modifications should be undertaken to control blood pressure and cholesterol by exercising more, smoking less or ideally not at all, consuming an appropriate diet, wearing diabetic socks, wearing diabetic shoes, and if necessary, taking any of several drugs to reduce blood pressure. Many type 1 treatments include combination use of regular or NPH insulin, and/or synthetic insulin analogs (e.g. Humalog, Novolog or Apidra) in combinations such as Lantus/Levemir and Humalog, Novolog or Apidra. Another type 1 treatment option is the use of the insulin pump (e.g. from Deltec Cozmo, Animas, Medtronic Minimed, Insulet Omnipod, or ACCU-CHEK). A blood lancet is used to pierce the skin (typically of a finger), in order to draw blood to test it for sugar levels.

In countries using a general practitioner system, such as the United Kingdom, care may take place mainly outside hospitals, with hospital-based specialist care used only in case of complications, difficult blood sugar control, or research projects. In other circumstances, general practitioners and specialists share care of a patient in a team approach. Optometrists, podiatrists/chiropodists, dietitians, physiotherapists, nursing specialists (e.g. DSNs (Diabetic Specialist Nurse)), nurse practitioners, or Certified Diabetes Educators, may jointly provide multidisciplinary expertise. In countries where patients must provide their own health care (i.e. in the developed world, the US and in much of the undeveloped world), the impact of out-of-pocket costs of adequate diabetic care can be very high. In addition to the medications and supplies needed, patients are often advised to receive regular consultation from a physician (e.g. at least every three to six months).

## Cure for Diabetes

### *Cures for Type I Diabetes*

There is no practical cure, at this time, for type 1 diabetes. The fact that type 1 diabetes is due to the failure of one of the cell types of a single organ with a relatively simple function (i.e. the failure of the beta cells in the Islets of Langerhans) has led to the study of several possible schemes to cure this form of diabetes mostly by replacing the pancreas or just the beta cells. Only those type 1 diabetic who have received either a pancreas or a kidney-pancreas transplant (often when they have developed diabetic kidney disease (i.e. nephropathy) and become insulin-independent) may now be considered 'cured' from their diabetes. A simultaneous pancreas-kidney transplant is a promising solution, showing similar or improved survival rates over a kidney transplant alone. Still, they generally remain on long-term immunosuppressive drugs and there is a possibility that the immune system will mount a host versus graft response against the transplanted organ. So diabetes is not treatable.

Transplants of exogenous beta cells have been performed experimentally in both mice and humans, but this measure is not yet practical in regular clinical practice partly due to the limited number of beta cell donors. Thus far, like any such transplant, it has provoked an inmune reaction and long-term immunosuppressive drugs have been needed to protect the transplanted tissue. An alternative technique has been proposed to place transplanted beta cells in a semi-permeable container, isolating and protecting them from the immune system. Stem cell research has also been suggested as a potential avenue for a cure since it may permit regrowth of Islet cells which are genetically part of the treated individual, thus perhaps eliminating the need for immuno-suppressants. This has been done in mice, and a 2007 trial of 15 newly diagnosed patients with type 1 diabetes treated with stem cells raised from their own bone marrow after immunosuppression showed that the majority did not require any insulin treatment for prolonged periods of time.

Microscopic or nanotechnological approaches are under investigation as well, in one proposed case with implanted stores of insulin metred out by a rapid response valve sensitive to blood glucose levels. At least two approaches have been demonstrated in vitro. These are, in some sense, closed-loop insulin pumps.

### *Cures for Type 2 Diabetes*

Type 2 has had no definitive cure, although recently it has been shown that a type of gastric bypass surgery can normalize blood glucose levels in 80–100 per cent of severely obese patients with diabetes. The precise causal mechanisms are being intensively researched; its results are not simply attributable to weight loss, as the improvement in blood sugars precedes any change in body mass. This approach may become a standard treatment for some people with type 2 diabetes in the relatively near future. This surgery has the additional benefit of reducing the death rate from all causes by up to 40 per cent in severely obese people. A small number of normal to moderately obese patients with type 2 diabetes have successfully undergone similar operations.

## Prognosis

Patient education, understanding, and participation are vital since the complications of diabetes are far less common and less severe in people who have well-controlled blood sugar levels. Wider health problems accelerate the deleterious effects of diabetes. These include smoking, elevated cholesterol levels, obesity, high blood pressure and lack of regular exercise. According to a study, women with high blood pressure have a threefold risk of developing diabetes.

Anecdotal evidence suggests that some of those with type 2 diabetes who exercise regularly, lose weight and eat healthy diets may be able to keep some of the disease or some of the effects of the disease in 'remission'. Certainly, these tips can help prevent people predisposed to type 2 diabetes and those at prediabetic stages from actually developing the disorder as it helps restore insulin sensitivity. However, patients should talk to their doctors about this for real expectations before undertaking it (esp. to avoid hypoglycemia or other complications); few people actually seem to go into total 'remission', but some may find they need less of their insulin medications since the body tends to have lower insulin requirements during and shortly following exercise. Regardless of whether it works that way or not for an individual, there are certainly other benefits to this healthy lifestyle for both diabetics and nondiabetics.

The way diabetes is managed changes with age. Insulin production decreases because of age-related impairment of pancreatic beta cells. Additionally, insulin resistance increases because of the loss of lean tissue and the accumulation of fat, particularly intra-abdominal fat, and the decreased tissue sensitivity to insulin. Glucose tolerance progressively declines with age, leading to a high prevalence of type 2 diabetes and postchallenge hyperglycemia in the older population. Age-related glucose intolerance in humans is often accompanied by insulin resistance, but circulating insulin levels are similar to those of younger people. Treatment goals for older patients with diabetes vary with the individual and take into account health status, as well as life expectancy, level of dependence, and willingness to adhere to a treatment regimen.

## Diabetes Diet

Diet plays a significant role in controlling the diabetes. The diabetic diet may be used alone or else in combination with insulin doses or with oral hypoglycemic drugs. Main objective of diabetic diet is to maintain ideal body weight, by providing adequate nutrition along with normal blood sugar levels in blood. The diet plan for a diabetic is based on height, weight, age, sex, physical activity and nature of diabetes. While planning diet, the dietician has to consider complications such as high blood pressure, high cholesterol levels.

With respect to the above factors, a dietician will assess calories to be given, like scheming the carbohydrates, proteins, fats, type of carbohydrate, amount of fiber and so on.

Exchange meal plan is a diet programme which balances the amount of carbohydrate that we intake per day. Glucose is a sugar released from carbohydrate so, if we want to control blood sugar we have to limit the consumption of simple carbohydrate. Carbohydrate foods are given as value per portion, known as the exchange. This plan helps us to decide on the type of food to be taken, the amount of food and also the time to eat. We can plan for more flexible meals as we get more knowledge about the diet for a diabetic, may be like the counting carbohydrate meal plan or constant carbohydrate. But there is no common diet that works for everyone. Nor is there any particular diet that works perfectly for any diabetic over a long period. While planning diabetes diet we should adhere to certain important factors; they are as follows:

- Fiber should be at least 1.4 oz/day
- Instead of 3 heavy meals, we should go for 4–5 small mid-intervals
- Replace bakery products and fast foods by simple whole cooked cereals, and don't eat carbohydrates 2 hours before bedtime
- Consume fresh fruit and vegetables at least 5 exchange/day

Diabetics always need to take care of their diet and also about the food they eat. Care has to be taken because all foods contain not only carbohydrate, but also some energy value. Protein and fat available in the food are converted to glucose in the body. This glucose has some effect on the blood sugar level, which has to be taken care of. Furthermore, we needn't have to eat only the bland boring diet. Instead, we can eat more fruits, vegetables and whole grains. All it means is that we need to select foods that are high in nutrition and low in calories.

## Diabetes Care

- Eat food at fixed hours
- Do not overeat
- Do not eat immediately after a workout
- Make sure to have three proper meals and light snacks in between
- Eat about the same amounts of food each day
- Eat meals and snacks at about the same times each day
- Make sure the gaps between meals are short
- Do not eat fast; masticate and munch food well before swallow
- Drink a lot of water that will help flush the toxins off system
- Avoid fried foods and sweetmeats
- Include fresh vegetable salad in every meal
- Include sprouts in the diet

- Take medicines at the same time each day
- Exercise at about the same time each day
- Avoid smoking. Smoking leads to heart disease and poor circulation
- Check feet for cuts, blisters and swelling which are likely to result from diabetes-related nerve damage
- Take good sleep daily
- Check blood sugar level regularly
- Try to stick up to the plan made up for sugar control
- Check the other tests such as kidney function, liver function, heart function, etc.
- Check weight periodically and maintain ideal body weight.

# 8

# Obesity

Obesity is from the Latin 'obesitas', which means 'stout, fat, or plump'. Obesity is a condition in which excess body fat has accumulated to such an extent that health may be negatively affected. It is commonly defined as a Body Mass Index (BMI) of 30 $kg/m^2$ or higher. This distinguishes it from being overweight as defined by a BMI of 25 $kg/m^2$ or higher. Excessive body weight is associated with various diseases, particularly cardiovascular diseases, diabetes mellitus type 2, obstructive sleep apnea, certain types of cancer, and osteoarthritis. As a result, obesity has been found to reduce life expectancy. The primary treatment for obesity is dieting and physical exercise. If this fails, anti-obesity drugs and (in severe cases) bariatric surgery can be tried.

A combination of excessive caloric intake, lack of physical activity and genetic susceptibility is thought to explain most cases of obesity, with a limited number of cases due solely to genetics, medical reasons, or psychiatric illness. As obesity is one of the leading preventable causes of death worldwide and with rates of adult and childhood obesity increasing, authorities view it as one of the most serious public health problem of the 21st century. Obesity is often stigmatized in the modern Western world. It has, however, been perceived as a symbol of wealth and fertility at other times in history and still is in many parts of Africa.

The Greeks were the first to recognize obesity as a medical disorder. Hippocrates states that 'Corpulence is not only a disease itself, but the harbinger of others'. It was known to the Indian surgeon Sushruta (6th century BCE), who related obesity to diabetes and heart disorder. He recommended physical work to help cure it and its side effects. For most of human history, mankind struggled with food scarcity. With the onset of the industrial revolution it was realized that the military and economic might of nations were dependent on both the body size and strength of their soldiers and workers. Increasing the average body mass index from underweight to the normal range played a significant role in the development of industrialized societies. Height and weight, thus, both increased through the 19th century in the developed world. During the 20th century, as populations reached their genetic potential for height, weight began increasing much more than height, resulting in obesity. In the 1950s, increasing wealth in the developed world decreased child mortality, but as body weight increased heart and kidney disease became more common. During this time period, insurance companies realized the connection between weight and life expectancy and increased premiums for the obese.

Many cultures throughout history have viewed obesity as a flaw. The *obesus* or fat character in Greek comedy was a glutton and figure of mockery. During Christian times, food was viewed as a gateway to the sins of sloth and lust. In modern Western culture, excess weight is often regarded as unattractive and obesity is commonly associated with various negative stereotypes. All ages can face social stigmatization and may be targeted by bullies or shunned by their peers. In Western culture, obesity is once again seen as a sign of a low socio-economic status.

How weight is viewed has changed over the last 100 years. The weight that is viewed as an ideal has become lower since the 1920s. This is illustrated by the fact that the average height of Miss America pageant winners increased by 2 per cent from 1922 to 1999, while their average weight decreased by 12 per cent. People's perceptions of what is a healthy weight, however, have changed in the opposite direction. In Britain the weight at which people considered themselves to be overweight was significantly higher in 2007 than in 1999. These changes are believed to be due to increasing rates of adiposity leading to increased acceptance of extra body fat as being normal.

## Classification

Obesity, in absolute terms, is an increase of body adipose tissue (fat tissue) mass. In a practical setting it is difficult to determine this directly. Therefore, obesity is typically assessed by BMI (Body Mass Index) and in terms of its distribution via the waist circumference. In addition, the presence of obesity needs to be evaluated in the context of other risk factors such as medical conditions that could influence the risk of complications.

## Body Mass Index

Body Mass Index or BMI is a simple and widely used method for estimating body fat mass. BMI was developed in the 19th century by the Belgian statistician and anthropometrist Adolphe Quetelet. BMI is an accurate reflection of body fat percentage in the majority of the adult population. It is less accurate in people such as bodybuilders and pregnant women in whom body composition is affected.

BMI is calculated by dividing the subject's mass by the square of his or her height, typically expressed either in metric or US 'Customary' units:

Metric: $BMI = kilograms/metres^2$

US/Customary and imperial: $BMI = lb * 703/in^2$

where *lb* is the subject's weight in pounds and *in* is the subject's height in inches.

| BMI | Classification |
|---|---|
| Less than 18.5 | underweight |
| 18.5–24.9 | normal weight |
| 25.0–29.9 is | Overweight |
| 30.0–34.9 is | class I obesity |
| 35.0–39.9 | class II obesity |
| Over 40.0 | class III obesity |

The most commonly used definitions, established by the WHO in 1997 and published in 2000; provide the values listed in the table above.

Some modifications to the WHO definitions have been made by particular bodies. The surgical literature breaks down 'class III' obesity into further categories.

- Any BMI > 40 is *severe obesity*
- A BMI of 40.0–49.9 is *morbid obesity*
- A BMI of >50 is *super obese*

As Asian populations develop negative health consequences at a lower BMI than Caucasions, some nations have redefined obesity. The Japanese have defined obesity as any BMI greater than 25 while China uses a BMI of greater than 28.

### Waist Circumference and Waist-hip Ratio

The absolute waist circumference (>102 cm in men and >88 cm in women) and the waist-hip-ratio (the circumference of the waist divided by that of the hips of >0.9 for men and >0.85 for women) are both used as measures of central obesity.

In those with a BMI under 35, intra-abdominal body fat is related to negative health outcomes independent of total body fat. Intra-abdominal or visceral fat has a particularly strong correlation with cardiovascular disease. In a study of 15,000 subjects, waist circumference also correlated better with metabolic syndrome than BMI. Women who have an abdominal obesity have a cardiovascular risk similar to that of men. In people with a BMI over 35, measurement of waist circumference however adds little to the predictive power of BMI as most individuals with this BMI have an abnormal waist circumferences.

### Body Fat Percentage

Body fat percentage is total body fat expressed as a percentage of total body weight. It is generally agreed that men with more than 25 per cent body fat and women with more than 33 per cent body fat are obese. Body fat percentage can be estimated from a person's BMI by the following formula:

*Body fat* per cent = (1.2 * *BMI*) + (0.23 * *age*) - 5.4 - (10.8 * *gender*)

where gender is 0 if female and 1 if male

This formula takes into account the fact that body fat percentage is 10 per cent greater in women than in men for a given BMI. It recognizes that a person's percentage body fat increases as they age even if their weight remains constant. The results have an accuracy of 4 per cent.

Direct attempts to determine body fat percentage are difficult and often expensive. One of the most accurate methods is to weigh a person underwater which is known as hydrostatic weighing. Two other simpler and less accurate methods for measuring body fat, therefore, have historically been used. The first is the skinfold test, in which a pinch of skin is precisely measured to determine the thickness of the subcutaneous fat layer. It has not, however, been adequately evaluated in obese subjects. The other is bioelectrical impedance analysis which uses electrical resistance. Bioelectrical impedance, however, has not been shown to provide an advantage over BMI. Therefore, the routine use of these tests is discouraged.

Body fat percentage measurement techniques used mainly for research include computed tomography (CT scan), magnetic resonance imaging (MRI), and dual energy X-ray absorptiometry (DEXA). These techniques provide very accurate measurements, but it may be difficult to scan the severely obese due to weight limits of the equipment and insufficient diameter of the CT or MRI scanner.

### Risk Factors and Comorbidities

The presence of risk factors and diseases associated with obesity are also used to establish a clinical diagnosis. Coronary heart disease, type 2 diabetes and sleep apnea are possible complications that would indicate a need to commence or intensify treatment for obesity. Smoking, high blood pressure, age and family history are other risk factors that in combination with obesity, may indicate an additional reason for treatment.

### Childhood Obesity

The healthy BMI range varies with the age and sex of the child. Obesity in children and adolescents is defined as a BMI greater then the 95th percentile. The reference data that these percentiles are based on is from 1963 to 1994 and thus has not been affected by the recent increases in rates of obesity.

Childhood obesity has reached epidemic proportions in 21st century with rising rates in both the developed and developing world. Rates of obesity in Canadian boys have increased from 11 per cent in 1980s to over 30 per cent in 1990s, while during this same time periods rates increased from 4 per cent to 14 per cent in Brazilian children.

As with obesity in adults, many different factors contribute to the rising rates of childhood obesity. Changing diet and decreasing physical activity are believed to be the two most important, in causing the recent increase in the rate of obesity. Treatments used in children are primarily lifestyle interventions and behavioural techniques as medications are not approved for use in this age group.

### Effects on Health

#### *Mortality*

Obesity is one of the leading preventable causes of death worldwide. Large scale American and European studies have found that mortality risk varies with BMI; the lowest risk is found at a BMI of 21–24 kg/m$^2$ in nonsmokers and at a BMI of 24–27 kg/m$^2$ in current smokers and increases with changes in either direction. Obesity increases the risk of death in current and former smokers as well as in those who have never smoked. A BMI of over 32 is associated with doubling the risk of death and obesity is estimated to cause an excess 1,11,909 to 3,65,000 death per year in the United States. Obesity on average reduces life expectancy by 6–7 years. Severe obesity (BMIs >40) reduces life expectancy by 20 years for men and 5 years for women.

### *Morbidity*

A large number of physical and mental conditions have been associated with obesity. These commodities are reflected predominately in metabolic syndrome. Metabolic syndrome is a combination of medical disorders which often includes diabetes mellitus type 2, high blood pressure along with high blood cholesterol and triglyceride levels.

Obesity is related to a variety of other complications as well. Some of these are directly caused by obesity and others are indirectly related through mechanisms sharing a common cause such as poor diet or a sedentary life style. The strength of the link between obesity and specific conditions varies. One of the strongest is the link with type 2 diabetes. Excess weight is behind 64 per cent of cases of diabetes in men and 77 per cent of cases in women.

Health consequences can be categorized by the effects of increased fat mass or by the increased number of fat cells (diabetes, cancer, cardiovascular disease, non-alcoholic fatty liver disease). Increases in body fat alter the body's response to insulin, potentially leading to insulin resistance. Increased fat also creates a pro-inflammatory state, increasing the risk of thrombosis.

## Obesity Survival Paradox

Although the negative health consequences of obesity in the general population are well supported by the available evidence, health outcomes in certain subgroups seem to be improved at an increased BMI, a phenomenon known as the obesity survival paradox. The paradox was first described in 1999 in overweight and obese patients undergoing hemodialysis. Since then it has been found in a few other subgroups and explanations for its occurrence have been put forward.

In people with heart failure, those with a BMI between 30.0–34.9 had lower mortality then those with a normal weight. This has been attributed to the fact that people often lose weight as they become progressively more ill. Similar findings have been made in other types of heart disease. People with class I obesity and heart disease do not have greater rates of further heart problems than people of normal weight who also have heart disease. In people with greater degrees of obesity, however, risk of further events is increased. Even after cardiac bypass surgery, no increase in mortality is seen in the overweight and obese. One study found that the increased survival could be explained by the more aggressive treatment obese people receive after a cardiac event.

## Causes of Obesity

Most researchers agree that a combination of excessive calorie consumption and a sedentary lifestyle are the primary causes of obesity. In a minority of cases, increased food consumption can be attributed to genetic, medical or psychiatric illness. Generally, however, the rising prevalence of obesity is attributed to the availability of an easily accessible and palatable diet, car culture and mechanized manufacturing. A 2006 review identifies ten other possible contributors to the recent increase of obesity:

- Insufficient sleep,
- Endocrine disruptors – food substances that interfere with lipid metabolism,
- Decreased variability in ambient temperature,
- Decreased rates of smoking as smoking suppresses appetite,
- Increased use of medication that leads to weight gain,
- Increased distribution of ethnic and age groups that tend to be heavier,
- Pregnancy at a later age,
- Intrauterine and intergenerational effects,
- Positive natural selection of people with a higher BMI,
- Assortative mating, heavier people tending to form relationships with each other.

### *Medical and Psychiatric Illness*

Certain physical and mental illnesses and the pharmaceutical substances used to treat them can increase risk of obesity. Medical illnesses that increase obesity risk includes several rare genetic syndromes (listed above) as well as some congenital or acquired conditions: hypothyroidism, Cushing's syndrome, growth hormone deficiency and the eating disorders: binge eating disorder and night eating syndrome. However, obesity is not regarded as a psychiatric disorder, and therefore is not listed in the Diagnostic and Statistical Manual of Mental Disorders, Fourth Edition (DSM-IV) as a psychiatric illness.

Certain medications may cause weight gain or changes in body composition; these include insulin, sulfonylureas, thiazolidinediones, atypical antipsychotics, antidepressants, steroids, certain anticonvulsants (phenytoin and valproate), pizotifen and some forms of hormonal contraception.

### *Socio-economic*

While genetic influences are important to understanding obesity, they cannot explain the current dramatic increase seen within specific countries or globally. Though it is accepted that calorie consumption in excess of calorie expenditure leads to obesity on an individual basis, the cause of the shifts in these two factors on the societal scale is much debated. There are a number of theories as to the cause but most believe it is a combination of various factors.

The correlation between social class and BMI varies globally. A review in 1989 found that in developed countries women of a high social class were less likely to be obese. No significant differences were seen among men of different social classes. In the developing world, women, men and children from high social classes had greater rates of obesity. An update of this review carried out in 2007 found the same relationships, but they were weaker. The decrease in strength of correlation was felt to be due to the effects of globalization.

Many explanations have been put forth for associations between BMI and social class. It is thought that in developed countries, the wealthy are able to afford more nutritious food; they are under greater social pressure to remain slim and have more opportunities along with greater expectations for physical fitness. In undeveloped countries the ability to afford food, high energy expenditure with physical labour and cultural values favouring a larger body size are believed to contribute to the observed patterns. Attitudes toward body mass held by people in one's life may also play a role in obesity. A correlation in BMI changes over time has been found between friends, siblings and spouses.

Smoking has a significant effect on a individual's weight. Those who quit smoking gain an average of 4.4 kg for men and 5.0 kg for women over ten years. Changing rates of smoking, however, have had little effect on the overall rates of obesity.

In the United States the number of children a person has is related to their risk of obesity. A woman's risk increases by 7 per cent per child, while a man's risk increases by 4 per cent per child. This could be partly explained by the fact that having dependent children decreases physical activity in Western parents.

### *Early Malnutrition*

Malnutrition in early life is believed to play a role in the rising rates of obesity in the developing world. Endocrine changes that occur during periods of malnutrition may promote the storage of fat once more calories become available.

## Treatment and Management for Obesity

The main treatment for obesity consists of dieting and physical exercise. Diet programmes may produce weight loss over the short term, but keeping this weight off can be a problem. It often requires making exercise and a lower calorie diet a permanent part of a person's lifestyle. In the general population only 20 per cent are successful at long-term weight loss maintenance. In a more structured setting, however, 67 per cent of people who lost greater then 10 per cent of their body mass maintained or continued to lose weight one year later. An average maintained weight loss of more than 3 kg or 3 per cent of total body mass could be sustained for five years. There are significant benefits to weight loss. In a prospective study, intentional weight loss of any amount was associated with a 20 per cent reduction in all-cause mortality.

The most effective, but also most risky treatment for obesity is bariatric surgery. Due to its cost and risk of complications, researchers are fervently searching for new obesity treatments.

### *Dieting*

Diets to promote weight loss are generally divided into four categories: low-fat, low-carbohydrate, low-calorie and very low calorie. A meta-analysis of six randomized controlled trials found no difference between the main diet types (low calorie, low carbohydrate and low fat), with a 2–4 kilogramme weight loss in all studies.

### *Low-fat Diets*

Low-fat diets involve the reduction of the percentage of fat in one's diet. Calorie consumption is reduced but not purposely so. Diets of this type include NCEP Step I and II. A meta-analysis of 16 trials of 2–12 months' duration found that low-fat diets resulted in weight loss of 3.2 kg over eating as normal.

### *Low-carbohydrate Diets*

Low-carbohydrate diets such as Atkins and Protein Power are relatively high in fat and protein. They are very popular in the press but are not recommended by the American Heart Association. A review of 107 studies did not find that low-carbohydrate diets cause weight loss, except when calorie intake was restricted. No adverse affect from low-carbohydrate diets were detected.

### *Low-calorie Diets*

Low-calorie diets usually produce an energy deficit of 500–1,000 calories per day, which can result in a 0.5 kilogramme weight loss per week. They include the DASH diet and Weight Watches among others. The National Institutes of Health reviewed 34 randomized controlled trials to determine the effectiveness of low-calorie diets. They found that these diets lowered total body mass by 8 per cent over 3–12 months.

### *Very low-calorie Diets*

Very low-calorie diets provide 200–800 kcal/day, maintaining protein intake but limiting calories from both fat and carbohydrates. They subject the body to starvation and produce an average weekly weight loss of 1.5–2.5 kilogrammes. These diets are not recommended for general use as they are associated with adverse side effects such as loss of lean muscle mass, increased risks of gout and electrolyte imbalances. People attempting these diets must be monitored closely by a physician to prevent complications.

### *Exercise*

With use, muscles consume energy derived from both fat and glycogen. Due to the large size of leg muscles, walking, running and cycling are the most effective means of exercise to reduce body fat. Exercise affects macronutrient balance. During exercise, there is a shift to greater use of fat as a fuel.

A meta-analysis of 43 randomized controlled trials by the Cochrane Collaboration found that exercising alone led to limited weight loss. In combination with diet, however, it resulted in a 1 kilogramme weight loss over dieting alone. A 1.5–kilogram loss was observed with a greater degree of exercise. Even though exercise as carried out in the general population has only modest effects, a dose response curve is found, and very intense exercise can lead to substantial weight loss. During 20 weeks of basic military training with no dietary restriction, obese military recruits lost 12.5 kg. High levels of physical activity seem to be necessary to maintain weight loss.

A systematic review found that people who use pedometers, during on average an 18-week period, increased their physical activity by 27 per cent and subsequently decreased their BMI by 0.38.

The city of Bogota, Colombia blocks of 113 kilometres (70 miles) of roads every Sunday and on holidays to make it easier for it citizens to get exercise. These car-free zones are part of an effort to combat chronic diseases, including obesity.

### *Medication*

Only two anti-obesity medications are currently approved by the Food and Drug Administration (FDA) for long-term use. One is orlistat (Xenical), which reduces intestinal fat absorption by inhibiting pancreatic lipase; the other is sibutramine (Meridia), which acts in the brain to inhibit deactivation of the neurotrasmitters norepinephrine, serotonin and dopamine (very similar to some anti-depressants), therefore, decreasing appetite. Rimonabant (Acomplia), a third drug, works via a specific blockade of the endocannabinoid system. It has been developed from the knowledge that cannabis smokers often experience extreme hunger pangs, which are often referred to as 'the munchies'. It has been approved in Europe for the treatment of obesity but has not yet received approval in the United States or Canada due to safety concerns.

Weight loss with these drugs is modest; over the longer term, average weight loss on orlistat is 2.9 kg, sibutramine is 4.2 kg and rimonabant is 4.7 kg. Orlistat and rimonabant lead to a reduced incidence of diabetes, and all three drugs have some effect on cholesterol. There is, however, little data on how these drugs affect the long-term complications or outcomes of obesity.

There are number of less commonly used medication. Some are approved for only short-term use, others are used off label, and still others are used illegally. Most are appetite suppressants that act on either one or more neurotransmitters. Phendimetrazine (Bontril), diethylpropion and phentermine are approved by the FDA for short-term use; bupropion, topiramate and zonisamide are sometimes used off label.

Certain drugs are useful depending on the comorbities present. Metformin is preferred in overweight diabetics as it may lead to mild weight loss in comparison to sulfonylureas or insulin. Well the thiazolidinediones, on the other hand, may cause weight gain, but decrease central obesity. Diabetics also achieve modest weight loss with fluoxetine (Prozac), orlistat and sibutramine over 12–57 weeks. The long-term health benefits of theses treatments, however, remain unclear.

Fenfluramine and dexfenfluramine were withdrawn from the market in 1997; ephedrine (Ma Huang) was removed from the market in 2004. Dexamphetamines are not approved by the FDA for the treatment of obesity due to concerns regarding addiction. These drugs are all not recommended due to potential side effects. People, however, do occasionally get these drugs illegally.

### *Surgery*

Bariatric surgery ('weight loss surgery') is the use of surgical interventions in the treatment of obesity. As every operation may have complications, surgery is only recommended for severely obese people (BMI >40) who have failed to lose weight with dietary modification and pharmacological treatment. Weight loss surgery relies on various principles; the most common approaches are reducing the volume of the stomach, producing an earlier sense of satiation (e.g. by adjustable gastric banding and vertical banded gastroplasty) and reduce the length of bowel that food will be in contact with, directly reducing absorption (gastric bypass surgery). Band surgery is reversible, while bowel shortening operations are not. Some procedures can be performed laparoscopically. Complications from weight loss surgery are frequent.

Surgery for severe obesity is associated with long-term weight loss and decreased overall mortality. One study found a weight loss of between 14 per cent and 25 per cent at 10 years, depending on the type of procedure performed and a 29 per cent reduction in all cause mortality when compared to standard weight loss measures. A marked decrease in the risk of diabetes mellitus, cardiovascular disease and cancer has also been found after bariatric surgery. Weight loss is marked in the first few months after surgery and is sustained in the long term. In one study there was an unexplained increase in deaths from accidents and suicide but this did not outweigh the benefit in terms of disease prevention. When the two main techniques are compared gastric bypass procedures are found to lead to 30 per cent more weight loss than banding procedures one year after surgery.

The effects of liposuction, however, are less well determined, with some small studies showing benefits and others showing none.

### Non-Medical Effects of Obesity

In addition to its health impacts, obesity leads to many problems including social stigmatization, disadvantages in employment and increased business costs. These effects are felt by all levels of society from individuals, to corporations, to governments.

Obesity and its health effects create sizable economic costs. In 1998 in the US, the medical costs attributable to obesity were $78.5 billion USD, or 9.1 per cent of all medical expenditures. Obesity prevention programmes have been found to reduce the cost of treating obesity-related disease. Those reductions, however, are offset by medical costs incurred during the additional years of life gained. The authors, therefore, conclude that reducing obesity may improve the public's health, but it is unlikely to reduce overall health spending.

Obese workers have higher rates of absenteeism from work and take more disability leave, thus increasing costs for employers and decreasing productivity. A study examining Duke University employees found that people with a BMI over 40 filed twice as many worker's compensation claims as those whose BMI was 18.5–24.9. They also had more than 12 times as many lost work days. The most common injuries in this group were due to falls and lifting, thus affecting the lower extremities, wrists or hands, and backs. The US state of Alabama Employees' Insurance Board approved a controversial plan to charge obese workers $25 per month if they do not take measures to reduce their weight and improve their health. These measures are set to start Jan. 2010 and apply to those with a BMI of greater than 35 kg/m who fail to make improvements in their health after one year.

Obese people are less likely to be hired for a job and are less likely to be promoted. Obese people are also paid less than their non-obese counterparts for an equivalent job. Obese women on average make 6 per cent less and obese men make 3 per cent less.

Specific industries, such as the airline and food industries, have special concerns. Due to rising rates of obesity, airlines face higher fuel costs and pressures to increase seating width. In 2000, the extra weight of obese passengers cost airlines US$275 million. Costs for restaurants are increased by litigation accusing them of causing obesity. In 2005, the US Congress discussed legislation to prevent civil law suits against the food industry in relation to obesity; however it did not become law.

# 9

# Social Epidemiology

Social epidemiology is a branch of epidemiology that studies the distribution and determinants of health and disease in populations. Social epidemiology focuses particularly on the effects of socio-structural factors on states of health. The major premise of social epidemiology is that each society forms its own distribution of health and disease. In other words, social epidemiology assumes that the distribution of health and disease in a society reflects the distribution of advantages and disadvantages in that society. Based on this premise, social epidemiology examines which socio-structural factors affect the distribution of health and disease, as well as how these factors influence individual and population health. Social epidemiology proposes to identify societal characteristics that affect the pattern of disease and health distribution in a society and to understand its mechanisms. Although social epidemiology has developed recently, the idea that social conditions affect health already existed at the beginning of the 19th century.

Social epidemiology is a branch of epidemiology that focuses particularly on the effects of social-structural factors on states of health. Social epidemiology assumes that the distribution of advantages and disadvantages in a society reflects the distribution of health and disease. It proposes to identify societal characteristics that affect the pattern of disease and health distribution in a society and to understand its mechanisms. The central and initial question of social epidemiology to be answered is: What effect do social factors have on individual and population health? However, the new focus on this theme using current epidemiological methods is a relatively recent phenomenon. There are several significant concepts in the field of social epidemiology: (1) the bio-psychosocial paradigm, (2) the population perspective, (3) use of new statistical approaches such as multilevel analysis and (4) significance of theory. The relationship between social class and health has been a major research field since the beginning of public health history. Many studies have identified the disparities in health among social classes and developed several theories, such as social selection theory and socio-biological translation theory. However, despite the long history of this research field, the effect of social class on health is not yet fully understood.

## Meaning and Definitions

The basic theme of social epidemiology that social conditions affect population health, is not new; several investigations based on the idea were conducted in the 19th century. As a branch of epidemiological study, however, social epidemiology is relatively new. Over the last few decades, the discipline of social epidemiology has developed by refocusing on its traditional perspective with contemporary epidemiological methods in order to understand disease etiology that includes social experiences as direct causes of diseases.

In *Social Epidemiology*, Berkman and Kawachi (2000) defined social epidemiology as 'the branch of epidemiology that studies the social distribution and social determinants of states of health'.

Social epidemiology may focus on individual-level measures, or on emergent social properties that have no correlation at the individual level; simultaneous analysis at both levels may be warranted. Use of such multilevel models (also known as hierarchical and mixed effects models) has grown in recent years but suffers from theoretical and practical concerns.

Social epidemiology overlaps with fields in the social sciences, most notably medical sociology and medical geography. However, these latter fields often use health and disease in order to explain specifically social phenomenon (such as the growth of lay health advocacy movements), while social epidemiologists generally use social concepts in order to explain patterns of health in the population.

Social epidemiology is the systematic and comprehensive study of health, well-being, social conditions or problems along with diseases and their determinants, using epidemiology and social science methods to develop interventions, programmes, policies, and institutions that may reduce the extent, adverse impact, or incidence of a health or social problem and promote health. This definition provides evidence-based methods for public health activism. Social problems are specifically included in this definition because many of today's challenges in public health, including obesity, infectious diseases, violence, child abuse and drug use are associated with both personal behaviour and macro trends in the social structure such as the distribution of wealth, social resources with exposure to media and market forces. Furthermore, those who specifically study social problems can enrich their research and practice through the methods of social epidemiology, revealing how social problems are intrinsically linked to the health status of populations. Social epidemiology is the combination of epidemiology (the study of the distribution and determinants of disease and injury in human populations) with the social and behavioural sciences.

This definition of social epidemiology emphasizes that determining the distribution of disease and social problems and understanding the relevant risk factors and their interrelationship are only one part of social epidemiology. Risk factors are the behaviours, attributes, inherited characteristics and exposures that increase the probability of a specific outcome such as a health or social condition, problem or disease (Last, 1995). In addition to determining distribution and identifying risk factors, a central focus of social epidemiology is implementing what we know about a particular condition in order to maintain and improve health and well-being. Inherent in this definition is the equal emphasis given to the psycho-social and the biological or medical determinants of disease and well-being. This definition emphasizes the use of multidisciplinary approaches to analyse complex social problems.

Some theorists have proposed an alternative definition of social epidemiology as 'the branch of epidemiology that studies the social distribution and social determinants of states of health' (Berkman and Kawachi, 2000: 6). This approach to social epidemiology contrasts with classic epidemiology in its explicit emphasis on investigating social factors such as poverty and gender through the judicious use of theories, concepts, and methods instead of merely assuming their effects as background variables in biomedical research (Krieger, 2001).

For example, alcohol consumption and driving are common activities among young people. However, their occurrences together in time and place make them risk factors that increase the likelihood of a motor vehicle accident. Numerous community groups, lawmakers and policymakers have applied this knowledge to the development of programmes and policies to combat driving under the influence of alcohol. Activities range from educating youth and police about the dangers of drinking and driving to providing alcohol-free events for youth and changing the legal drinking age. Although alcohol consumption has been illegal for those under twenty-one years of age since 1988, according to the 1998 national Household survey on Drug abuse an estimated 10.5 million current drinkers were twelve to twenty years old (Center for Mental Health Services, 1999). There have been no statistically significant changes in the rates of underage drinking since 1994, which reinforces the conclusion that simply enacting laws does not necessarily change behaviour.

The approach of social epidemiology reflects the understanding that social variables or conditions can lie on either side of the equation determining which factors affect health and illness. They can be independent variables, which are the characteristics hypothesized to explain the phenomena of health and disease. They can also be the social condition or outcome that we are trying to understand, or the dependent variable. For example, depression can be a risk factor for some diseases or social conditions, such as alcohol abuse or child neglect. It can also be the illness outcome of interest in its own right, measured by either reported symptoms or psychiatric diagnoses. Similarly, homelessness can be a risk factor for contracting an infectious disease or becoming the victim of violent crime, and it can also be a social condition that we seek to elucidate.

## Socio-Cultural Factors Bearing on Health in India

Health is multifactoral. The factors which influence health lie both within the individual and externally in the society in which he or she lives. It is a truism to say that what man is and to what disease he may fall victim depends on a combination of two sets of factors – his genetic factor and the environment factors to which he is exposed. These factors interact and the result of these interactions may be health of individuals and whole communities may be considered to be the result of many interaction. According to the WHO (1946), 'Health is state of complete physical, mental and social well-being and not merely the absence of disease or infirmity'. Providing conditions for achieving normal health for all is the duty of the state and society. In fact, it is the deepest urge of humanity to be healthy. Health is one of the essentials of life without which nothing can be achieved. The sick and hungry child cannot learn and the sick and hungry adult cannot produce.

Health is a means of social development and vice versa. The success of any health care delivery system to meet health needs of a society is dependent upon the extent of people's participation or utilization of services by the people. Various factors social, economic and psychological have important significance in Health Care Service. On the basis of some of the studies by sociologists, anthropologists, social workers and medical scientists it has been advocated that health and diseases are not merely biological phenomena. The socio-cultural and economic environment, faith in supernatural powers and other related belief style, nature of medical profession and services, and their utilization also affect the health and disease profile of a community. It indicates that the consideration of such factors is indispensable to planning, organizing, implementing and monitoring the medical and health care programmes in any community for far-reaching results.

## Social Factors

There are several social factors which determine the health and disease profile in a community. The social factors are various, like religion, caste, education, occupation, family, lifestyle, income and living conditions. The health status of a social group cannot really be maintained and safeguarded unless the importance and interrelationship of these factors with health and disease is understood. The study of religion and caste in a community is relevant to ensure people's participation in comprehensive community health care programmes. Various infections and respiratory diseases occur more in particular religious and caste groups because of their lifestyles. It is due to certain rituals and religious observances which people practice, out of belief and faith in their cult. This factor renders particular religious groups unable to prevent illness. For example, when small-pox was widespread, Hindus used to refuse taking small-pox vaccination due to the fear of Mata Maiya (*Bari Mata*) a goddess who was considered to cause this epidemic; Muslims, for example, are reluctant to accept family planning for obvious religious reasons. Similarly, there are certain occupations which are still caste specific. The unhygienic conditions related with these occupations are responsible for appended diseases more prevalent in these castes. Education is supposed to generate understanding which facilitates utilization of health and social welfare facilities and accomplishes people's accessibility and participation in such programmes. Education again prepares individual to make proper choices of therapeutic alternatives, appropriate medical technologies, physicians and institution. The lifestyle components such as proper path, proper rest, exercises, smoking, alcoholism, etc. also affect health accordingly.

### Economic Factors

Economic conditions have long been known to influence human health. For the majority of the world's people, health status is determined primarily by their level of economic development, e.g. per capita GNP, education, nutrition, employment, housing, the political system of the country, etc. The per capita GNP is the most widely accepted measure of general economic performance. No doubt that in many developing countries, it is the economic progress that has been the major factor in reducing morbidity, increasing life expectancy and improving the quality of life. The economic status determines the purchasing power, standard of living, quality of life, family size along with the pattern of disease and deviant behaviour in the community. It is also an important factor in seeking health care. Ironically, affluence may also be a contributory cause of illness as exemplified by the high rates of coronary heart disease, diabetes and obesity in the upper socio-economic groups. Family income is the prime determinant of social status and there are certain diseases which mostly occur in lower socio-economic class. The diseases which occur most in lower income group according to Park (1983) are chronic bronchitis, tuberculosis, gastroenteritis, leprosy, cervical cancer, etc. The upper classes essentially have lower morbidity and mortality in relation to the diseases indicated.

### Psychological Factors

Various psychological factors play an important role in one's health. The living conditions, hectic lifestyle, lack of rest and sleep, lack of recreation and entertainment leads to mental stress, anxiety and depression – thus it leads to mental illness. Sometimes, people start smoking and consuming alcohol in order to reduce their mental stress and develop addiction which affect the dependants of the earning member. Besides due to negligence and lack of faith in staffs of hospitals, people do not go there for treatment. Hospital staffs, including doctors have no sympathetic attitude towards patients and the patients try to avoid going to hospital. Medical social worker understands the feeling, pain and condition of the patient and can motivate the patients towards their treatment.

In 1977, the Government of India launched a Rural Health Scheme, based on the principle of 'Placing people's health in people's hands'. It is a three-tier system of health care delivery in rural areas based on the recommendation of the Srivastav committee in 1975. The Government of India is committed to achieving the goal of health for all, through primary health care approach which seeks to provide universal comprehensive health care at a cost which is affordable. In 1983, India evolved a National Health Policy based on Primary health care approach. Steps are already underway to implement the National Health Policy objectives towards achieving 'Health for All'.

# 10

# Common Occupational Diseases and their Prevention

An occupational disease is any chronic ailment that occurs as a result of work or occupational activity. An occupational disease is typically identified when it is seen to be more prevalent in a given body of workers than in the general population, or in other worker populations. Occupational hazards that are of a traumatic nature (such as falls by roofers) are not considered to be occupational diseases. Under the law of worker's compensation in many jurisdictions, there is a presumption that specific diseases are caused by the worker being in the work environment and the burden is on the employer or insurer to show that the disease came about from another cause.

Some well-known occupational diseases include:

- Asbestosis among asbestos miners and those who work with friable asbestos insulation.
- Black lung (coal worker's pneumoconiosis) among coal miners.
- Carpal tunnel syndrome among persons who work in the poultry industry and who do data entry.
- Radiation sickness.
- Phossy jaw.
- Radium jaw.
- Squamous cell carcinoma of the skin of the scrotum.
- Byssinosis among workers in parts of the cotton textile industry.

### Asbestosis

Asbestosis is a chronic inflammatory medical condition affecting the parenchymal tissue of the lungs. It occurs after long-term, heavy exposure to asbestos, e.g. in mining, and is, therefore, regarded as an occupational lung disease. Sufferers have severe dyspnea (shortness of breath) and are at an increased risk regarding several different types of lung cancer. As clear explanations are not always stressed in non-technical literature, care should be taken to distinguish between several forms of relevant diseases. According to the World Health Organization (WHO), these may be defined as; asbestosis (the subject of this article), lung cancer and mesothelioma (generally a very rare form of cancer but increasing in frequency as people exposed to asbestos age).

### *Signs and Symptoms*

The primary symptom of asbestosis is generally the slow onset of shortness of breath on exertion. In severe, advanced cases, this may lead to respiratory failure. Coughing is not usually a typical symptom, unless the patient has other, concomitant respiratory tract diseases.

People with extensive occupational exposure to the mining, manufacturing, handling or removal of asbestos are at a risk of developing asbestosis. There is also an increased risk of lung cancer and mesothelioma. Asbestosis and lung cancer require prolonged exposure to asbestos. However, cases of mesothelioma have been documented with even 1–3 months of exposure with only indirect exposure (through air ventilation system.) Most cases of asbestosis do not become apparent until 5–10 years after the initial exposure to the material.

### *Pathogenesis*

Asbestosis is the scarring of lung tissue (around terminal bronchioles and alveolar ducts) resulting from the inhalation of asbestos fibres There are two types of fibres, amphibole (thin and straight) and serpentine (curved). The former is primarily responsible for human disease as they are able to penetrate deeply into the lungs. When such fibres reach the alveoli (air sacs) in the lung, where oxygen is transferred into the blood, the foreign bodies (asbestos fibres) cause the activation of the lung's local immune system and provoke an inflammatory reaction. This inflammatory reaction can be described as chronic rather than acute, with a slow ongoing progression of the immune system in an attempt to eliminate the foreign fibres. Macrophages phagocytose (ingest) the fibres and stimulate fibroblasts to deposit connective tissue. Due to the asbestos fibres' natural resistance to digestion, the macrophage will die off, releasing certain cytokines and attracting further lung macrophages and fibrolastic cells to lay down fibrous tissue, which eventually forms a fibrous mass. The result is interstitial fibrosis. The fibrotic scar tissue causes alveolar walls to thicken, which reduces elasticity and gas diffusion, reducing oxygen transfer to the blood as well as the removal of carbon dioxide.

Asbestosis presents as a restrictive lung disease. The total lung capacity (TLC) may be reduced through alveolar wall thickening. In the more severe cases, the drastic reduction in lung function due to the stiffening of the lungs and reduced TLC may induce right-sided heart failure.

More than 50 per cent of people affected with asbestosis develop plaques in the parietal pleura, in the space between the chest wall and lungs. Clinically, patients present with dry inspiratory crackles, clubbing of the fingers and a diffuse fibrotic pattern in the lower lung lobes (where asbestosis is most prevalent).

#### Treatment

There is no curative treatment. Oxygen therapy at home is often necessary to relieve the shortness of breath. Supportive treatment of symptoms includes respiratory physiotherapy to remove secretions from the lungs by postural drainage, chest percussion and vibration. Nebulized medications may be prescribed in order to dilute secretions.

### Black Lung/Coalworker's Pneumoconiosis

Black lung disease, also known as coal workers' pneumoconiosis (CWP), is caused by long exposure to coal dust. It is a common affliction of coal miners and others who work with coal, similar to silicosis from inhaling silica dust, and to the long-term effects of tobacco smoking. Inhaled coal dust progressively builds up in the lungs and is unable to be removed by the body, leading to inflammation, fibrosis and, in the worst case necrosis.

Coal workers' pneumoconiosis, in its most severe state, develops after the initial, milder form of the disease known as anthracosis (anthrac – coal, carbon). This is often asymptomatic and is found, to at least some extent, in all urban dwellers due to air pollution. Prolonged exposure to large amounts of carbon dust can result in more serious forms of the disease, simple coal workers' pneumoconiosis and complicated coal workers' pneumoconiosis.

#### History and Prevention Efforts

There are currently about 42,000 underground coal miners actively working in the United States. The mining and production of coal is a major part of the economy in several developed countries. In the past 10 years, over 10,000 American miners have died from CWP. Although this disease is preventable, many miners are still developing advanced and severe cases.

In the 40 years since the Federal Coal Mine Health and Safety Act of 1969 became law, the proportion of miners with black lung disease has gone down by about 90 per cent. But the downward trend of this disease in coal miners has stopped. Rates of black lung are on the rise and have almost doubled in the last 10 years. From 2000 to 2004, over 4,000 miners died from black lung disease in the United States.

The National Institute for Occupational Safety and Health (NIOSH), with support of the Mine Safety and Health Administration (MSHA), has started a Mobile Health Screening Programme. This Mobile Unit travels to mining regions around the United States. Miners who participate in the programme receive health evaluations once every five years, at no cost to themselves. Chest X–rays can detect the early signs of and changes in CWP, often before the miner is aware of any lung problems. The screening programme is only available to current miners.

### *Pathogenesis*

Coal dust that enters the lungs can neither be destroyed nor removed by the body. The particles are engulfed by resident alveolar or interstitial macrophages and remain in the lungs, residing in the connective tissue or pulmonary lymph nodes. Aggregations of carbon-laden macrophages can be visualized under a microscope as granular, black areas. In serious cases, the lung may grossly appear black. These aggregations can cause inflammation and fibrosis, as well as the formation of nodular lesions within the lungs. The centres of dense lesions may become necrotic due to ischaemia, leading to large cavities within the lung.

### *Appearance*

Simple CWP is marked by the presence of 1–2 mm nodular aggregations of anthracotic macrophages, supported by a fine collagen network, within the lungs. Those 1–2 mm in diameter are known as coal macules, with larger aggregations known as coal nodules. These structures occur most frequently around the initial site of coal dust accumulation – the upper regions of the lungs around the respiratory bronchioles.

Continued exposure to coal dust following the development of simple CWP may result in its progression to complicated CWP, which generally requires a number of years to develop. Large, black, fibrotic scars 2–10cm in diameter are present, with accompanying decreased lung function. The lung itself appears blackened. A minority of these cases progresses to progressive massive fibrosis (PMF), the most serious form of CWP.

#### *Symptoms*

Both CWP and mild complicated CWP are often asymptomatic or only affect lung function slightly. Shortness of breath and pain may be felt. However, progression to PMF is marked by lung dysfunction, pulmonary hypertension, and cor pulmonale.

### Carpal Tunnel Syndrome

Carpal tunnel syndrome (CTS), or median neuropathy at the wrist, is a medical condition in which the median nerve is compressed at the wrist, leading to paresthesias, numbness and muscle weakness in the hand. The diagnosis of CTS is often misapplied to patients who have activity-related arm pain.

Most cases of CTS are idiopathic (without known cause), genetic factors determine most of the risk, and the role of arm use and other environmental factors is disputed.

Night symptoms and waking at night – the hallmark of this illness – can be managed effectively with night-time wrist splinting in most patients. The role of medications, including corticosteroid injection into the carpal canal, is unclear. Surgery to cut the transverse carpal ligament is effective at relieving symptoms and preventing ongoing nerve damage, but established nerve dysfunction in the form of static (constant) numbness, atrophy or weakness are usually permanent and do not respond predictably to surgery.

#### *History*

Although the condition was first noted in medical literature in the early 20th century, the first use of the term 'carpal tunnel syndrome' was in 1939. The pathology was identified by physician Dr George S. Phalen of the Cleveland Clinic after working with a group of patients in the 1950s and 1960s. CTS became widely known among the general public in the 1990s because of the rapid expansion of office jobs.

#### *Anatomy*

The median nerve passes through the carpal tunnel, a canal in the wrist that is surrounded by bone on three sides, and a transverse carpal ligament on the fourth. Nine tendons – the flexor tendons of the hand – pass through this canal. The median nerve can be compressed by a decrease in the size of the canal, an increase in the size of the contents (such as the swelling of lubrication tissue around the flexor tendons), or both. Simply bending the wrist at 90 degrees will decrease the size of the canal.

Compression of the median nerve as it runs deep to the transverse carpal ligament (TCL) causes wasting of the thenar eminece, weakness of the flexor pollicis brevis, adductor pollicis, opponens pollicis, abductor pollicis brevis, as well as sensory loss in the distribution of the median nerve distal to the transverse carpal ligament, sparing the superficial sensory branch given that its branch point is normally proximal to the TCL and travels superficially thus avoiding compression.

### *Symptoms*

Many people that have carpal tunnel syndrome have gradually increasing symptoms over time. The first symptoms of CTS may appear when sleeping and typically include numbness and paresthesia (a burning and tingling sensation) in the thumb, index, and middle fingers, although some patients may experience symptoms in the palm as well. These symptoms appear at night because people tend to bend their wrists when they sleep, which further compresses the carpal tunnel.

Patients may note that they 'drop things'. It is unclear if carpal tunnel syndrome creates problems holding things, but it does increase sweating, which decreases friction between an object and the skin.

In early stages of CTS, individuals often mistakenly blame the tingling and numbness on restricted blood circulation. They may also be at ease in accepting of the symptoms and believe their hands are simply 'falling asleep'. In chronic cases, there may be wasting of the thenar muscles (the body of muscles which are connected to the thumb), weakness of palmar abduction of the thumb (difficulty bringing the thumb away from the hand).

Unless numbness or paresthesias are among the predominant symptoms, it is unlikely the symptoms are primarily caused by carpal tunnel syndrome. In effect, pain of any type, location or severity with the absence of significant numbness or paresthesia is not likely to fall under this diagnosis.

### *Causes*

Most cases of CTS are idiopathic. CTS is sometimes associated with trauma, pregnancy, multiple myeloma, amyloid, rhematoid arthritis, acromegaly, mucopolysaccharidoses or hypothyroidism.

### *Genetic*

The most important risk factors for carpal tunnel syndrome are structural and biological rather than environmental or activity-related. The strongest risk factor is genetic predisposition.

### *Work Related*

The international debate regarding the relationship between CTS and repetitive motion and work is ongoing. The Occupational Safety and Health Administration (OSHA) have adopted rules and regulations regarding cumulative trauma disorders. Occupational risk factors of repetitive tasks, force, posture and vibration have been cited. However, the American Society for Surgery of the Hand (ASSH) has issued a statement that the current literature does not support a causal relationship between specific work activities and the development of diseases such as CTS.

The relationship between work and CTS is controversial; in many locations, workers diagnosed with carpal tunnel syndrome are entitled to time off and compensation. Carpal tunnel syndrome results in billions of dollars of workers compensation claims every year.

Some speculate that carpal tunnel syndrome is provoked by repetitive grasping and manipulating activities, and that the exposure can be cumulative. It has also been stated that symptoms are commonly exacerbated by forceful and repetitive use of the hand and wrists in industrial occupations, but it is unclear if this refers to pain (which may not be due to carpal tunnel syndrome) or the more typical numbness symptoms.

A review of available scientific data by the National Institute for Occupational Safety and Health (NIOSH) indicated that job tasks that involve highly repetitive manual acts or specific wrist postures were associated with incidents of CTS, but causation was not established, and the distinction from work-related arm pains that are not carpal tunnel syndrome was not clear. It has been proposed that repetitive use of the arm can affect the biomechanics of the upper limb or cause damage to tissues. It has also been proposed that postural and spinal assessment along with ergonomic assessments should be included in the overall determination of the condition. While addressing these factors has been found to improve comfort in some studies, there is no evidence that they affect the natural history of carpal tunnel syndrome.

### *Psycho-social Factors*

Studies have related activity-related upper extremity pain with psychological and social factors, but most such pains are non-specific but commonly mislabelled as carpal tunnel syndrome. Psychological distress correlates with increased pain at work, as do other psychosocial stressors such as job demands, poor support from colleagues, and work dissatisfaction.

As mentioned elsewhere in this chapter, carpal tunnel is characterized by numbness, not pain. Therefore, any associations between stress and carpal tunnel syndrome are debatable.

### *Trauma Related*

- Fractures of one of the arm bones, particularly a Colles' fracture.
- Dislocation of one of the carpal bones of the wrist.
- Strong blunt trauma to the wrist or lower forearm, incurred for example by using arm extremity to cushion a fall or protecting oneself from falling heavy objects.
- Hematoma forming inside the wrist, because of internal haemorrhaging.
- Deformities from abnormal healing of old bone fractures.

### *Carpal Tunnel Syndrome Associated with Other Diseases*

Non-traumatic causes generally happen over a period of time, and are not triggered by one certain event. Many of these factors are manifestations of physiologic ageing.

*Examples Include:*

- Rheumatoid arthritis and other diseases that cause inflammation of the flexor tendons can create median nerve compression at the carpal tunnel.
- With pregnancy and hypothyroidism, fluid is retained in tissues, which swells the tenosynovium.
- Acromegaly, a disorder of growth hormones, compresses the nerve by the abnormal growth of bones around the hand and wrist.
- Tumours (usually benign), such as a ganglion or a lipoma, can protrude into the carpal tunnel, reducing the amount of space. This is exceedingly rare (less than 1%).
- Obesity also increases the risk of CTS with individuals who are classified as obese (BMI > 29) 2.5 times more likely than slender individuals (BMI < 20) to be diagnosed with CTS.
- Double crush syndrome is a speculative and debated theory which postulates that when there is compression or irritation of nerve

branches contributing to the median nerve in the neck or anywhere above the wrist, this then increases the sensitivity of the nerve to compression in the wrist. There is little evidence, however, that this syndrome really exists.

### *Diagnosis*

The reference standard for the diagnosis of carpal tunnel syndrome is electrophysiological testing. Patients with intermittent numbness in the distribution of the median nerve and positive Phalen's and Durkan's tests, but normal electrophysiological testing have – at worst – very mild carpal tunnel syndrome. A predominance of pain rather than numbness is unlikely to be due to carpal tunnel syndrome, no matter what the result of electrophysiological testing is.

Clinical assessment by history taking and physical examination can support a diagnosis of CTS.

- Phalen's manoeuvre is performed by flexing the wrist gently as far as possible, then holding this position and awaiting symptoms. A positive test is one that results in numbness in the median nerve distribution when holding the wrist in acute flexion position within 60 seconds. The quicker the numbness starts, the more advanced the condition.
- Tinel's sign, a classic, though less specific test, is a way to detect irritated nerves. Tinel's is performed by lightly tapping the area over the nerve to elicit a sensation of tingling or 'pins and needles' in the nerve distribution.
- Durkan test, carpal compression test or applying firm pressure of the palm over the nerve for up to 30 seconds to elicit symptoms has also been proposed.

Other conditions may also be misdiagnosed as carpal tunnel syndrome. Thus, if history and physical examination suggest CTS, patients will usually be tested electrodiagnostically with nerve conduction studies and electomyography. The goal of electrodiagnostic testing is to compare the speed of conduction in the median nerve with conduction in other nerves supplying the hand. When the median nerve is compressed, as in CTS, it will conduct more slowly than normal and more slowly than other nerves. There are many electro-diagnostic tests used to make a diagnosis of CTS, but the most sensitive, specific and reliable test is the Combined Sensory Index (also known as Robinson index). The role of MRI or Ultra sound imaging in the diagnosis of carpal tunnel syndrome is unclear.

### *Prevention*

Current best evidence suggests that carpal tunnel syndrome is an inherent, structural disease determined primarily by one's genes. Therefore, carpal tunnel syndrome is probably not preventable. Those who favour activity as a cause of carpal tunnel syndrome, speculate that activity-limitation might limit the risk of developing carpal tunnel syndrome, but there is little or no data to support these concepts and they stigmatize and demonize arm use in way that risks increasing illness. Recommendations for preventing carpal tunnel syndrome have poor scientific support. Several are listed here:

- Take frequent breaks from repetitive movement such as computer keyboard usage or use of browser-based games that encourage the user for excessive finger movement. Free software programs such as Workrave and Xwrits are available to remind users to take breaks and stretch their wrists.
- Reduce your force and relax your grip. Most people use more force than needed to perform many tasks involving the hands. If your work involves a cash register, for instance, hit the keys softly. For prolonged handwriting, use a big pen with an oversized, soft grip adapter and free-flowing ink. This way you will not have to grip the pen tightly or press as hard on the paper.
- Take frequent breaks. Every 15 to 20 minutes give your hands and wrists a break by gently stretching and bending them. Alternate tasks when possible. If you use equipment that vibrates or that requires you to exert a great amount of force, taking breaks is even more important.
- Watch your form. Avoid bending your wrist all the way up or down. A relaxed middle position is best. If you use a keyboard, keep it at elbow height or slightly lower.
- Improve your posture. Incorrect posture can cause your shoulders to roll forward. When your shoulders are in this position, your neck and shoulder muscles are shortened, compressing nerves in your neck. This can affect your wrists, fingers and hands.
- Keep your hands warm. You are more likely to develop hand pain and stiffness if you work in a cold environment. If you cannot control the temperature at work, put on fingerless gloves that keep your hands and wrists warm.

### *Treatment*

There has been much discussion as to the most effective treatment for CTS. It is important to distinguish palliative treatments (treatments that control symptoms) from disease modifying treatments. The only treatment established to be disease modifying is operative release of the transverse carpal ligament. All other treatments seem palliative, at best, according to current best evidence.

### *Reversible Causes*

Some causes of CTS are secondary to other conditions – metabolic disorders such as hypothyroidism, for example. Treatment of the primary disorder often resolves CTS symptoms.

### *Immobilizing Braces*

A wrist splint helps limit numbness by limiting wrist flexion. Night splinting helps in a patient's sleep. There is no evidence that wrist splinting is disease modifying.

The importance of wrist braces and splints in the carpal tunnel syndrome therapy is known, but many people are unwilling to use braces. In 1993, The American Academy of Neurology recommends a non-invasive treatment for the CTS at the beginning (except for sensitive or motor deficit or grave report at EMG/ENG): a therapy using splints was indicated for light and moderate pathology. Current recommendations generally do not suggest immobilizing braces, but instead, activity modification and non-steroidal anti-inflammatory drugs as initial therapy, followed by more aggressive options or specialist referral if symptoms do not improve.

Many health professionals suggest that, for best results, one should wear braces at night and, if possible, during the activity primarily causing stress on the wrists.

### *Localized Steroid Injections*

Steroid injections can be quite effective for temporary relief from symptoms of CTS for a short time-frame while a patient develops a long-term strategy that fits with his/her lifestyle. This treatment is not appropriate for extended periods, however. In general, medical professionals only prescribe to localized steroid injections until other treatment options can be identified. For most patients, permanent relief requires surgery.

### *Physiotherapy*

There is little evidence to support physiotherapy or occupational therapy as a disease modifying treatment. They seem to be oriented primarily towards non-specific activity-related pain, rather than the numbness of carpal tunnel syndrome.

Physiotherapy offers several ways to treat and control carpal tunnel syndrome. This procedure should be directed specifically towards the pattern of pain/symptoms and dysfunction assessed by the therapist. As such, it may include a range of modalities ranging from soft tissue massage, conservative stretches and exercises and techniques to directly mobilize the nerve tissue. It can also include the aforementioned immobilizing braces.

Clinically, sometimes a patient will present with a hand that is very inflamed and swollen with severe symptoms of pain, tingling and numbness and almost a fear of use because of the pain. In these cases a physiotherapist may focus on techniques to reduce the pain and inflammation, and exercises to encourage improved circulation. A comprehensive review of effectiveness of hand therapies in carpal tunnel management demonstrates that there is some valid scientific evidence for a range of therapeutic modalities. For instance, Body Awareness Therapy such as the Feldenkrais method has positive effects in relation to fibromyalgia and chronic pain. Structured exercise programmes using these therapies to reduce wrist pain have been developed.

### *Occupational Therapy*

Occupational therapy offers ergonomic suggestions to prevent worsening of the symptoms and occupational therapist facilitates hand functions through functional activities and helps to regain the functions which are necessary for the functional living through remedial adaptive approaches.

Any forceful and repetitive use of the hands and wrists can cause upper extremity pain. More frequent rest can be useful if it can be orchestrated into one's schedule. It has been shown that taking multiple mini breaks during the stressful activity is more effective than taking occasional long breaks. There are computer applications that aid users in taking breaks. All of these applications have recommended defaults, following the most effective average break configuration, which is a 30 sec. pause every 3 to 5 minutes (the more severe the pain, the more often one should take this break). There are also programmes that automatically click the mouse. Before investing in these types of programs, it is best to consult with a doctor and research whether computer use is causing or contributing to the symptoms, as well as getting a formal diagnosis.

More proactive ways to reducing the stress on the wrists which will alleviate wrist pain and strain involve adopting a more ergonomic work and life environment. Switching from a QWERTY computer keyboard layout to a more optimized ergonomic layout such as Dvorak was commonly cited as beneficial in early CTS studies; however, some meta analyses of these studies claim that the evidence that they present is limited.

It is also important that one's body be aligned properly with the keyboard. This is most easily accomplished by bending ones elbows to a 90-degree angle and making sure the keyboard is at the same height as the elbows. Also it is important not to put physical stress on the wrists by hanging the wrist on the edge of a desk, or exposing the wrists to strong vibrations (e.g. manual lawn mowing). Position the computer monitor directly in front of your seat, so the neck is not twisted to either side when viewing the screen.

Exercises that relax and strengthen the muscles of the upper back can reduce the risk of a double crush of the median nerve.

Massage is one of the most overlooked methods for treatment of the symptoms of CTS. The use of myofascial release and active stretch release can erase the pain, numbness, tingling and burning in minutes. Then, following up with the stretches and exercises aforementioned will lengthen the relief attained by these release techniques.

### *Medication*

Using an over-the-counter anti-inflammatory drug such as aspirin, ibuprofen or naproxen can be effective as well, for controlling symptoms. Pain relievers like paracetamol will only mask the pain, and only an anti-inflammatory will affect inflammation. Non-steroidal anti-inflammatory medications theoretically can treat the root swelling and thus the source of the problem. Oral steroids (prednisone) do the same, but are generally not used for this purpose because of significant side effects. The most common complications associated with long-term use of anti-inflammatory medications are gastrointestinal irritation and bleeding. Also, some anti-inflammatory medications have been linked to heart complications. Use of anti-inflammatory medication for chronic, long-term pain should be done with doctor's supervision.

A more aggressive pharmaceutical option is an injection of cortisone, to reduce swelling and nerve pressure within the carpal tunnel. Methylcobalamin (vitamin B12) has been helpful in some cases of CTS.

### *Carpal Tunnel Release Surgery*

Release of the transverse carpal ligament ('carpal tunnel release' surgery) is recommended when there is static (ever-present, not just intermittent numbness), weakness of palmar abduction, or atrophy and when night-splinting no longer controls intermittent symptoms. In general, milder cases can be controlled for months to years, but severe cases are unrelenting symptomatically and are likely to result in surgical treatment.

### *Procedure*

In carpal tunnel release surgery, the goal is to divide the transverse carpal ligament in two. This is a wide ligament that runs across the hand, from the base of the thumb to the base of the fifth finger. It also forms the top of the carpal tunnel, and when the surgeon cuts across it (i.e. in a line with the middle finger) it no longer presses down on the nerves inside, relieving the pressure.

There are several carpal tunnel release surgery variations: each surgeon has differences of preference based on their personal beliefs and experience. All techniques have several things in common, involving brief outpatient procedures; palm or wrist incision(s); and cutting of the transverse carpal ligament.

The two major types of surgery are open-hand surgery and endoscopic surgery. Most surgeons perform open surgery, widely considered to be the gold standard. However, many surgeons are now performing endoscopic techniques. Open surgery involves a small incision somewhere on the palm about an inch or two in length. Through this the ligament can be directly visualized and divided with relative safety. Endoscopic techniques involve one or two smaller incisions (less than half inch each) through which instrumentation is introduced including probes, knives and the scope used to visualize the operative field.

All of the surgical options typically have relatively rapid recovery profiles (days to weeks depending on the activity and technique), and all usually leave a cosmetically insignificant scar.

### *Efficacy*

Surgery to correct carpal tunnel syndrome has high success rate, especially using endoscopic surgery techniques. Up to 90 per cent of patients were able to return to their same jobs after surgery. In general, endoscopic techniques are as effective as traditional open carpal surgeries, though the faster recovery time typically noted in endoscopic procedures may be offset by higher complication rates. Success is greatest in patients with the most typical symptoms. The most common cause of failure is incorrect diagnosis, and it should be noted that this surgery will only fix carpal tunnel syndrome and will not relieve symptoms with alternative causes. Recurrence is rare, and apparent recurrence usually results from a misdiagnosis of another problem. Complications can occur, but serious ones are infrequent to rare.

Carpal tunnel surgery is usually performed by a hand surgeon, orthopaedic or plastic surgeon; some neuro-surgeons and general surgeons also perform the procedure.

### *Long-term Recovery*

Most people who find relief of their carpel tunnel symptoms with conservative or surgical management, find minimal residual or 'nerve damage'. Long-term chronic carpal tunnel syndrome (typically seen in the elderly) can result in permanent 'nerve damage', i.e. symptoms of numbness, muscle wasting and weakness.

While outcomes are generally good, certain factors can contribute to poorer results that have little to do with nerves, anatomy or surgery type. One study showed that mental status parameters, alcohol use, yield much poorer overall results of treatment.

Many mild carpal tunnel syndrome sufferers either change their hand use pattern or posture at work or find a conservative, non-surgical treatment that allows them to return to full activity without hand numbness or pain, and without sleep disruption. Some find relief by adjusting their repetitive movements, the frequency with which they do the movements, and the amount of time they rest between periods of performing the movements. Other people end up prioritizing their activities and possibly avoiding certain hand activities so that they can minimize pain and perform the essential tasks. Keyboard remapping software can help people whose condition is aggrevated by one-handed key strokes involving a combination of the Control, Shift or Alt keys and an alphanumeric key. Programs such as Autohotkey allow a person to disable key combinations while they train themselves to use two hands to perform the offending key strokes.

While recurrence after surgery is a possibility, true recurrences are uncommon to rare. Such recurrence can also be non-CTS hand pain. Such hand pain may have existed prior to the surgery, which is one reason it is very important to get a proper diagnosis.

## Radiation Poisoning

Radiation poisoning, also called 'radiation sickness' or a 'creeping dose', is a form of damage to organ tissue due to excessive exposure to ionizing radiation. The term is generally used to refer to acute problems caused by a large dosage of radiation in a short period, though this also has occurred with long-term exposure. The clinical name for 'radiation sickness' is acute radiation syndrome (ARS) as described by the Centres for Discase Control and Prevention (CDC). A chronic radiation syndrome does exist but is very uncommon; this has been observed among workers in early radium source production sites and in the early days of the Soviet nuclear programme. A short exposure can result in acute radiation syndrome; chronic radiation syndrome requires a prolonged high level of exposure.

The use of radionuclides in science and industry is strictly regulated in most countries (in the US by the Nuclear Regulatory Commission). In the event of an accidental or deliberate release of radioactive material, either evacuation or sheltering in place will be the recommended measures.

### *Measuring Radiation Dosage*

The rad is a unit of absorbed radiation dose defined in terms of the energy actually deposited in the tissue. One rad is an absorbed dose of 0.01 joules of energy per kilogramme of tissue. The more recent SI unit is the gray (Gy), which is defined as 1 joule of deposited energy per kilogramme of tissue. Thus, one gray is equal to 100 rad.

To accurately assess the risk of radiation, the absorbed dose energy in rad is multiplied by the relative biological effectiveness (RBE) of the radiation to get the biological dose equivalent in rems. Rem stands for 'Rontgen equivalent in man'. In SI units, the absorbed dose energy in grays is multiplied by the same RBE to get a biological dose equivalent in sieverts(Sy). The sievert is equal to100 rem.

The RBE is a 'quality factor', often denoted by the letter Q, which assesses the damage to tissue caused by a particular type and energy of radiation. For alpha particles Q may be as high as 20, so that one rad of alpha radiation is equivalent to 20 rem. The Q of neutron radiation depends on their energy. However, for beta particles, X–rays, and gamma rays, Q is taken as one, so that the rad and rem are equivalent for those radiation sources, as are the gray and sievert.

### *Acute (short-term) vs Chronic (long-term) Effects*

Radiation sickness is generally associated with acute exposure and has a characteristic set of symptoms that appear in an orderly fashion. The symptoms of radiation sickness become more serious (and the chance of survival decreases) as the dosage of radiation increases. These effects are described as the deterministic effects of radiation.

Longer term exposure to radiation, at doses less than that which produces serious radiation sickness, can induce cancer as cell-cycle genes are mutated. If a cancer is radiation-induced, then the disease, the speed at which the condition advances, the prognosis, the degree of pain, and every other feature of the disease are not functions of the radiation dose to which the sufferer is exposed.

Since tumours grow by abnormally rapid cell division, the ability of radiation to disturb cell division is also used to treat cancer and low levels of ionizing radiation have been claimed to lower one's risk of cancer.

### *Exposure: External vs Internal*

#### *External*

External exposure is exposure which occurs when the radioactive source (or other radiation source) is outside (and remains outside) the organism which is exposed. Below are a series of three examples of external exposure.

- A person who places a sealed radioactive source in their pocket.
- A space traveller who is irradiated by cosmic rays.
- A person who is treated for cancer by either tele-therapy or brachytherapy. While in brachytherapy the source is inside the person it is still external exposure because the active part of the source never comes into direct contact with the biological tissues of the person.

One of the key points is that external exposure is often relatively easy to estimate, and the irradiated objects do not become radioactive (except for a case where the radiation is an intense neutron beam which causes activation of the object). It is possible for an object to be contaminated on the outer surfaces, assuming that no radioactivity enters the object it is still a case of external exposure and it is normally the case that decontamination is easy (wash the surface).

*Internal*

Internal exposure is when the radioactive material enters the organism, and the radioactive atoms become incorporated into the organism. Below are a series of examples of internal exposure.

- The exposure due to 40 K present within a normal person.
- The exposure to the ingestion of a soluble radioactive substance, such as 89 Sr in cow's milk.
- A person who is being treated for cancer by means of an open source radiotherapy method where a radioisotope is used as a drug. A review of this topic was published in 1999. Because the radioactive material becomes intimately mixed with the affected object it is often difficult to decontaminate the object or person in a case where internal exposure is occurring. While some very insoluble materials such as fission products within a uranium dioxide matrix might never be able to truly become part of an organism, it is normal to consider such particles in the lungs as a form of internal contamination which results in internal exposure. The reasoning is that the particles have entered via an orifice and cannot be removed with ease from what the lay person (non-biologist) would regard as within the animal. It is important to note that, strictly speaking, the contents of the digestive tract and the air within the lungs are outside the body of a mammal.

### Nuclear Warfare and Bomb Tests

Nuclear warfare and bomb tests are more complex because a person can be irradiated by at least three processes. The first (the major cause of burns) is not caused by ionizing radiation.

- Thermal burns from Infrared heat radiation.
- Beta burns from shallow ionizing radiation (this would be from fallout particles; the largest particles in local fallout would be likely to have very high activities because they would be deposited so soon after detonation and it is likely that one such particle upon the skin would be able to cause a localized burn); however, these particles are very weakly penetrating and have a short range.
- Gamma burns from highly penetrating radiation. This would likely cause deep gamma penetration within the body, which would result in uniform whole body irradiation rather than only a surface burn. In cases of whole body gamma irradiation (circa 10 Gy) due to accidents involving medical product irradiators, some of the human

subjects have developed injuries to their skin between the time of irradiation and death.

The normal clothing that the woman was wearing would have been unable to attenuate the gamma radiation and it is likely that any such effect was evenly applied to her entire body. Beta burns would be likely all over the body due to contact with fallout, but thermal burns are often on one side of the body as heat radiation does not penetrate the human body. In addition, the pattern on her clothing has been burnt into the skin. This is because white fabric reflects more infrared light than dark fabric. As a result, the skin close to dark fabric is burned more than the skin covered by white clothing. There is also the risk of internal radiation poisoning by ingestion of fallout particles.

### *Nuclear Reactor Accidents*

Radiation poisoning was a major concern after the Chernobyl reactor accident. Thirty-one people died as an immediate result.

Of the 100 million curies (4 exabecquereles) of radioactive material, the short-life radioactive isotopes such as 131 I, Chernobyl released were initially the most dangerous. Due to their short half-life of 5 and 8 days they have now decayed, leaving the more long-life 137 Cs (with a half-life of 30.07 years) and 90 Sr (with a half-life of 28.78 years) as main dangers.

### *Other Accidents*

Improper handling of radioactive and nuclear materials leads to radiation release and radiation poisoning. The most serious of these, due to improper disposal of a medical device containing a radioactive source (teletherapy), occurred in Brazil in 1987.

### *Ingestion and Inhalation*

When radioactive compounds enter the human body, the effects are different from those resulting from exposure to an external radiation source. Especially in the case of alpha radiation, which normally does not penetrate the skin, the exposure can be much more damaging after ingestion or inhalation. The radiation exposure is normally expressed as a committed effective dose equivalent (CEDE).

### *Deliberate Poisoning*

On 23 November 2006, Alexander Litvinenko died due to suspected deliberate poisoning with polonium-210. His is the first case of confirmed death due to such a cause, although it is also known that there have been other cases of attempted assassination such as in the cases of KGB defector Nikolay Khokhlov and journalist Yuri Schkochikhin where radioactive thallium was used. In addition, an incident occurred in 1990, at Point Lepreu Nuclear Generaign Station where several employees acquired small doses of radiation due to the contamination of water in the office water cooler with tritium contaminated heavy water.

### *Prevention*

The best prevention for radiation sickness is to minimize the dose suffered by the human, or to reduce the dose rate.

### *Distance*

Increasing distance from the radiation source reduces the dose due to the inverse-square law for a point source. Distance can be increased by means as simple as handling a source with forceps rather than fingers.

### *Time*

The longer humans are subjected to radiation the larger the dose will be. The advice in the nuclear war manual entitled 'Nuclear War Survival Skills' published by Cresson Kearny in the US, was that if one needed to leave the shelter then this should be done as rapidly as possible to minimize exposure.

In peacetime, radiation workers are taught to work as quickly as possible when performing a task which exposes them to irradiation. For instance, the recovery of a lost radiography source should be done as quickly as possible.

### *Shielding*

By placing a layer of a material which will absorb the radiation between the source and the human, the dose and dose rate can be reduced. For instance, in the event of a nuclear war, it would be a good idea to shelter within a building with thick stone walls. During the height of the cold war, fallout shelters were identified in many urban areas. It is interesting to note that, under some conditions, shielding can increase the dose rate. For instance, if the electrons from a high energy beta source (such as $^{32}P$) strike a lead surface, X-ray photons will be generated (radiation produced in this way is known as bremsstahlung). It is best for this reason to cover any high Z materials (such as lead or tungsten) with a low Z material such as aluminium, wood, plastic. This effect can be significant if a person wearing lead-containing gloves picks up a strong beta source. Also, gamma photons can induce the emission of electrons from very dense materials by the photoelectric effect; again, by covering the high Z material with a low Z material, this potential additional source of exposure to humans can be avoided. Furthermore, gamma rays can scatter off a dense object; this enables gamma rays to 'go around corners' to a small degree. Hence, to obtain a very high protection factor, the path in/out of the shielded enclosure should have several 90 degree turns rather than just one.

### *Reduction of Incorporation into the Human Body*

Potassium iodide (KI), administered orally immediately after exposure, may be used to protect the thyroid from ingested radioactive iodine in the event of an accident or terrorist attack at a nuclear power plant, or the detonation of a nuclear explosive. KI would not be effective against a dirty bomb unless the bomb happened to contain radioactive iodine, and even then it would only help to prevent thyroid cancer.

### *Fractionation of Dose*

While Devair Alves Ferreira received a large dose during the Goiania accident of 7.0 Gy, he lived while his wife received a dose of 5.7 Gy and died. The most likely explanation is that his dose was fractionated into many smaller doses which were absorbed over a length of time, while his wife stayed in the house more and was subjected to continuous irradiation without a break, giving her body less time to repair some of the damage done by the radiation. In the same way, some of the people who worked in the basement of the wrecked Chernobyl plant received doses of 10 Gy, but in small fractions, so the acute effects were avoided.

It has been found in radiation biology experiments that if a group of cells are irradiated, then as the dose increases, the number of cells which survive decreases. It has also been found that if a population of cells is given a dose before being set aside (without being irradiated) for a length of time before being irradiated again, then the radiation causes less cell death. The human body contains many types of cells and the human can be killed by the loss of a single type of cells in a vital organ. For many short-term radiation deaths (3 days to 30 days), the loss of cells forming blood cells (bone marrow) and the cells in the digestive system (microvilli which form part of the wall of the intestine are constantly being regenerated in a healthy human) causes death.

### *Treatment*

Treatment reversing the effects of irradiation is currently not possible. Anaesthetics and antiemetics are administered to counter the symptoms of exposure, as well as antibiotics for countering secondary infections due to the resulting immune system deficiency.

There are also a number of substances used to mitigate the prolonged effects of radiation poisoning, by eliminating the remaining radioactive materials, post exposure.

### *Whole Body vs Part of Body Exposure*

In the case of a person who has had only part of their body irradiated then the treatment is easier, as the human body can tolerate very large exposures to the non-vital parts such as hands and feet, without having a global effect on the entire body. For instance, if the hands get a 100 Gy dose which results in the body receiving a dose (averaged over the entire body of 5 Gy) then the hands may be lost but radiation poisoning would not occur. The resulting injury would be described as localized radiation burn.

As described below, one of the primary dangers of whole-body exposure is immunodeficiency due to the destruction of bone marrow and consequent shortage of white blood cells. It is treated by maintaining a sterile environment, bone marrow transplants and blood transfusions.

Chelation therapy can be useful to an extent if radiation poisoning is caused by the presence of heavy fissionable materials (e.g. radium or plutonium) in the bloodstream.

### *Experimental Treatments Designed to Mitigate the Effect on Bone Marrow*

Neummune, an androstenediol was introduced as a radiation countermeasure by the US Armed Forces Radiobiology Research Institute, and was under joint development with Hollis Eden Pharmaceuticals until March 2007. Neumune is in Investigational New Drug (IND) status and Phase I trials have been performed.

Some work has been published in which Cordyceps sinensis, a Chinese Herbal Medicine has been used to protect the bone marrow and digestive systems of mice from whole body irradiation.

## Cutaneous Radiation Syndrome

The concept of cutaneous radiation syndrome (CRS) was introduced in recent years to describe the complex pathological syndrome that results from acute radiation exposure to the skin.

Acute radiation syndrome (ARS) usually will be accompanied by some skin damage. It is also possible to receive a damaging dose to the skin without symptoms of ARS, especially with acute exposures to beta radiation or X-rays. Sometimes, this occurs when radioactive materials contaminate skin or clothes.

When the bascal cell layer of the skin is damaged by radiation, inflammation, erythema and dry or moist desquamation can occur. Also, hair follicles may be damaged, causing hair loss. Within a few hours after irradiation, a transient and inconsistent erythema (associated with itching) can occur. Then, a latent phase may occur and last from a few days up to several weeks, when intense reddening, blistering and ulceration of the irradiated site are visible. In most cases, healing occurs by regenerative means; however, very large skin doses can cause permanent hair loss, damaged sebaceous and sweat glands, atrophy, fibrosis, decreased or increased skin pigmentation, and ulceration or necrosis of the exposed tissue.

### *History*

What may be the earliest confirmed cases of acute radiation poisoning occurred in 1879 in Barry County, Missouri, USA, where three men were fatally poisoned and a fourth permanently injured under mysterious circumstances. After chasing an animal they were hunting to the mouth of a cave, they discovered what the cave appeared to be several large veins of silver. They returned the next day to begin prospecting, but fled when they began to fall ill; by the time they had left, one of them was so ill that he was paralysed and had to be carried to aid. In 1912, after the discovery of radium was announced, a local entrepreneur who had recalled the story investigated the cave to find that the metal was in fact radium, the first isolated veins of the metal ever found (previously, radium was only known from samples extracted from uranium-bearing pitchblende ore). The mine would be the first in the world to be excavated specifically for radium.

Note that the above story is unbelievable, as radium has the half-life of 1,600 years and cannot form 'veins' in a cave. Two references point to the same article, which looks like an obvious fraud.

Although radiation was discovered in late 19th century, the dangers of radioactivity and of radiation were not immediately recognized. Acute effects of radiation were first observed in the use of X-rays when the Serbo-Croatian-American electric engineer Nikola Tesla intentionally subjected his fingers to X-rays in 1896. He published his observations concerning the burns that developed, though he attributed them to ozone rather than to X-rays. His injuries healed later.

The genetic effects of radiation, including the effects on cancer risk, were recognized much later. In 1927, Hermann Joseph Muller published research showing genetic effects, and in 1946 was awarded the Nobel Prize for his findings.

Before the biological effects of radiation were known, many physicians and corporations had begun marketing radioactive substances as patent medicine and radioactive quackery. Examples were radium enema treatments, and radium-containing waters to be drunk as tonics. Marie Curie spoke out against this sort of treatment, warning that the effects of radiation on the human body were not well understood. (Curie later died from aplastic anaemia assumed due to her work with radium, but later examination of her bones showed that she had been a careful laboratory worker and had a low burden of radium. A more likely cause was her exposure to unshielded X-ray tubes while a volunteer medical worker in WWI.) Eben Byers, a famous American socialite, died in 1932 after consuming large quantities of radium over several years; his death drew public attention to dangers of radiation. By the 1930s, after a number of cases of bone necrosis and death in enthusiasts, radium-containing medical products had nearly vanished from the market.

Nevertheless, dangers of radiation were not fully appreciated by scientists until later. In 1945 and 1946, two US scientists died from acute radiation exposure in separate criticality accidents. In both cases, victims were working with large quantities of fissile materials without any shielding or protection.

Atomic bombings of Hiroshima and Nagasaki resulted in a large number of incidents of radiation poisoning, allowing for greater insight into its symptoms and dangers.

# 11

# Health Professionals and Health Care Organizations

The social importance of the medical function and the limited number of people with the training to perform as physicians are not the only criteria explaining their professional dominance. A particularly important factor is the organization of the medical profession. Many physicians and surgeons work long, irregular hours; more than one-third of full-time physicians worked 60 hours or more a week. Acceptance to medical school is highly competitive. Formal education and training requirements are among the most demanding of any occupation, but earnings are among the highest. Job opportunities should be very good, particularly in rural and low-income areas.

Physician, medical practitioner or medical doctor practices medicine, is concerned with maintaining or restoring human health through the study, diagnosis, and treatment of disease and injury. This is accomplished through a detailed knowledge of anatomy, physiology, diseases and treatment – the science of medicine and its applied practice – the art or craft of medicine. Physicians and surgeons diagnose illnesses and prescribe and administer treatment for people suffering from injury or disease. Physicians examine patients, obtain medical histories order, perform and interpret diagnostic tests. They counsel patients on diet, hygiene and preventive health care.

## Professional Qualities of Physician

The word 'physician' (*physis*) and its derived adjective *physikos*, meaning 'nature' and 'natural'. From this, amongst other derivatives came the Vulgar Latin *physicus*, this meant a medical practitioner. After the Norman Conquest, the word entered Middle English via Old French *fisicien*, as early as 1100. Originally, physician meant a practitioner of physic (pronounced with a hard C). This archaic noun had entered Middle English by 1300 (via Old French *fisique*). Physic meant the art or science of treatment with drugs or medications (as opposed to surgery), and was later used both as a verb and also to describe the medications.

In English, there have been many synonyms for physician, both old and new, with some semantic variation. The noun phrase 'medical practitioner' is perhaps the most widely understood and neutral synonym. Medical practitioner is lengthy but inclusive: it covers both medical specialists and general practitioners (family physician, family practitioner), and historically would include physicians (in the narrow sense), surgeons or apothecaries. In England, apothecaries historically included those who now would be called general practitioners and pharmacists. The term doctor (medical doctor) is older and shorter can be confused with holders of other academic doctorates.

Doctor means teacher in Latin and is an agentive noun derived from the verb *docere* (teach). In French, *medecin* (doctor, physician) is a contraction of *docteur médecin*, a direct equivalent of doctor of medicine.

### *Nature of Work*

There are two types of physicians: MD: Doctor of Medicine and DO: Doctor of Osteopathic Medicine. MDs also is known as allopathic physicians. While both MDs and DOs may use all accepted methods of treatment, including drugs and surgery, DOs place special emphasis on the body's musculoskeletal system, preventive medicine and holistic patient care. DOs are most likely to be primary care specialists although they can be found in all specialities. About half of DOs practise general or family medicine, general internal medicine, or general pediatrics.

Physicians work in one or more of several specialties, including, but not limited to, anaesthesiology, family and general medicine, general internal medicine, general pediatrics, obstetrics and gynaecology, psychiatry, and surgery

Anaesthesiologists focus on the care of surgical patients and pain relief. Like other physicians, they evaluate and treat patients and direct the efforts of their staffs. Through continual monitoring and assessment, these critical care specialists are responsible for maintenance of the patient's vital life functions – heart rate, body temperature, blood pressure, breathing – during surgery. They also work outside of the operating room, providing pain relief in the intensive care unit, during labour and delivery, and for those who suffer from chronic pain. Anaesthesiologists confer with other physicians and surgeons about appropriate treatments and procedures before, during, and after operations.

Family and general practitioners often provide the first point of contact for people seeking health care, by acting as the traditional family doctor. They assess and treat a wide range of conditions, from sinus and respiratory infections to broken bones. Family and general practitioners typically have a base of regular, long-term patients. These doctors refer patients with more serious conditions to specialists or other health care facilities for more intensive care.

General internists diagnose and provide non-surgical treatment for a wide range of problems that affect internal organ systems, such as the stomach, kidneys, liver and digestive tract. Internists use a variety of diagnostic techniques to treat patients through medication or hospitalization. Like general practitioners, general internists commonly act as primary care specialists. They treat patients referred from other specialists, and, in turn they refer patients to other specialists when more complex care is required.

General pediatricians care for the health of infants, children, teenagers and young adults. They specialize in the diagnosis and treatment of a variety of ailments specific to young people and track patients' growth to adulthood. Like most physicians, pediatricians work with different health care workers, such as nurses and other physicians, to assess and treat children with various ailments. Most of the work of pediatricians involves treating day-to-day illnesses, minor injuries, infectious diseases and immunizations – that are common to children, much as a general practitioner treats adults. Some pediatricians specialize in pediatric surgery or serious medical conditions, such as autoimmune disorders or serious chronic ailments.

Obstetricians and gynecologists (OB/GYNs) specialize in women's health. They are responsible for women's general medical care, and they also provide care related to pregnancy and the reproductive system. Like general practitioners, OB/GYNs attempt to prevent, diagnose and treat general health problems, but they focus on ailments specific to the female anatomy, such as cancers of the breast or cervix, urinary tract and pelvic disorders, and hormonal disorders. OB/GYNs also specialize in childbirth, treating and counselling women throughout their pregnancy, from giving prenatal diagnoses to assisting with delivery and providing postpartum care.

Psychiatrists are the primary caregivers in the area of mental health. They assess and treat mental illnesses through a combination of psychotherapy, psychoanalysis, hospitalization, and medication. Psychotherapy involves regular discussions with patients about their problems; the psychiatrist helps them find solutions through changes in their behavioural patterns, the exploration of their past experiences, or group and family therapy sessions. Psychoanalysis involves long-term psychotherapy and counselling for patients. In many cases, medications are administered to correct chemical imbalances that cause emotional problems. Psychiatrists may also administer electroconvulsive therapy to those of their patients who do not respond to, or who cannot take medications.

Surgeons specialize in the treatment of injury, disease and deformity through operations. Using a variety of instruments, and with patients under anaesthesia, a surgeon corrects physical deformities, repairs bone and tissue after injuries, or performs preventive surgeries on patients with debilitating diseases or disorders. Although a large number perform general surgery, many surgeons choose to specialize in a specific area. One of the most prevalent specialties is orthopaedic surgery: the treatment of the musculoskeletal system. Others include neurological surgery (treatment of the brain and nervous system), cardiovascular surgery, otolaryngology (treatment of the ear, nose, and throat), and plastic or reconstructive surgery. Like other physicians, surgeons also examine patients, perform and interpret diagnostic tests, and counsel patients on preventive health care.

Other physicians and surgeons work in a number of other medical and surgical specialists, including allergists, cardiologists, dermatologists, emergency physicians, gastroenterologists, ophthalmologists, pathologists and radiologists.

### *Work Environment*

Many physicians – primarily general and family practitioners, general internists, pediatricians, OB/GYNs, and psychiatrists – work in small private offices or clinics, often assisted by a small staff of nurses and other administrative personnel. Increasingly, physicians are practising in groups or health care organizations that provide backup coverage and allow for more time off. Physicians in a group practice or health care organization often work as part of a team that coordinates care for a number of patients; they are less independent than the solo practitioners of the past. Surgeons and anaesthesiologists usually work in well-lighted, sterile environments while performing surgery and often stand for long periods. Most work in hospitals or in surgical outpatient centres.

Many physicians and surgeons work long, irregular hours. Over one-third of full-time physicians and surgeons worked 60 hours or more a week in 2006. Only 8 per cent of all physicians and surgeons worked part-time, compared with 15 per cent for all occupations. Physicians and surgeons must travel frequently between office and hospital to care for their patients. While on call, a physician will deal with many patients' concerns over the phone and make emergency visits to hospitals or nursing homes.

### *Education and Training*

Formal education and training requirements for physicians are among the most demanding of any occupation – four years of undergraduate school, four years of medical school, and three to eight years of internship and residency, depending on the specialty selected. A few medical schools offer combined undergraduate and medical school programmes that last six years rather than the customary eight years.

Premedical students must complete undergraduate work in physics, biology, mathematics, English, and inorganic and organic chemistry. Students also take courses in the humanities and the social sciences. Some students volunteer at local hospitals or clinics to gain practical experience in the health professions.

The minimum educational requirement for entry into medical school is three years of college; most applicants, however, have at least a bachelor's degree, and many have advanced degrees. There are 146 medical schools in the United States–126 teach allopathic medicine and award a Doctor of Medicine (MD) degree; twenty teach osteopathic medicine and award the Doctor of Osteopathic Medicine (DO) degree.

Acceptance to medical school is highly competitive. Applicants must submit transcripts, scores from the Medical College Admission Test, and letters of recommendation. Schools also consider an applicant's character, personality, leadership qualities and participation in extracurricular activities. Most schools require an interview with members of the admissions committee.

Students spend most of the first 2 years of medical school in laboratories and classrooms, taking courses such as anatomy, biochemistry, physiology, pharmacology, psychology, microbiology, pathology, medical ethics, and laws governing medicine. They also learn to take medical histories, examine patients, and diagnose illnesses. During their last 2 years, students work with patients under the supervision of experienced physicians in hospitals and clinics, learning acute, chronic, preventive and rehabilitative care. Through rotations in internal medicine, family practice, obstetrics and gynaecology, pediatrics, psychiatry and surgery, they gain experience in the diagnosis and treatment of illness.

### *Other Qualifications*

People who wish to become physicians must have a desire to serve patients, be self-motivated, and be able to survive the pressures and long hours of medical education and practice. Physicians also must have a good bedside manner, emotional stability and the ability to make decisions in emergencies. Prospective physicians must be willing to study throughout their career to keep up with medical advances

### *Social Role*

Physicians are traditionally considered to be members of a learned profession, because of the extensive training requirements, and also because of the occupation's special ethical and legal duties. Physicians are often members, or fellows of professional organizations such as the Royal College of Physicians in the United Kingdom.

The practice of medicine has ancient associations with religion and magic.

Physicians commonly enjoy high social status, often combined with expectations of a high and stable income and job security. However, medical practitioners often work long and inflexible hours, with shifts at unsociable times, and may earn less than other professionals whose education is of comparable length.

Some commentators have argued that physicians have duties to serve as role models for the general public in matters of health, for example, by not smoking cigarettes.

### *Education and Training*

Medical education and career pathways for doctors vary considerably across the world. In all developed countries, entry-level medical education programmes are tertiary-level courses, undertaken at a medical school medical school attached to a university. Depending on jurisdiction and university, entry may follow directly from secondary school or require prerequisite undergraduate education. The former commonly take five or six years to complete. Programmes that require previous undergraduate education (typically a three or four-year degree, often in Science) are usually four or five years in length. Hence, gaining a basic medical degree may typically take from five to eight years, depending on jurisdiction and university.

Following completion of entry-level training, newly graduated medical practitioners are often required to undertake a period of supervised practice before full registration is granted, typically one or two years. This may be referred to as 'internship' or 'conditional registration'. Some jurisdictions (like the United States) require residencies for practice.

Medical practitioners hold a medical degree specific to the university from which they graduated. This degree qualifies the medical practitioner to become licensed or registered under the laws of that particular country, and sometimes of several countries, subject to requirements for internship or conditional registration.

### *Specialists in Internal Medicine*

After graduation, medical practitioners often undertake further training in a particular field, to become a medical specialist. In North America, this is often referred to as residency training; in Commonwealth countries, such trainees are often called registrars.

This further training typically takes from three to six years, but can be longer depending on specialty and jurisdiction. Primary care is increasingly recognized as a specialty, and residency programmes in this field are becoming common. A medical practitioner who completes specialist training in internal medicine (or in one of its sub-specialties) is an internist or a physician in the older, narrower sense.

In some jurisdictions, specialty training is begun immediately following completion of entry-level training, or even before. In other jurisdictions, junior medical doctors must undertake generalist (unstreamed) training for one or more years before commencing specialization. Hence, depending on jurisdiction, a specialist physician (internist) often does not achieve recognition as a specialist until twelve or more years after commencing basic medical training – five to eight years at university to obtain a basic medical qualification, and up to another six years to become a specialist.

Most countries have some method of officially recognizing specialist qualifications in all branches of medicine, including internal medicine. Sometimes, this aims to promote public safety by restricting the use of hazardous treatments. Other reasons for regulating specialists may include standardization of recognition for hospital employment and restriction on which practitioners are entitled to receive higher insurance payments for specialist services.

### Professionalization of Physician

Professionalism has been described by the American Board of Internal Medicine (1989) as 'constituting those attitudes and behaviours that serve to maintain patient interest above physician self-interest.' The word profession is derived from *profess* which means 'to proclaim something publicly'. The act of 'profession' of commitment to an ideal to which the professional should conform is the essence of a profession. Physicians profess two things: to be competent to help the patients and to have the patient's best interests in mind. Such commitment invites trust from their patients. Physicians profess in two ways: the first is the public act of 'oath taking' during medical graduation ceremonies. This is truly the moment of transition – from being a student to becoming a professional. The oath, not the medical degree, professes the way the newly acquired competencies are to be employed. Without the oath, the doctor is just a skilled worker. The second way of professing is implicit in the doctor-patient encounters: Whenever a physician asks the patient, 'What can I do for you?' they commit themselves to having adequate technical expertise and to using that in the best interests of the patients. Such tacit commitment occurs every day between a physician and a patient. Otherwise, the patient would never willingly consult the physician.

In the early 20th century, professionalism included issues like maintaining technical expertise and self-regulation of medical practice. Formulated by Talcott Parsons in the 1920s, these tenets formed the foundation of professionalism. In the developed world, technical expertise improved with the Flexner's report of 1910 on Medical Education, but quality of education is still a matter of concern in developing countries. Self-regulation by the profession has always been its Achilles' heel: Most professional bodies do not effectively discipline their members; most do not publish records of their disciplinary actions, if any. Such shortcomings make it clear that effective self-regulation is nonexistent and needs to be created.

The demystification of the medical profession in the 1970s and 1980s, resulted in two great upheavals. First, medicine changed from an autonomous, publicly respected profession to one vilified in the public press. Doctors, once the 'perfect angels', had fallen from the pedestal of public adulation. Second, health managers appeared to be potent rivals for the authority that physicians thought they owned. Sociologist Paul Starr (1988) commenting on the growing privatization and monetarization of medicine, described medicine as a 'sovereign profession', that once had reigned supreme, but was now threatened by the 'coming of the corporation'. Today, medical professionalism is in peril as several factors have weakened it. Increasingly, physicians encounter perverse financial incentives as well as restrictions, fierce market competition, and the resultant erosion of patients' trust. Professionalism has virtually vanished in the battle between market competition of the 'health care industry' and ineffective government regulation of health care services

### *Perspectives of Professionalism*

Professionalism in medicine can be viewed from the perspective of professional virtues or that of professional obligations. Professional virtues are the desirable qualities and traits a physician ought to possess and professional obligations are what a responsible physician needs to understand and do.

### *Professional Virtues*

Medicine has always been considered a 'noble profession'. The image of a doctor has always suggested integrity, loyalty and compassion – key aspects of a physician's professional identity. The world over, communities have always acknowledged medicine's vital role in healing the sick and permitted unique powers and privileges to those who practised it. In turn, the societies expected medical professionals to altruistically serve the sick and suffering. Some of the virtues a physician needs to commit to possess are:

- Fidelity to trust – essential for establishing rapport and for healing to occur.
- Benevolence – action taken for patient's welfare and avoiding all avoidable harm.
- Intellectual honesty to accept when one does not know, having the humility to admit it and obtain assistance and specialist help.
- Courage to face the dangers of contagion, to possibilities of physical harm and political retribution, and deceptions of various

kinds; courage to be the patient's advocate in a commercialized health care setting.

- Compassion – empathize and feel something of the patient's plight in order to make scientific judgements that are morally defensible and suited to the life-world of a particular patient.
- Truthfulness – enables the patient to make informed choices, on treatment modalities.

These are virtues obligated by the dyadic nature of the medical encounter between a physician and an individual patient.

However, the social importance of the medical function and the limited number of persons with the training and talent to perform as physicians are not the only criteria explaining the professional dominance of the physician group. A particularly important factor is the organization of the medical profession itself. William Goode (1957, 1960) after eliminating such occupational traits as prestige, power and income has noted that two basis characteristics are sociologically relevant in explaining professionalism: prolonged training in a body of specialized abstract knowledge and on orientation toward providing a service.

Moreover, once a professional group becomes established, Goode indicates that it begins further to consolidate its power by formalizing social relationships that govern the interaction of the professionals with their clients, their colleagues and with official agencies outside the profession. Recognition on the part of both clients, outside agencies and the wider society of the profession's claim to competence as well as the profession's ability to control its own membership, is necessary if professional decisions are not to be reviewed by outside authorities. Once this situation occurs, Goode believes that additional features of the profession can be established. Goode described these features as follows:

- The profession determines its own standards of education and training.
- The student professional goes through a more stringent socialization experience than the learner in other occupations.
- Professional practice is often legally recognized by some form of licensure.
- Licensing and admission boards are manned by members of the profession.
- Most legislation concerned with the profession is shaped by that profession.

- The occupation gains income, power and prestige ranking, and can demand high caliber students.
- The practitioner is relatively free of lay evaluation and control.
- The norms of practice enforced by the profession are more stringent than legal controls.
- Members are more strongly identified and affiliated with the profession than are members of other occupations.
- The profession is more likely to be a terminal occupation. Members do not care to leave it, and a higher proportion asserts that if they had it to do over again, they would again choose that type of work.

What Goode has accomplished for our purposes, is the development of guidelines for analysing the development of the medical profession in American society. While physicians in the US have traditionally shared a basic service orientation, the second requirement that of lengthy training in a specialized and abstract body of knowledge, was initially lacking. Most American medical practitioners in the period before the American Revolution were ship's surgeons, apothecaries, or clergy who had obtained a familiarity with medical knowledge in Europe. Few practitioners had been educated in either a university setting or a medical school. Anyone who wanted to practise medicine could do so and could claim the title of 'doctor', which in Europe was reserved exclusively for persons educated at a university. The most distinguished early American physicians were those trained at the University of Edinburgh, Great Britain's foremost medical school in that era. From this small group of British trained physicians came the impetus for establishment of the first American medical school in 1765, at the College of Philadelphia. This medical school, which later becomes part of the University of Pennsylvania, was subsequently joined in the years prior to 1800 by the organization of other medical schools at King's College (Columbia), Harvard and Dartmouth.

After 1800, American medical schools virtually mushroomed, and an impressive body of scientific knowledge was formulated, both in Europe and the United States. Louis Pasteur's germ theory of disease, advanced during the mid-1800s provided the foundation for the discovery, classification and treatment of numerous health problems. Other significant medical improvements during the 1800s included Rene Laennec's (1816) invention of the stethoscope; the work of Crawford Long (1842), Robert Liston (1846) and William Morton (1846) on ether as an anaesthetic; Claude Bernard's (1849) discovery of glycogen and the development of a theory of hormonal secretion providing the basis for endocrinology; Rudolf Virchow's (1858) investigation of cellular pathology; Joseph Lister's (1866) use of antiseptic procedures in surgery; Robert Koch's work in bacteriology leading to the discovery of the bacillus for anthrax (1876), tuberculosis (1882), and cholera (1883); Roentgens's (1895) development of the X-ray; and Ronald Ross (1895) research on the cause of malaria. Thus, by the beginning of the twentieth century, American medical doctors were clearly able to claim the two core characteristics of a profession as outlined by Goode – a service orientation and a body of specialized knowledge.

### *Doctor-Nurse Relationship*

It might be presumed from the literature examined thus for that nurses have generally been powerless and dependent practitioners. Some studies clearly suggest that nurses perceive themselves as pawns in most power struggles that they have perhaps internalized the attitudes of subordination projected by physicians and hospital administrators. The attitudes of all participants are no doubt reinforced by the stereotypical roles of male dominance and female passivity. Mauksch (1972) has suggested, for example, that physician-nurse interaction 'might be the last vestigial remains of the nineteenth century relationship between the sexes'.

Sex roles, however, are not the only social psychological factors affecting the physician-nurse relationship. As Barbara Bates (1970) has noted, the full development of the nursing role has been limited both by pressures from without (physicians) and by timidity from within. In her review of the literature, Bates observed that few nurses have openly rebelled against physicians' authoritarianism and most have accepted a position of deference toward the physician. This attitude is also prevalent in nursing traditions where obedience to the physician has been emphasized (Straus, 1966; Bates, 1970; Mauksch, 1972). Additionally, significant in this regard is that physicians are often older than the nurses they work with, come from a higher socio-economic background, are the socially recognized 'experts' on medicine, and have been accorded greater rewards and higher prestige by the general public (Bates, 1970; Fesidson, 1970). Nor have medical schools provided experiences for medical students concerning the potential contribution of nurses (Becker et al., 1961).

The relationship between doctor and nurse is to some extent affected by what the patients think of them. Radcliffe (2000) argued that the power within it is mediated by the patient: 'If in doubt ask the patient who is in control. The public may love its angels but it holds its medics in awe'. This reflects the traditional, popular view of doctor's and nurse's roles. However, patients' expectations of what nurses and doctors do or do not do, are changing very quickly. Increasing publicity of medical and nursing fallibility and use of the internet has removed some of the magical aura and gloss from these professions (Stein et al., 1990).

Patients and their families are also major players in the current culture of litigation, and the consequent emphasis on risk management can induce defensive practices on the part of both doctors and nurses.

### *Role of Doctor and Nurse in Decision-making*

Traditional relationships have been slow to change in the in-patient environment. Institutional and professional norms still defer to medical decision-making, the nurses' code of conduct and management lines of accountability. The in-patient setting highlights an essential aspect of the doctor-nurse relationship: its mutual interdependence. Neither can function independently of the other. If the psychiatrist is the responsible medical officer and a patient is on section under the Mental Health Act, that psychiatrist is dependent on the nurses for the containment and safe care of the patient while in hospital care. Nurses rely on aspects of the doctor's authority and medico-legal responsibility to support them and help contain the situation.

Nevertheless, doctors in psychiatry still hold essential powers and responsibilities that have an impact on this interdependence: for example, doctors are the ones who decide, either formally or informally, whether a patient is admitted and discharged. Under Section 12 of the Mental Health Act 1983, doctors have specific responsibilities that are not shared with other professional groups.

Daily decisions such as agreeing to a patient's leave or the need for close observation are rarely delegated to nurses, even though in these areas doctors may have no more knowledge than their nursing colleagues. If anything, they are probably less able to make appropriate judgments because of their more distant contact with in-patients, and yet, deference is paid to their 'expertise'.

Current pilot studies delegating some of these responsibilities to nurses have shown no major difficulties and have, in fact, reduced the need for expensive close nursing observations and reliance on agency staff (T. Reynolds and L. Dimery, personal communication, 2003).

The closer relationship with community mental health centres has produced some shifts in the balance of power. Community staff, whether associated with community mental health teams, assertive outreach or home treatment teams, now have more say in admission and discharge arrangements, altering what was once the exclusive province of doctors.

Although the decision to admit rests finally with doctors, it is helpful to make explicit that different staff will be able to contribute different knowledge to the decision-making process.

Senior doctors appointed to cover a catchment area are likely to be more familiar with past events in a patient's life than most other members of the team, simply by virtue of having worked in that catchment area for longer. They, therefore, use experience of previous psychiatric interventions to guide their thinking when a new episode occurs. There is some suggestion that nursing turnover, especially in metropolitan districts, is increasing, making it even more likely that doctors will 'hold the history' of patients. Conversely, in the 'here and now' of an in-patient stay, nurses will be much more in touch with a patient's current state and preoccupations. Depending on the attitudes of those involved, the nurses' knowledge can contribute to clinical care or can become a source of contention in the battle about who knows the patient best and whose decision should prevail.

Traditionally, doctors have been seen as the repositories of clinical knowledge and have been charged with keeping abreast of recent advances and imparting this knowledge not only to their own apprentices, but also to nurses within the team. University education as opposed to hospital experience accounts for the public view that doctors 'are educated whilst nurses are trained' (Warelow, 1996). Purported knowledge, therefore, is a source of the differential power that underpins the doctor-nurse relationship. To some extent this differential has been reduced by increasing university training for nurses, as envisioned in the Department of Health's Project 2000 (United Kingdom Central Council for Nursing, Midwifery and Health Visiting, 1986). However, some critics have observed a gap between theory and practice and the creation of a training deficit at graduation, as it does not meet the practical nature of service demand (Department of Health, 1997). Shared learning (with doctors and other professional groups) is beginning to happen in areas such as Mental Health Act legislation, Health of the Nation Outcome Scales (HoNOS) and ethical issues.

### *Conflict between Nurse and Doctor*

When conflict arises between nurses and doctors on communication and decision-making, the nurses' objections are often buttressed by 'You are not here as much as we are' a familiar clinical situation. The 'parental' couple of doctor and nurse are in a conflict generated (or exacerbated) by the pathology of the patient, who has a propensity to idealize paternal figures and vilify maternal ones. Such situations tend to reinforce stereotypical roles and require successful clinical management with some insight into psychodynamic interaction.

### *Family Roles, Patients' Projections and Gender Issues*

The doctor-nurse pairing, not surprisingly, also becomes a potent target for patient projection. Father/mother fantasies are often mentioned, particularly by patients in vulnerable and regressive states. They expect the same total, unconditional care that they expected from their real parents. The relationship that doctors and nurses have with patients is also of an intimate nature, not only because details of the patients' lives are shared, but also because physical contact is often required during treatment and care, and the patients' illnesses might bring to the fore discussion of life and death. This is a domain that is not often shared with others in the team. In this setting the 'specialness' is regularly confirmed.

These projections are affected to some extent by gender. In contrast to general nursing, psychiatric nursing was traditionally a male domain, as working in asylums with potentially violent patients emphasized the need for physical containment. Although this is not the case today, in the UK male nurses are still relatively overrepresented in psychiatry (40%) compared with general nursing (1%) (Royal College of Nursing, 2003). For obvious reasons, male nurses are still identified as those who will have a central role in control and restraint procedures when patients are agitated and at risk to themselves or others. In fact, anxiety can become palpable when there are not enough male nurses on a particular shift, especially when the unit is disturbed. These different roles and assignations have an impact on relationships between nurses as well as with doctors and patients.

Traditional sociological studies of the doctor-nurse relationship describe its patriarchal nature (Dingwall and McIntosh, 1978), understood in terms of sexual stereotypes, with gender assignations of nurturance and passivity to the female role, and decisiveness and competitiveness to the male role (Savage, 1987). Drawing parallels with family roles, doctors assumed the position of the head of the family, deciding where and how the important work had to be done, while nurses (their 'wives') looked after the physical and emotional needs of those dependent on them, whether they be patients, junior nurses or inexperienced doctors (Oakley, 1984; Willis and Parish, 1997; Gaze, 2001). Although this model still carries some validity, modern changes in nurses' roles, particularly the introduction of clinical nurse specialists, nurse consultants and modern matrons, indicate major shifts in influential positions which are now fairly well established (Department of Health, 2003a, 2003b; NHS Modernisation Board, 2003). The replacement of the ward sister with the ward manager in the 1980s has had a profound impact, some say by 'selling nursing to management rather than being led by clinical imperatives' (V. Franks, personal communication, 2004). Changes in the status of doctors have followed public airings of their fallibility, requirements to make them accountable for their actions and an increase in the general population's medical knowledge owing to widespread use of the internet. Despite such changes, which reflect parallel shifts in all occupations, trust in the medical profession persists. Militant nurses are advocating a radical move from the status quo in terms of power relationships, and have raised awareness of their potential as agents for change in the medico-political arena.

While all of this may seem silly to persons unfamiliar with the physician-nurse relationship, it nonetheless represents a significant social mechanism by which the physician is able to utilize the nurse as a consultant and the nurse is able to gain self-esteem and professional satisfaction from her work. A successful game creates a doctor-nurse alliance and allows the doctor to have a good 'score' by gaining the respect and admiration of the nursing staff; the nurse, in turn scores by being identified by the physician as 'a damn good nurse'. If the doctor fails to play the game well, pleasant working relationship with the nurses may become difficult and the doctor may have problems of trivial, yet annoying nature when it comes to getting his work done. Nurses who do not play the game well are either terminated from employment if they also lack intelligence, or are tolerated but not 'loved' if they are bright. Nurses who do not play the game at all, according to Stein, are defined as dull and are relegated to the background in the social lift of the hospital.

### *Doctor-Patient Relationship*

There is a common belief among the public that a medical practitioner is at the beck and call of anyone who chooses to send for him, but it must be remembered that there is no law to compel a medical practitioner to attend a patient except in a case where he has previously bound himself by contractual obligations or has already undertaken the treatment. A contractual doctor-patient relationship is established when the patient makes a request for medical examination, diagnosis, opinion, advice or treatment and the doctor undertakes to provide these. There are situations when a request by the patient is not necessary. Treatment of an infant, where the parents make the request, or those of a comatose victim of an accident are examples. The sanctity of such a relationship safeguards the interest of the patient, the doctor assuming all responsibility for providing health care.

The patient has every right to terminate a relationship with his doctor at any time and seek the help of another. A reciprocal right rests with the doctor. The formal relationship may be brought to an end when the patient gives notice of intent to terminate it or when the doctor withdraws his undertaking.

A doctor can, at any time, request the help of a colleague or specialist in the best interests of his patient. Such a request must be specific and made in writing, all relevant medical details being provided to the other doctor. In an emergency, the request may be made and details provided orally on the understanding that as soon as time permits, a written note will follow. This step precludes any the consultant misunderstanding of intention or fact by the consultant. The consultant, in turn, is duty-bound to return the patient to the referring doctor with a note bearing details of facts elicited, diagnosis made and treatment advised.

Talcott Parsons's (1951) concept of the sick role provided some basic guidelines for understanding doctor-patient interaction. Parsons explains that the relationship between a physician and his or her patient is one that is oriented toward the doctor helping the patient to deal effectively with a health problem. The physician has the dominant role since he or she is the one invested with medical knowledge and expertise, while the patient holds a subordinate position oriented toward accepting, rejecting or negotiating the recommendations for treatment being offered. In the case of a medical emergency, however, the options of rejection or negotiation on the part of the patient may be quickly discarded as the patient's medical needs require prompt and decisive action from the doctor.

Parsons's concept of the sick role details the obligation of patients and physicians toward each other. Patients cooperate with doctors and doctors attempt to return patients to as normal a level of functioning as possible; when people visit doctors for treatment and medical advice, doctors usually take some type of action to satisfy the patient's expectations. Eliot Freidson (1970a) suggests that physicians tend to have a bias in favour of finding illness in their patients. He cites the medical decision rule as the guiding principle behind everyday medical practice. The medical decision rule, described by Thomas Scheff (1966) is the notion that since the work of the physician is for the good of the patient, physicians tend to impute illness to their patients rather than to deny it and risk overlooking or missing it. Although this approach may promote tendencies to prescribe drugs and order laboratory tests and X-rays, such consequences should not be surprising. Patients desire and demand services, and physicians are trained to meet these demands. As Freidson (1970) points out: 'While the physician's job is to make decisions, including the decisions not to do anything, the fact seems to be that the everyday practitioner feels impelled to do something when (patients) are in distress'.

### *Models of Interaction*

Since Parsons formulated his concept of the sick role, two additional perspectives on physician-patient interaction has added to our understanding of the experience. These are the views of Szasz and Hollender and Hayes-Bautista. Thomas Szasz and Mark Hollender (1956), both physicians, take the positions that the seriousness of the patient's symptoms is the determining factor in doctor-patient interaction. Depending on the severity of symptoms, Szasz and Hollender argue that physician-patient interaction falls into one of three possible models:

- Activity-passivity model
- Guidance-cooperation model
- Mutual participation model

*Activity-passivity model:* This model applies when the patient is seriously ill or being treated on an emergency basis in a state of relative helplessness due to severe injury or lack of consciousness. Typically, the situation is desperate as the physician works in a state of high activity to stabilize the patient's condition. Decision-making and power in the relationship are all on the side of the doctor, as the patient is passive and contributes little or nothing to the interaction.

*Guidance-cooperation model:* This model arises most often when the patient has an acute, often infectious illness, like the flue or measles.

The patient knows what is going on and can cooperate with the physician by following his or her guidance in the manner, but the physician makes the decisions.

*Mutual participation model:* This model applies to the management of chronic illness in which the patient works with the doctor as a full participant in controlling the disease. Often the patient modifies his or her lifestyle by making adjustments in diet or giving up cigarettes and that is responsible.

### Misunderstandings in Communication

The interaction that takes place between doctor and patient is an exercise in communication. Medical treatment usually begins with a dialogue. As is the case in any face-to-face situation, the effectiveness of doctor-patient interaction depends upon the ability of the participants to understand each other. However, a major barrier to effective communication lies in the differences between physicians and their patients with respect to status, education, professional training and authority. Several sources report that a failure to explain a patients' condition to the patient in terms easily understood is a serious problem in medical encounters (Allman, Yoels and Clair, 1993; Coe, 1978; Davis, 1972). Physicians, in turn, state that an inability to understand or the potentially negative effect of threatening information are the two most common reasons for not communicating fully with their patients. (Davis, 1972).

Yet, some doctors are very effective communicators and as Eric Cassell (1985) explains, information can be an important therapeutic tool in medical situations if it meets three tests: (1) reduces uncertainty (2) provides a basis for action, and (3) strengthens the physician-patient relationship.

### Patient Compliance

Another important aspect of physician-patient interaction is patient compliance with medical regimens (Svarstad, 1986). Physicians prescribe medications, diets and the like and expect patients to follow them faithfully. Many, perhaps most patients comply with a physician's instructions, but other patients do not; in fact, some patients may pay little attention to a doctor's guidance, and this is especially the case when they begin to feel better or when symptoms are not obvious.

Compliance requires comprehension by the patient, and communication is the key for avoiding noncompliance. The motivation to be healthy, a perceived vulnerability to an illness, the potential for negative consequences, effectiveness of the treatment, sense of personal control and effective communications are the strongest influences on compliance.

### *Doctor-Patient Relations and Technology*

An important factor likely to have profound implications for the doctor-patient relationship in the future is new medical technology. The forthcoming development of computerized information highways connecting a patient's personal home computer to those of doctors, hospitals, drug companies, medical suppliers, health insurers and medical databases will allow patients to obtain health information directly from their own computer rather than visiting a physician. Electronic monitoring devices will allow the patient to keep track of his or her physical and mental state and report these to physicians or databases by computer. Physicians may be consulted via home computers, electronic mail or teleconferencing rather than in person. A computer can be used to diagnose the patient's ills and determine treatment. Prescription drugs may be ordered electronically and delivered to the patient.

Other measures like the use of robotics and computer guided imagery of a patient's body may increase efficiency and precision in surgery and reduce the need for extensive hospitalization. Doctors may have little direct involvement in certain surgeries as robots and terms of nurses handle most of the tasks. Also, gene therapy may anticipate an individual's susceptibility to various chronic diseases and eliminate many health problems in early stages. It may be the patient, however, who discovers the requirement for treatment through self-monitoring and computer assisted analysis of his or her medical history. This situation significantly changes the traditional doctor-patient relationship because patients, not doctors will cause health care to take place. Doctors will be responding to what patients themselves decide they need, rather than the other way around. Doctors and patients will still have contact, but much of that contact may be through computers. A new doctor-patient relationship is likely to emerge in which the patient's initiative, determines and controls much of the health services he or she consumes.

## Hospital as a Social Organization

A hospital is an institution for health care, providing patient treatment by specialized staff and equipment, and often but not always providing for longer-term patient stay.

Today, hospitals are usually funded by the state, health organizations (for profit or non-profit), health insurances or charities, including direct charitable donations. In history, however, they were often founded and funded by religious orders or charitable individuals and leaders. Similarly, modern-day hospitals are largely staffed by professional physicians, surgeons and nurses, whereas in history, this work was usually done by the founding religious orders or by volunteers.

During the middle ages the hospital could serve other functions, such as almshouse for the poor, hostel for pilgrims or hospital school. The name comes from Latin *hospes* (host), which is also the root for the English words hotel, hostel, and hospitality.

The development of the hospitals as institutions providing medical services for the general public proceeded in pace with the prevailing needs, beliefs, values and attitudes of the societies they served (Coe, 1978; Rosenberg, 1987). Historically, hospitals have passed through four distinct phases of development:

- As centres of religious practice
- As poor houses
- As death houses
- As centres of medical technology.

## Hospitals as Centres of Religious Practice

Although the Romans were the first to establish separate medical facilities that have been described as hospitals, the origin of the institution we know today as the hospital has usually been associated with the rise of Christianity. Christian theology emphasized that human beings were duty bound to provide assistance to the sick and needy; this belief was reinforced by the notion that spiritual salvation could be obtained by whoever provided such a service. Consequently, the Roman Catholic Church encouraged its clergy to found hospitals and to locate these hospitals near churches as an integral feature of Christian religious endeavour.

The medieval hospital, however, was not a hospital by any modern standard. True, these hospitals were community centres for the care of the lower-class sick yet the medical care, supervised and largely performed by clergy and nuns, consisted primarily of a rudimentary form of nursing. The primary functions of the medieval hospital were the exercise of religious practices and the extension of charity and welfare services to the poor, including both the able-bodied and the sick. These early hospitals, therefore, provided a wide spectrum of social tasks for the benefit of the lower classes, especially the provision of food, shelter, and sanctuary and prayer as well as nursing.

### Hospitals as Poor Houses

The secular control of hospitals marked a period of decline for the development of Europe's hospital system. Even though monks and nuns continued to work in hospitals, the removal of the centralized authority of the church left hospitals under many separate administrations, usually those of municipal governments. Without general regulations pertaining to hospital administration, individual hospitals were free to pursue any course of action they desired. This situation encouraged abuse, particularly in regard to neglect of facilities, misappropriations of funds, and the lowering of prevailing standards of patient care.

However, by the end of the sixteenth century, the economic and social conditions of the poor worsened to a considerable degree. Unemployment, higher prices and the loss of land created a serious problem of vagrancy throughout Europe. Many vagrants claimed to be sick or crippled, and they crowded whatever hospital facilities were available. In accordance with the new definitions of social welfare as a community rather than a church responsibility, measures were eventually taken by city and national authorities to provide public assistance. Many hospitals were reopened, but they soon acquired the characteristics of boarding houses because they offered food and shelter to the poor, regardless of whether they were sick or healthy. Those persons living in hospitals who could work were required to pay for their lodging. While hospitals received further financial support through public taxation, hospitals became little more than social 'warehouses', where invalids, the aged, orphans and the mentally defective could be sent and thus removed from the mainstream of society.

### Hospitals as Death Houses

Following the renaissance and the reformation, the outward character of hospitals appeared to change very little from that of public institutions whose purpose was to provide welfare services for the lower social classes on behalf of the communities in which they were located. Nonetheless, changes were taking place as physicians discovered that hospitals contained large numbers of sick and injured people whose health problems could be studied and upon whom the various evolving techniques of medical treatment could be practised.

Physicians had first begun to associate themselves with hospitals during the fourteenth century; initially they had little influence because they were not members of the hospital's staff and provided their services on a purely voluntary basis. By the seventeenth century, however, physicians acquired a virtual monopoly over the existing body of medical knowledge that placed them in the position of first advising and eventually directing all patient care within the hospitals. As physicians became increasingly influential, non-medical hospital tasks gradually disappeared; by the early nineteenth century, hospitals had clearly assumed their present-day role as institutions for medical care, for medical research and for the education of medical students.

Although medical treatment was recognized as the primary function of the hospital in the eighteenth century, the primitive level of that treatment produced few cures. Trained physicians were unable to achieve consistent results with their techniques and accordingly neither they nor hospitals were held in high esteem by the general population. Because so few patients survived treatment despite occasional heroic efforts, hospitals acquired images as places where the poor went to die.

According to Coe (1978), the high death rate in hospitals was also related to the appalling living conditions provided to the patients. Typically, hospitals were dirty, poorly ventilated and filled to capacity. Often more than one patient was placed in a single bed regardless of the patient's disorder, and treatment was usually carried out publicly in the ward itself. Surgery, which Coe points out was limited at that time mostly to amputations and childbirth, plus the purging of fevers with various potions, blood-letting to eliminate 'excess' blood, and the removal of the dead all occurred in the same general area where patients ate and slept. Nor did the attending physicians and surgeons practise even the most rudimentary standards of sanitation, moving from bed to bed and treating a great variety of diseases, including those that were infectious, without washing their hands or changing their clothes. Thus, it is not surprising that hospitals were regarded by most people as places where only the lower social classes went to die.

### Hospitals as Centres of Medical Technology

Since the end of the nineteenth century, a new image of hospitals evolved as institutions where patients of all social classes could generally expect to fund the highest quality medical care and could reasonably expect to be cured of their disorders. Three major factors were responsible for this change. First was the fact medicine had indeed become a science in terms of employing the scientific method to seek out accurate medical knowledge and to develop successful techniques that could be employed in a consistent manner. Of particular importance were increased knowledge about human physiology and the development of the science of bacteriology; also important was the perfection of ether as and anaesthetic, which allowed surgery to be performed in a relatively painless fashion. Since the new medical technology required extensive and often expensive facilities, these facilities were centralized in hospitals so that they could be available to most physicians. Hospitals eventually became places where physicians also referred their upper and middle class patients, since the most advanced medical technology was located there. While the poor generally remained in a charity status as hospital patients, a new type of patient came into being – the private patient who required private accommodations, usually had a private physician and who paid for hospital services.

A second important factor, concomitant with the development of medical technology was the discovery and use of antiseptic measures in the hospital to help curtail infection. The use of surgical masks, rubber gloves, and sterilized surgical instruments became common place. These procedures not only reduced the number of deaths among hospital patients but also reduced the amount of time required for patient's recovery.

Third, there was a significant improvement in the quality of hospital personnel. Especially important was the entry on the scene of the trained nurse and the laboratory technician, whose specialized skills were able to support the physician in his or her primary role of diagnostician and practitioner. As Charles Rosenberg (1987) points out in his historical analysis of the development of American hospital, no single change has transformed the day-to-day work in a hospital more than trained nurses. In the twentieth century, the hospital has become the major institutional resource available to society for coping with problems of health and illness.

# 12

# Structure and Functions of a Hospital

## Organization of the Hospital

Certainly not all hospitals are alike in their organization of service, but general hospital, as the most common single type of hospital in the United States, exhibit organizational features similar to most other types of hospital. As a social organization, the general hospital has been described as being formal, highly satisfied, quasi-bureaucratic, and quasi-authoritarian. General hospitals have also been described as 'multipurpose institution' in that they provide a variety of health-related functions for society such as (1) treating patients, (2) conducting medical research, (3) training health practitioners, (4) providing laboratories and other medical facilities to the community and (5) sponsoring health education and preventive medicine programmes for the general public. The primary goal of the hospital, however, is that of providing medical knowledge and technology and the hospital's available resources. The hospital thus qualifies as a formal organization in that it has developed to coordinate scarce resources to achieve stated goals in as efficient a manner as possible.

In order to accomplish its tasks and coordinate its various activities, the hospital relies upon a prescribed hierarchy of authority, which is operationalized through formal rules, regulations and administrative procedures. The key to hospital efficiency and overall effectiveness is coordination of the various departments and individuals. They represent a complex and highly specialized division of labour that is both interlocking and interdependent.

Consider what happens when a staff doctor prescribes medication for a patient. The doctor's order for medication is written in the patient medical records by a floor clerk, and the clerk, or a nurse's aide or orderly, takes the request to the pharmacy. When the medication is sent by the pharmacy, it is most likely administered by a nurse. A record is then forwarded to the accounting office so that the proper charges for the drug can be entered upon the patient's bill; another written order might be sent from the pharmacy to purchasing to reorder the medication and replace it for future use by another patient. So the rather routine activity of one particular member of the hospital staff (in this case doctor) initiates a chain of events that affects the work of several other hospital employees.

The overall supervision of the general hospital comes under the auspices of its governing body. In most nonfederal hospitals, that governing body is aboard of trustees. Whereas the medical director and the hospital administrator are linked to the governing body by a direct line of responsibility, they are only indirectly responsible to each other. What this type of arrangement indicates is that the authority system of the general hospitals operates on a dual level. This system is an outgrowth of the organizational conflict in the hospital between bureaucracy and professionalism.

The occupational group in the hospital most affected by its system of dual authority are the nurses and auxiliary nursing workers who perform health care tasks on the hospital's wards. Nurses are responsible to the physician for carrying out the physician's orders, but they also are responsible to the nursing supervisions and the upper echelons of the hospital's administration.

Some patients in a hospital come just for diagnosis and/or therapy and then leave ('out-patients'); while others are 'admitted' and stay overnight or for several weeks or months ('in-patients'). Hospitals are usually distinguished from other types of medical facilities by their ability to admit and care for in-patients.

### *General*

The best-known type of hospital is the general hospital, which is set up to deal with many kinds of disease and injury, and typically has an emergency department to deal with immediate threats to health and the capacity to dispatch emergency medical services. A general hospital is typically the major health care facility in its region, with large numbers of beds for intensive care and long-term care; and specialized facilities for surgery, plastic surgery, childbirth, bioassay laboratories, and so forth. Larger cities may have many different hospitals of varying sizes and facilities.

### *Specialized*

Types of specialized hospitals include trauma centres, rehabilitation hospitals, children's hospitals, seniors' (geriatric) hospitals, and hospitals for dealing with specific medical needs such as psychiatric problems, certain disease categories, and so forth.

A hospital may be a single building or a campus. (Many hospitals with pre-20th-century origins began as one building and evolved into campuses.) Some hospitals are affiliated with universities for medical research and the training of medical personnel. Worldwide, most hospitals are run on a non-profit basis by governments or charities.

### *Teaching*

A teaching hospital (or university hospital) combines assistance to patients with teaching to medical students and is often linked to a medical school.

### *Clinics*

A medical facility smaller than a hospital is generally called a clinic, and is often run by a government agency for health services or a private partnership of physicians (in nations where private practice is allowed). Clinics generally provide only out-patient services.

### *Departments*

Hospitals may have any of the following departments or units:

- Behavioural health services
- Burn unit
- Cancer centre
- Cardiology
- Coronary care unit
- Dentistry
  - — Oral and Maxillofacial Surgery
- Dermatoly
- Dispensary
- Emergency department
  - — Trauma Centre
- Gastroenterology
- Intensive Care Unit
- Internal Medicine

- — Endocrinology
- — Epidemiology
- — Immunology
- Laboratory services
- Neurology
- Nursing unit
- OB/GYN
  - — Neonatal Intensive Care Unit
- Orthopaedic Services
- Outpatient department
- Pathology
- Pediatrics
- Pharmacy
- Plastic Surgery
- Psychiatric ward
- Rehabilitation service
- Physical Therapy
- Post anaesthesia care unit
- Radiology
- Respiratory Therapy
- Surgery
- Urgent care
- Urology
- Non-medical departments include:
  - — Medical records department
  - — Release of information department

### Cost of Hospitalization

Any discussion of hospitals would be incomplete without considering the financial cost of hospitalization, which has risen more sharply in recent years than any other aspect of medical care. For purposes of comparison, John Knowles (1973) indicates that in 1925, the cost of one day's stay as a patient at the Massachusetts General Hospital in Boston was $3.00 and the bill was paid entirely by the patient. By 1977, however, the average one day cost of hospitalization had risen to nearly $225, with most of the expense paid by a third party such as a private health insurance company Blue Cross, Blue Shield or some other hospital medical plan – Medicare, Medicaid or a state welfare agency. Not only did costs increase significantly but the manner of payment has also changed, as about 90 per cent of all expenses for hospital services are now paid by third party sources. In some cases, third party coverage has led to increased hospital admission rates, since health needs which are met in the physicians office are often not covered by insurance. Hospitalization can, therefore, reduce the patient's direct cost of health care.

But this does not mean that patients escape paying hospital bills. Government expenditures are paid out of tax revenues, while private health insurance costs must also be covered, and private companies are set up to make a profit. In 1969, health insurance companies paid $ 14 billion in benefit payments in return for $ 17 billion they received in insurance premiums from policy holders. In 1974, health insurance companies paid nearly $ 28 billion out of approximately $ 50 billion in premiums.

About sixty-one cents of every dollar insurance claim goes for hospital bills, thirty-one cents for physician's services, three cents for dentists, three cents for drugs and drug sundries, and the remaining two cents for private duty nursing, eye care, nursing home care, visiting nurse service and other types of care.

What does the hospital do with its income? Knowles explains that hospital expenses are categorized as either routine or ancillary costs. Routine costs are those expenses of providing room and board, including the provision of several different diets of three meals a day served in bed; the cost of non-medical supplies and equipment; the salaries of all members of the hospitals' non-medical staff; and the salaries of medical technicians, nurses, auxiliary nursing workers, interns, and residents who are available to patients on a twenty-four hour basis, seven days a week. Ancillary expenses include the host of laboratories, the pharmacy and operating rooms, X-ray rooms, cast rooms and other specialized hospital facilities, plus the cost of all medical supplies. Even though patients do not get to see or even utilize all of the hospital's facilities, the cost of maintaining and operating these facilities for those patients, who do use them, continues regardless.

It has also been found that one of the most significant factors affecting costs is the structure of the decision-making process. Edward Morse and his associates (1974) argue that decentralization of decision-making tends to facilitate a hospital's adoption of modern medical technology. But while the application of new technology usually reduces the average length of stay and may increase the average occupancy rate, it has little direct impact upon the hospital's total expenses. Instead, Morse suggests that the more centralized the hospital's decision-making structure, the more efficient it will be in controlling expenses by selecting those organizational practices that facilitate goal achievement at the lowest cost. Inefficient hospital management has, needless to say, been a major factor in the rise in hospital costs.

Two other factors contributing to higher hospital expenses have been inflation and increased costs of hospital labour. Between 1967 and 1974, the overall cost of medical care in the United States rose by 50.5 per cent, which ranked third behind the rise in the cost of food (61.7%) and the increase in the cost of housing. The increase in the cost of all consumer items combined was 47.7 per cent. Moreover, inflation has not only affected the cost of medical equipment, supplies and new construction, but it has also served to intensify the demands of hospital employees for higher salaries to meet the rise in the cost of living. Labour constitutes about 70 per cent of a hospital's total expenses and increased labour costs are, therefore, a highly significant component of rising hospital expenses.

Herman Somers (1970) points out; it would be illusory to believe that health care costs can be prevented from rising. So long as the prices of goods and services in general continue to increase, the cost of health care and hospitalization may be expected to proceed apace. The principle issue is whether or not increase can be contained in such a way that hospital care is kept within a reasonable relationship to the rest of the economy and that the highest quality of care can be provided for all peoples for the amount of money spent for that care.

## Medical Social Service in a Hospital

Health care embraces all the goods and services designed to promote health, including preventive, curative and palliative interventions, whether directed to individuals or to populations. Health is multifactoral. The factors which influence health lie both within the individual and externally in the society in which he/she lives. It is a truism to say that, what man is and to what disease he may fall victim to depends on a combination of two sets of factors – his genetic factor and the environment factors to which he is exposed. These factors interact and the result of these interactions may be health of individuals and whole communities may be considered to be the result of many interaction.

A century ago, the individual practitioner was likely to be responsible for all aspects of the health care of the people in his community. Today, however, the requirements for providing health and medical care services have become so complex that a wide variety of individuals and organizations are now needed to perform and/or support these services. For example, one study of health-related organizations of a small rural country reported that not less than eighty-three separate agencies were involved in the provision of medical care, and this did not include fifty-four others concerned with preventive medicine.

Since adequate hospital facilities are among a community's most important resources, it is likely that the functions of the contemporary hospital are well known to nearly everyone. Nonetheless, it may be useful to restate them briefly here. A hospital is first and foremost a place in which members of the community can obtain services designed to restore them to good health. More recently, it has become a place for rehabilitation of the physically disabled and a setting in which especially older members of the community can obtain services to restore partially the use of enfeebled limbs or vital organs worn from age. The modern hospital is also a place of earning, a centre for the practical training of physicians and surgeons to be, as well as other practitioners. At the same time, advances in scientific knowledge of disease are often made in research conducted in the hospital setting. Yet the hospital is also a very large complex organization in the sociological sense of a recognizable hierarchy of statuses and roles, rights and obligations, attitudes, values and goals.

# 13

# Health Planning in India

## Health Policies Before 1970

Medical planning in India has a number of objectives. Among the three important objectives are: (a) keeping up with modern development in the field of allopathic and other medicines, (b) making medical care and medical education relevant to India's needs and (c) increasing the access of the masses to the modern and other medicines. The progress made in the health planning in all its aspects has been periodically reviewed by several committees appointed by the central government since Independence. The purpose of this chapter is to review, briefly, certain important aspects of health planning of the country on the basis of valuable guidelines suggested by various committees. The second section contains a series of alternative viewpoints for a health policy which is more relevant to the local conditions and has a wider access to the people. The last section contains the main conclusions drawn by this paper.

### *Reports of the Health Commission and Committees*

The process of health planning in India began with the work initiated by the well-known Bhore Committee in 1946. The Bhore Committee reviewed the state of health care in the mid-1940s and suggested valuable guidelines for its future development. In the following years, several other committees were set up by the central government to review the implementation of various aspects of health policy in the country. The committees that deserve mention are: Mudaliar Committee (1961), Chadah Committee (1963), Mukherjee Committee (1965), Jungalwala Committee (1967), Jain Committee (1968), Kartar Singh Committee (1973) and Shrivastava Committee (1975). Besides these committees, some studies on health policy were conducted by autonomous institutions like the Indian Council of Social Science Research (ICSSR) and the Indian Council of Medical Research (ICMR). The important recommendations by these various committees can be thematically grouped under the following: (a) to improving the existing structure of health care delivery system, (b) to improving the supporting services for a proper and quick delivery of Medicare facilities and (c) to improving the quality of the delivery system thereby improving the health standard of the masses. We shall discuss the important features of some of these committees, starting with the Bhore committee, and then go on to how health care planning has undergone changes in its structure, personnel and in its access of the populace. The review mostly highlights the modem system of medicine.

### *The Bhore Committee (1946) (The Health Survey and Development Committee)*

The Government of India appointed the Bhore Committee in October, 1943 to survey the state of the health organizations in the country and to make recommendations for their future development. The committee submitted its report in 1946. It was published in the year when India gained its Independence. The committee had to confine itself mainly to statistics of ill-health and death in the absence of data on positive health. The committee reviewed the nation's health (British India) under:

1. Public health,
2. Medical relief,
3. Professional education with special reference to professional training of hospital social workers,
4. Medical research and
5. International health.

The proposals for the health programmes were formulated and their contents remain valid even today. They are: (i) no one should fail to secure adequate medical care because of an inability to pay for it; (ii) the health programmes from their inception must lay emphasis on preventive work; (iii) health services should be placed as close to the people as possible; (iv) the doctor of the future – the basic doctor as the report called him – should be a social physician; (v) medical services should be free to all without any exceptions and the contribution from those who can afford to pay should be through general and local taxation; (vi) full-time salaried staff should be employed by government to ensure that doctors served in areas where they were most needed; (vii) greatest attention should be paid to environmental sanitation, nutrition and health education.

To achieve the above objectives the committee has suggested both, short-term and long-term measures. The short-term measures consist of the setting up of primary units covering a population of 40,000 and secondary units with as many as 16 doctors covering a population of 6,00,000 at a sub-district level. It requires two medical doctors and 36 non-medical staff per primary unit. The long-term measures suggested include the setting up of a district headquarter staffed with 269 medical officers and 1,398 non-medical staff, the raising of the bed-population ratio to 2 per thousand and the establishment of more medical colleges having training centre for nurses. The Bhore Committee also suggests the setting up of primary units covering a population of ten to twenty thousand which could be manned by six medical officers and 78 non-medical staff per unit. Secondary units have been conceived of at the sub-divisional staff level with as many as 140 medical officers and 358 non-medical staff. It also suggested the raising of the bed-population ratio from 0.24 per 1,000 to 1.03 at the end of 10 years, providing for travelling dispensaries to supplement the health services rendered by primary health centre and the promotion of hygiene.

### *The Mudaliar Committee (1961)*

The Government of India, Ministry of Health set up a committee in June 1959 to undertake a review of the developments that had taken place during late 1940s and 1950s. This committee was essentially formed with a view to formulating new health programmes in the country for the third time following Five-Year Plans. The terms of reference of this committee were:

1. The assessment of developments in the field of medical relief and health centre, and submission of the Health Survey and Development Committee Report.
2. Review of the aspects relating to health projects in the Second Five-Year Plan and
3. Formation of recommendations for the future health development projects in the country.

The committee known as the Health Survey and Planning Committee (Mudaliar Committee) submitted its report in October 1961. The major recommendations of the committee in respect to the future organization of health in the country are as follows: (i) the consolidation of advances, efforts and achievements made during the first two five-year plans in the field of health; (h) equipping district level hospitals with specialist services; (iii) regionalizing health services by setting up of regional structures between the state and district headquarters; (iv) ensuring that each primary health centre does not serve more than 40,000 people, (v) improving the quality of care provided by the PHC, (vi) the integration of medical and health services as suggested by the Bhore committee and (vii) the constitution of an all-India Health Service on the lines of the Indian Administrative Service.

The Mudaliar Committee analysed the extent to which the Bhore Committee targets had been realized. The committee noted that though there had been a large increase (from 7,400 in 1946 to 12,000 in 1958) in the number of hospitals and dispensaries, it was still proving difficult to provide proper health care services to the people due to the 'large increase in population', and because of an unbalanced distribution of the trained personnel. The Bhore Committee desired a ratio of one doctor for 2,000 population by 1971. In 1960, only one doctor for 4,850 population and one nurse for 14,300 population could be achieved. The realization of the doctor population ratio was slowed down because of the, Planning Commission's decision to sanction a PHC per community development block with populations varying from 60,000 to one lakh. Since, many villages were still waiting 9.6 miles away from the nearest hospital. The Mudaliar Commission strongly recommended the readaptation of the Bhore Committee short term plan for the establishment of PHCs for a population of 40,000 and a staff of two doctors and 36 non-medical staff per unit. In addition, the committee suggested the setting up of town level hospitals manned by 3 doctors each and a district level hospital providing specialty services in at least nine areas.

The committee found the quality of services provided by the Primary Health Centre (PHC) inadequate and stressed the need to strengthen the capabilities of existing PHC before new centres were created. It also stressed the need to strengthen sub-divisional and district hospitals so that these could effectively function as referral centres. The committee also emphasized the fact that since children formed a sizeable proportion of the population, it is essential to focus more attention on their health. The committee also observed that as compared to the rural areas, the urban areas had better and more antenatal, midwifery, post-natal infant and child care services. The committee also noticed that there was little coordination and follow up from one stage to another. It recommended that this work should be systematically organized, at least in urban areas, so as to serve as demonstration projects. Stressing the urgency of the problem of maternal and child health in India, the committee recommended that a network of primary health centre should be developed and expanded in such a way that within a period of ten years, there is one midwife for 5,000 to 6,000 rural people supported by a public health nurse and an auxiliary health worker for twice that number.

In short, the Mudaliar committee emphasized the consolidation, integration of the health infrastructure with more attention to child and maternal health. Even though there was an increase in the basic health care facilities during the 1950s, preventive aspects of many diseases were not dealt with proper care, it observed. In other words, these aspects were not given proper attention. In order to improve this aspect the government set up Chadah committee.

### *The Chadah Committee (1963)*

This committee was set up by the Government of India in 1963 under the chairmanship of Dr M.S. Chadah, the Director General of Health Services, to study the arrangements for the maintenance phase of the National Malaria Eradication Programme. The committee recommended that: (i) the vigilance operation of National Malaria Eradication Programme should be the responsibility of the general health services, that is, PHC at the block level; (ii) the vigilance operations through monthly home visits should be implemented through basic health workers. The norm of one basic health worker per 10,000 populations was recommended; (iii) the basic health workers should look after additional duties of collecting vital statistics on family planning, in addition to malaria vigilance. Three to four workers may be supervised by a family planning health assistant; and (iv) the general health services at the district level should undertake the responsibility for the maintenance phase.

It was realized in the early 1960s that the growth in the population of the country was eating away the fruits of development in the health sector as in other sectors of the country. It was felt that the rapid growth in population should be checked systematically so that given the resources the quality of life could be improved. In order to plan the growth of population, top priority was given to family planning methods. To take care of this particular aspect in detail, the central government set up a committee in 1965 known as the Mukherjee Committee.

### *The Mukherjee Committee (1965)*

The Mukherjee Committee was appointed in 1965 to review the strategy for the Family Planning Programme (FPP). The FPP up to 1961 was being implemented as a part of the health programme. However, the census of 1961 revealed that the Family Planning Programme, though being run for nearly a decade, has not made much headway and hardly any appreciable reduction has been achieved during the last decade in the growth rate. India invited a UN Mission on population activities to visit the country to chart out steps to be taken for greater acceptance of the small family norms by the population. The recommendations of UN Mission were considered by a committee appointed by the Government of India. Based on the recommendations of this committee, it was decided to have the FPP as a vertical programme with separate workers of *family planning*. Considering the direct relationship between infant mortality and acceptance of small family norms, it was also decided to integrate the Mother and Child Health Programme with Family Planning. The Mukherjee Committee felt that the FPP should be a priority based on-going programme. The major recommendations of the committee were: (i) a separate staff for the FPP; (ii) that the basic health worker not to be utilized for the FPP; and (iii) the malaria eradication activities be separated from the family planning, so that the latter could concentrate on the FPP.

This committee also emphasized on voluntary participation, training programmes for the personnel of various categories and urgent changes at the district level in rural and urban areas. Because of the earnest implementation of the FPP, by 1980, the total number of men who had undergone vasectomy operations totalled 4,71,283 and the number of women who had undergone tubectomy operations stood at 13,01,757. In other words, of the total population, around 17,73,040 men and women had undergone operations for sterilization. Besides, various other methods of family planning were also made popular. However, despite these efforts the population of India continued to grow. In 1981, the population stood at 68,38,10,000. As a result there began a considerable rethinking on the subject of health services to ensure that they were suitable to Indian conditions. It was also beginning to be realized, that the western models of medicine was not proving to be a correct decision because the population of rural India was not receiving adequate attention. It was underlined that to provide adequate health services for the rural population, specially designed rural health schemes suited to the needs would be required.

The future of the country's well-being depends on the all-round development of the rural areas. But these have not benefited eighty per cent of the population living in rural areas. The PHC, started way back in 1932, should have been the major vehicle for the delivery of health care services to the rural population. However, a committee which was constituted by the government of India recommended that additional staff be recruited for the various agencies administering the health services in the country to overcome the shortcomings in the existing infrastructure. The suggestions were (a) At the level of the PHC – one basic health worker for a population of 1,000, one health inspector for every four basic health workers, one clerk and one laboratory technician. (b) At the level of the District Health Organization – upgradation of the post of administrative officer sanctioned under the FPP, one health supervisor for every PHC subject to a maximum of one per district, one public health engineer for 2 or 3 districts and one sanitary inspector. (c) At the level of the district hospitals – one administrative officer. (d) In urban areas – one basic health worker for a population of 15,000 and one health inspector for 5 basic health workers.

The scheme for establishing the PHCs was launched in India in 1952. By March 1978, 5,400 PHCs and 38,115 subcentres had been established in 5,228 blocks. Out of these, 4,568 PHCs are being served by two doctors per centre, while the remaining 771 PHCs are without any doctor. 'The PHC has not made the kind of impact expected of them. The basic objectives of these health centres are to create delivery system of health service which reaches out to the grassroots level in rural areas. "Of the 4,500 PHCs, 700 are without any buildings while 2,620 have no staff quarters". Of the 39,000 subcentres functioning today, 15,000 have no buildings'. This shows how inadequate these services are in terms of staff and facilities.

Thus, this committee deals with the 'basic health services' which should be provided at the block level and the measures required at higher levels of administration.

### *The Jungalwala Committee (1967)*

The committee on integration of health services was appointed in 1964 under the chairmanship of Dr N. Jungalwala, who was then the

Director of the National Institute of Health Administration and Education, New Delhi, to examine the various problems including those of service conditions. The major recommendations made by the committee included the integration of organizations and personnel in the field of health from highest to the lowest level through a unified cadre, common seniority, recognition of extra qualifications, equal pay for equal work, special pay for specialized work and no private practice but good service conditions. The committee did not spell out steps or programmes for the integration recommended by it but left the matter entirely in the hands of individual states. It, however, defined the integrated health services as (i) a service with a unified approach for all problems instead of a segmented approach for different problems, (ii) a system of medical care for the sick and conventional public health programmes functioning under a single administrator and operating in a unified manner at all levels of hierarchy with due priority to each programme.

Thus, this committee tries to integrate the personnel of the health organizations by defining their work and service conditions. To review the development of the health infrastructure and manpower, Government of India once again set up a committee in 1968.

### *The Jain Committee (1968)*

The Government of India appointed the Jain Committee in 1968 to review the development in the health infrastructure and health manpower. This committee observed that for the period 1961–66 'the doctor-population ratio has remained more or less stationery at 1:16,000 in 1961 and 1:11,000 in 1966'. According to this committee 'in spite of the considerable progress made during the last twenty years since Independence, the country has remained short of medical men, nurses and other para-medical personnel. This deficiency makes the work of establishing comprehensive health services extremely difficult'. This committee noted that the recommendations of the Mudaliar Committee could not be accepted (by the Central Council of Health in 1962) due to the shortage of trained personnel and funds. The development of PHCs was, therefore, to continue as envisaged by the Planning Commission. The committee remarked that 'complete' integration of medical and health services even in the PHCs was still to be achieved.

The national programmes in the field of Health and Family Planning and Nutrition have been in operation in the country for many years. In general, these programmes are run independently of each other by their respective staff. There had been little or no coordination between the field workers or supervisory personnel of these programmes. They are separate and independent functionaries. This state of affairs came into existence because the various health programmes and the family planning programme were launched at different times and each was conceived as a vertical project to be run with its own staff. A debate on whether the same objectives could be achieved by coordinating these programmes and pooling personnel spurred the organization of the committee on multipurpose workers under the Health and Family Planning Programme.

## Health Policy after 1970–2000

### *Committee on Multipurpose Workers Under Health and Family Planning Programmes (1972–73)*

The first meeting of the executive committee of the Central Family Planning Council held on 20 September, 1970 recommended that steps should be taken for the integration of medical, public health and family planning services at the peripheral level. It was also suggested that a committee should be set up to examine and make detailed recommendations on the (i) structure of integrated services at the peripheral and supervisory levels; (ii) feasibility of having multipurpose/dual-purpose workers in the field; (iii) training: requirements for such workers; and (iv) utilization of mobile service units set up under family planning programme for integrated medical, public health and family planning services.

After its suggestions on the feasibility of having multipurpose workers in the health care delivery systems and their expected training requirements, another committee known as Kartar Singh Committee was set up to pursue the recommendations made by executive committee of the Central Family Planning Service (1972).

### *The Kartar Singh Committee (1973)*

The Government of India constituted a committee in October 1972 on 'Multipurpose Workers under Health and Family Planning' under the chairmanship of Kartar Singh, the then Additional Secretary Ministry of Health, and Government of India.

The committee's terms of reference were to study and make recommendations on:

1. The structure for integrated services at the periphery and supervisory levels;
2. The feasibility of having multipurpose dual-purpose workers in the field;
3. The training requirements for such workers; and
4. The utilization of public mobile units, set up under family planning services operating in the field.

The Kartar Singh committee submitted its report in September 1973. The multipurpose health worker scheme of the committee was a significant development favouring grass-root level integration of several vertical health programmes. The main recommendations of the committee were: (i) the Auxiliary Nurse Midwives be replaced by newly designated Female Health Workers and the existing basic health workers, malaria eradication assistants and family planning health assistants be replaced by 'Male Health Workers'; (ii) the programmes for having multipurpose workers be first introduced in areas where there is malaria in the maintenance phase, and where small pox has been controlled, and later in other areas; (iii) for a proper coverage there should be one PHC for a population of 80,000; (iv) each PHC should be divided into 16 subcentres each having a population of about 3,000–3,500 depending upon topography and means of communication; (v) each subcentre should be staffed by a team of one male and one female health worker; (vi) there should be a male health supervisor to supervise the work of 3–4 male health workers and a female health supervisor to supervise the work of four female health workers; (vii) the post of lady health visitor should be redesignated as female health supervisor; and (viii) the doctor in charge of a PHC should have charge over all the supervisors and health workers in his area.

Certain practical difficulties surfaced at three levels, namely, at the administrative, training and at the level of attitude during the actual implementation of these recommendations. For many other reasons too the scheme of multipurpose health workers could not gain momentum. The failure of these schemes could be attributed to (i) the quick changeover of the doctors at various centres; (ii) the failure on the part of the state government to sort out basic bureaucratic details like pay scale of these workers, what kits they were to carry with them and how they were to be replenished. Despite these major shortcomings, the government expected to complete the training of multipurpose workers by 1983.

### *The Shrivastava Committee (1975)*

The government of India in 1974 appointed the Shrivastava Committee known also as the 'group of medical education and support manpower' under the chairmanship of J.B. Shrivastava, the then Director General, Health Services, Government of India, to review the progress in the field of medical education and identify the reasons for its failure to make an impact on the health needs of the masses. The terms of reference of the group were;

1. To design a suitable curriculum for training a cadre of health assistants who could be made conversant with basic medical aid, preventive welfare activities so that they could serve as an effective link between the qualified medical practitioners and multipurpose workers, thus forming an effective team to deliver health care, family welfare and nutritional services to the people,
2. To suggest suitable ways and means for implementation of the recommendations of the earlier committees on medical education especially the medical education committee (1968) and the medical education conference (1970), and to suggest steps for improving the existing medical educational processes so as to provide due emphasis on the problems particularly relevant to national requirements, and
3. To make any other suggestions to realize the above objectives and matters.

After examining various reports and papers relevant to the subject, the recommendations of the group were: (i) to evolve a national-wide network of efficient and effective services suitable for our conditions, limitation and potentialities, (ii) to take steps to create a band of para-professional or semi-potentialities, health workers from the community itself to provide simple protective, preventive and curative services which are needed by the community; (iii) these workers should interact as mediators between the community and PHC, and should be trained and equipped to give simple specified remedies for day-to-day illness. Health assistants should work as intermediaries between the health workers and the PHC. The health assistants should be located at the subcentres. Like the health workers, they should also be trained and equipped to give specific remedies for simple day-to-day health problems. While they are a supervisory role over the health workers, they should also function as health workers in their own areas and carry out the same duties and responsibilities but as a higher level of technical competence; (iv) the PHCs should be provided with an additional doctor and a nurse to look after the maternal and child health services; (v) the possibility of utilizing the services of senior doctors at medical college should be explored; regional medical college hospitals should each develop direct links with the community around them, as well as with one another within a total referral services complex; (vii) the Government of India should constitute a medical and a Health Education Commission for co-coordinating and maintaining standards in medical and health education based on the pattern of the UGC.

This committee opined that 'it will be financially impracticable to increase the number of primary health centres, except perhaps marginally'. The committee advocated the creation of a 'Health Assistant' cadre to affect curative programmes amongst others, and suggested that ultimately there should be one health assistant (male/female) for every two health workers (male/female). It envisaged that by the end of the sixth plan there should be one male and one female worker for every 5,000 population. The committee recommended 'the creation of local para-professional workers in the community itself to provide simple specified medicines for day-to-day illness'. Thus, a major contribution of the Shrivastava Committee was the involvement of the community health workers. There were approximately one lakh community health volunteers in the field as on 1 April 1980. By 1985, the Government of India hopes to have 3.60 lakh community health volunteers.

The Government of India is fully aware that an in-depth evaluation of the centrally sponsored community health volunteer scheme is necessary to make the programme effective. The decision to recruit para-professional from the community itself, like the Chinese model of barefoot doctors, indicates that the policy shift was made with the hope of creating active community participation.

After the Shrivastava Committee's action plan and the creation of the village level workers by the government, there were more changes implemented. Compulsory sterilization and family planning camps during Emergency rule in the country led to widespread hostility among the people leading to the overthrow of the Congress party by the Janta regime and this resulted in altered approach in health services. Besides giving importance to family planning, Mr Raj Narain, the then Health Minister encouraged the scheme of the village level workers as suggested by the Shrivastava Committee. The recommendations of a Shrivastava Committee and the inspiration from the

Chinese Scheme of barefoot doctors formed the basis for the introduction of the Community Health Volunteer (CHV) scheme in India by Mr Raj Narain. This scheme, now renamed as Village Health Guide scheme, provides for one village guide for a population of 1,000 The need to revive the earlier multipurpose worker scheme for the effective functioning of the primary health centre was underlined. Besides, large mobile vans fully equipped for the village-level health services were operated under the instructions of the health minister with a view to create mobile clinic services. These were under the control of the government and municipal hospitals. An objective analysis, however, reveals that these mobile clinic services extended through the preventive and social medicines departments of hospitals in urban areas and slums have not made any positive impact.

### Health for All by the Year 2000 AD

The low access to the basic health care facilities is a common phenomenon in most of the developing countries. In order to provide minimum basic health facilities, it was decided by the Health Assembly of the WHO to launch a movement known as 'Health for All' by the year 2000 AD. In 1978, the Alma Ata conference reaffirmed health for all, as the major social goal of all governments. In 1981, a global strategy for this programme was adopted by the WHO, which was later endorsed by the United Nations Central Assembly. India is a signatory to those declarations and has made efforts to extend health facilities to the vulnerable sections of its society. Health for all has been defined as attainment of 'a level of health that will enable every individual to lead a socially and economically productive life'. To achieve the goal of 'Health for All by the year 2000 AD', the Ministry of Health and Family Welfare, Government of India convened a national conference to discus national strategies and action plans. The Planning Commission appointed a working group on 'Health for All' to suggest and monitor the progress of this programme on a regular basis.

Thus, as working group submitted its report in 1981, the goals recommended by the working group are:

1. Reduction of infant mortality from the present level of 125 to below 60 by 2000 AD.
2. To raise the expectation of life at birth from the present level of 52 years to 64 by 2000 AD.
3. To reduce the crude birth rate from the present level of 33 per 1,000 population to 21 by 2000 AD.

4. To reduce crude death rate from the present level of 14 per 1,000 population to 9 per 1,000 by 2000 AD.
5. To achieve a net reproduction rate of one by 2000 AD.
6. To provide potable water to the entire rural population by 1990.

The concept of 'Health for All by 2000 AD', implies a substantial change in basic health policies and in the approaches to health care. In order to provide minimum health facilities, the Government of India, along with state governments has increased the allocation to the health sector and has started some additional programme to boost its success in this field. The Minimum Need Programme which was first launched in the Fifth Five-Year Plan was reformulated in 1978 to provide minimum facilities to the poor which includes education, health, food, water and shelter. Under this programme, one subcentre for a population of 5,000, one PHC for 30,000 people and one community health centre with specialization in four areas for a population of 1,00,000 has been targeted. The Sixth Plan provision for the minimum need programme for the state amounted to ₹ 5,807 crore which was increased to ₹ 10,081.72 crore in the Seventh Plan. In order to achieve the goal of this programme, the concept of PHC, that is, the active participation of the people individually and collectively was promoted. Primary health care includes these eight elements – promotion of food supply and proper nutrition; an adequate supply of safe drinking water, basic sanitation, education, methods of preventing and controlling the maternal and child care including family planning, immunization against major infectious diseases, prevention and control of locally endemic diseases, appropriate treatment of common diseases and injuries, and the provision of essential drugs.

Thus, the important operational components of primary care should be formulated as:

1. It should be need-based.
2. It should be accessible to all.
3. It should conform to the cultural and the economic set-up of the community.
4. It should involve people actively and ultimately makes them self-reliant in health.
5. It should have appropriate linkages with other health services.
6. It should be accompanied by necessary socio-economic development of the community.

The measures undertaken by the government for providing health care include the introduction of the rural health scheme based on the principle of placing people's health in people's hands. Under the rural health scheme, there are two functionaries at the village level, namely, a village health guide and a trained *dai* who are entrusted with the delivery of primary health care. Special emphasis was laid under this programme on the health status of mothers and children which stipulated an acceleration of programmes for the welfare for women and children and nutritional programmes for pregnant women, nursing mothers and children. The national health policy also gave great importance to maternal and child health programmes by extending more services in rural and urban areas, through primary health centre, rural family welfare centre, subcentre, urban family welfare centre and postpartum centre. Stress was also laid on the control of communicable diseases. The immunization programme also considered as important with its objectives to reduce the incidence of diphtheria, whooping cough, tetanus, poliomyelitis childhood, tuberculosis and typhoid fever.

On the whole, it appears that there has been a tremendous investment in widening the health infrastructure which include within its purview a variety of programmes and views health and humans a vital components of overall socio-economic development. For the realization of the various objectives, the policy lays down that specified goals are to be achieved by 1985, 1990, 1995 and the year 2000.

## An Overall View of the Preceding Reports

The Health Services and Development Committee known also as the Bhore Committee (1946) pointed out the link between the socio-economic conditions and health of the people. It also suggested the establishment of PHCs for providing health care. The Health Survey and Planning Committee (Mudaliar Committee) in its report (1961) pointed out that the doctors were concentrating on curative work and suggested that they should instead share responsibilities with the auxiliary health personnel. The committee also recommended that vertical programmes be scrapped. The Chadah Committee took care of malaria vigilance in addition to family planning services at all levels. In 1965, the Mukherjee Committee recommended the extension of the educational approach to the family planning programme in place of the clinic-dominated functioning in the field. The Jungalwala Committee (1967) recommended the integration of organizations and personnel in the field of health through a unified cadre, common seniority, recognition of extra qualifications, equal pay for equal work and no private practice but good service conditions. In 1968, the Jain Committee suggested the need to integrate the medical and health services in the field of the PHCs. The Committee on the multipurpose workers (1973) pointed out, among other things, the unsatisfactory functioning of the PHCs and noted that 60 per cent of the times of the medical officers at the PHCs were not accounted for. It recommended an integrated approach to the PHC services with the health supervisors providing guidance to the multipurpose workers. The Kartar Singh Committee defined the feasibility of the multipurpose workers and their training requirements. To make the health services community based, the CHV scheme recommended by the Srivastava Committee (group on Medical Education and Supporting Manpower, 1975) was launched on 2 October 1977. 'Health for All by 2000 AD' was a substantial shift in the basic health policies practised and was a healthy improvement in the approach to health care and, in laying stress on the 'provision of basic health facility to each, and every citizen'. The alternative strategy also suggested health for all based on the principle 'of integrating promotive, preventive and curative aspects.

In the above pages, we have highlighted the, significant aspects of the official reports available on the health committees and commission. Since we are concerned with the health situation in independent India, we started off with the Bhore Committee report (1946) and ended with the report on alternative strategy (1981).

The Bhore Committee identified two aspects of social policy which was subsequently accepted and pursued in free India. This related to the social role of medicine and the doctor, as well as the quality of the training and personnel. 'The first recommendation of the Bhore committee underlines that every person suffering from a disease should get immediate medical attention irrespective of his socio-economic status'. Oommen (1955) commenting on the same theme says: 'health problems should not remain the private worry of diseased individuals but should be recognized as a public issue to be tackled by the government'. Another recommendation of the committee was the doctor of the future should be a social physician... It may be viewed that a social physician is one who has an altruistic outlook towards the community he *serves.* In fact, this is the real task of a doctor, the report enumerates. In a country, like ours, there is a need for health professionals to serve in rural areas rather than concentrate in the urban sectors. The government should draft a policy that motivates trained physicians to work in rural areas.

To review the health scene between the second and third five-year plans, a period spanning almost fifteen years, the Mudaliar Committee was appointed in 1961. This committee found that though noteworthy progress had been made in many directions, even the short-term targets of the Bhore Committee were far from accomplished and this committee revised the targets in a more realistic manner. While working in the area of communicable diseases, it was realized that the health services for maternal and child welfare were fragile and their reach was limited. This committee spoke against the revival of short-term courses even as a traditional measure. The committee found that the medical profession and all the associations connected with professional bodies were against it.

There were two reasons for this:

1. The proper development of the country in the field of health can take place only if the doctor possesses the minimum qualifications.
2. India is no longer alienated from the international health scene and is participating in all problems of international health. The world health organizations have laid down certain minimum standards of qualifications. In view of India being an active member, and participating in all public health measures at the international level, we think that it will be unfortunate if at this stage recourse is taken in short-term measures.

The Mudaliar Committee defended its position by forwarding two arguments. First, the committee felt that its recommendation for training several categories of para-medical personnel would justifiably meet the demand and, therefore, the need for short-term medical course would be redundant. Second, those with short-term training are usually the ones who go to rural areas. This would amount to a different treatment accorded to rural areas in matters relating to health care.

An analysis of the recommendations of the Bhore Committee and the Mudaliar Committee relating to the policy of training medical personnel indicates that these were based on the following considerations: (1) a concern for qualitative medical services; (2) a belief in facing resistance from the medical profession; (3) an anxiety to maintain international standards in medical education; (4) the belief that para-medical personnel can serve as a functional alternative to medical personnel in some contexts; and (v) a concern for maintaining parity in the quality of medical services between rural and urban areas.

After the Bhore Committee and the Mudaliar Committee, came the Jain Committee (1968) to review the situation of the health infrastructure and health manpower. This committee noted that the recommendations of the Mudaliar Committee could not be accepted mainly because of the shortage of trained personnel and funds. Therefore, the Planning Commission envisaged the development of PHCs. The Jungalwala Committee (1967) recommended the integration of health services. Over a period of time, the Government of India has come to recognize 'the urban orientation of medical education in India which relies heavily on curative methods and sophisticated diagnostic aides, with little emphasis on the preventive and promotional aspects, or the needs of the country, primarily because of the emphasis on community health rather than institutional care'. A committee of allopathic experts known as the Srivastava Committee (1975) attempted to evolve a framework for organizing a 'nationwide network of efficient and effective health services for the country'. The committee advocated the principle that 'health services should be provided within the community itself'. It maybe explained that the concept that the community-level health workers should essentially provide the 'links between the people at large and the multipurpose workers functioning at the subcentres and doctors at the PHC level was being this rationale. The committee admitted that the modern system of medicine (that is allopathy), although manned by the fully trained and competent persons, lacked the emotional, psychological and social angle in its interaction with the community. In contrast, the practitioners of indigenous system, while not sufficiently trained or competent according to the committee, had the necessary rapport with the community. To remedy the situation, the committee recommended the creation of a cadre of para-professionals to be designated as health assistants who could provide the essential and day-to-day health and medical services with an emphasis on promotive and preventive functions'.

The committee, however, concludes that what we need even for rural areas is a better trained doctor 'and it found no justification to make any change in the present policy of producing an adequately trained general practitioner, both for rural and urban areas'.

It is a fact that India lives in its villages (8%) hence, the delivery of health services in those areas is of paramount importance. However, the reports and recommendations of various committees on developing a community based delivery system failed to make an impact on the ultimate consumers of the health services that is the people of the rural areas. The only targets reached by the health sector were the production of doctors and urban hospitals. Therefore, the government seriously considered an alternative machinery and constituted a committee on multipurpose workers under health and family planning programmes (1972–73) followed by the Kartar Singh Committee (1973). A few other committees have been appointed by Government of India to review the National Malaria Eradication Programme (the Chadah Committee, 1963) and the Family Planning programme (the Mukherjee Committee, 1965).

It has been seen that the various reports lined up different programmes of action and are different in their emphasis. Top priority has been given to the control of communicable diseases, medical education, training of health personnel, medical research, services for promoting health of children and mothers, nutrition and national malaria eradication. It was this urgency in the situation that prompted the government to evolve the National Health Policy. The NHP aims at taking the health services to the doorsteps of the people and ensuring a fuller participation of the community in the health development process. It has been recognized that if the quality of life of the people is to be improved their health status must be raised. In this perspective, health development is to be viewed as an integral part of the overall human resources development. Consequently, a coordinated approach is sought to be established among all the health related programmes, for example, protected water supply, environmental sanitation and hygiene, nutrition, housing and education.

There have been some new strategies recommended by social scientists and by those medical scientists who are keen to promote a social sciences perspective. The Ramalingaswami Committees' health policy document entitled, 'Health for All' is a comprehensive report. This committee notes that in the last thirty years, the reproduction of institutions based on western models, services and values have increased tremendously. It pleads for the abandoning of these western models of health-care services which have been actually imposed on us 'and also impresses the fact that health for all cannot be achieved through a linear expansion of the existing system or by tinkering with it through minor reforms. The committee advocated nothing short of a radical change and called for a comprehensive national health policy'.

The above reviews of the health planning process in India clearly indicates the enormous efforts made by the various committees to chart out the growth of health manpower in India, The work of these committees have, however, been subject to serious data limitations. Information on different categories of health personnel, their profiles and distribution (especially in respect to professionals outside the public sectors) has been rather scanty. The various committees and even institutions like the ICSSR/ICMR group, have been focusing on their attention providing expert opinion rather than garnering hard statistical data. No committee has been able to take into account the contribution of non-governmental health institutions and that of professionals in rendering health care services. Also, perhaps more importantly, the committees have been unable to assess the health care needs of the people through field surveys and ascertain the extent of utilization of health care institutions and practitioner.

No concerted effort has yet been made to develop a health care system that encompasses both theory and practice. Today, we need a comprehensive National Health Policy for the developmental health programmes. This policy should be essentially Indian and distinct from the western Chinese models and strategies developed in other countries. The new model should attempt to integrate health plans with the socio-economic development. It implies that the human environment has to be conducive to health, that food should be available to all and that everyone should have the means to get sufficient food. Other implications are also involved that people must be aware of health as a right and a responsibility and they must be willing to participate in plans and programmes to promote their own health and the health of the community as a whole.

The National Health Policy lays down an integrated and comprehensive approach as envisaged above for the development of health services in the country, including family planning services. The policy is aimed at providing 'health for all' by 2000 AD through primary health care approach as recommended by the Alma-Ata declaration. The stress in the National Health Policy is on the provision of preventive, promotive and rehabilitative health services to the people representing a shift from medical care to health care and in short, from the urban to rural population. This includes substantial augmentation and provision of primary health care facilities and family welfare services on a universal basis in every village, town and urban community; acceleration of programmes for the welfare of women and children, including family planning; control of leprosy, tuberculosis and blindness and nutrition programmes for pregnant women, nursing mothers and children, especially in the more remote, hilly and backward areas. Quantitative targets have been fixed for each of these areas. At this point, it is clear that if the adequacy of care, that is, the distribution of health services, could be improved, these should result in considerable savings to the economy of the nation, not only in strict economic terms, but also in a general social and psychological sense of well-being of the society. Improvement in the health status of the population then may be less dependent upon increasing the amount of health services than it is on reorganizing them to improve their availability and accessibility.

Given the health planning structure in the country as inherited from the 1950s, it is unlikely that the alternative strategies suggested will be incorporated in the health planning in the country. The health care plans for the near future is to be centred around the expansion of the existing facilities to the areas/groups who have no access to them. In view of this, one has to find ways and means to improve the existing health delivery system for the masses. Even in this area a number of problems are faced by the people which include doctor's attitudes, organizational difficulties, people's beliefs, cost effectiveness and the inaccessibility of life saving drugs. However, the existing literature on health care has either neglected these or hardly highlighted them while framing the policies in the health field for the masses.

## Health Policy 2002

### *Health Policy*

The main objective of this policy is to achieve an acceptable standard of good health amongst the general population of the country. The approach would be to increase access to the decentralized public health system by establishing new infrastructure in deficient areas and by upgrading the infrastructure in the existing institutions. Overriding importance would be given to ensuring a more equitable access to health services across the social and geographical expanse of the country. Emphasis will be given to increasing the aggregate public health investment through a substantially increased contribution by the Central Government. It is expected that this initiative will strengthen the capacity of the public health administration at the State level to render effective service delivery. The contribution of the private sector in providing health services would be much enhanced, particularly for the population group which can afford to pay for services. Primacy will be given to preventive and first-line curative initiatives at the primary health level through increased sectoral share of allocation. Emphasis will be laid on rational use of drugs within the allopathic system. Increased access to tried and tested systems of traditional medicine will be ensured. Within these broad objectives, National Health Policy, 2002 (NHP-2002) will endeavour to achieve the time-bound goals mentioned as follows.

### *Goals to be Achieved by 2000–2015*

| | |
|---|---|
| Eradicate Polio and Yaws | 2005 |
| Eliminate Leprosy | 2005 |
| Eliminate Kala Azar | 2010 |
| Achieve Zero level growth of HIV/AIDS | 2007 |
| Reduce mortality by 50 per cent on account of TB, Malaria and other Vector and water-borne diseases | 2010 |
| Reduce prevalence of blindness to 0.5 per cent | 2010 |
| Reduce IMR to 30/1,000 and MMR to 100/Lakh | 2010 |
| Increase utilization of public health facilities from current level of <20 to >75 per cent | 2010 |
| Establish an integrated system of surveillance, National Health Accounts and Health Statistics | 2005 |
| Increase health expenditure by Government as a percentage of GDP from the existing 0.9 per cent to 2.0 per cent | 2010 |
| Increase share of Central grants to constitute at least 25 per cent of total health spending | 2010 |
| Increase State Sector Health spending from 5.5 per cent to 7 per cent of the budget | 2005 |
| Further increase to 8 per cent | 2010 |

## Equity in Health

To meet the objective of reducing various types of inequities and imbalances – inter-regional; across the rural-urban divide; and between economic classes – the most cost-effective method would be to increase the sectoral outlay in the primary health sector. Such outlets afford access to a vast number of individuals, and also facilitate preventive and early stage curative initiative, which are cost effective. In recognition of this public health principle, NHP-2002 sets out an increased allocation of 55 per cent of the total public health investment for the primary health sector; the secondary and tertiary health sectors being targeted for 35 per cent and 10 per cent respectively. The Policy projects of the increased aggregate outlays for the primary health sector will be utilized for strengthening existing facilities and opening additional public health service outlets, consistent with the norms for such facilities.

This policy envisages a key role for the Central Government in designing national programmes with the active participation of the State Governments. Also, the Policy ensures the provisioning of financial resources, in addition to technical support, monitoring and evaluation at the national level by the Centre. However, to optimize the utilization of the public health infrastructure at the primary level, NHP-2002 envisages the gradual convergence of all health programmes under a single field administration. Vertical programmes for control of major diseases like TB, malaria, HIV/AIDS, as also the Reproductive and Child Health (RCH) and Universal Immunization Programmes, would need to be continued till moderate levels of prevalence are reached. The integration of the programmes will bring about a desirable optimization of outcomes through a convergence of all public health inputs. The Policy also envisages that programme implementation be effected through autonomous bodies at State and district levels. The interventions of State Health Departments may be limited to the overall monitoring of the achievement of programme targets and other technical aspects. The relative distancing of the programme implementation from the State Health Departments will give the project team greater operational flexibility. Also, the presence of State Government officials, social activists, private health professionals and MLAs/MPs on the management boards of the autonomous bodies will facilitate well informed decision-making.

The Policy also highlights the need for developing the capacity within the State Public Health administration for scientific designing of public health projects, suited to the local situation.

The Policy envisages that apart from the exclusive staff in a vertical structure for the disease control programmes, all rural health staff should be available for the entire gamut of public health activities at the decentralized level, irrespective of whether these activities relate to national programmes or other public health initiatives. It would be for the Head of the District Health administration to allocate the time of the rural health staff between the various programmes, depending on the local need. NHP-2002 recognizes that to implement such a change, not only would the public health administrators be required to change their mindset, but the rural health staff would need to be trained and reoriented.

The health needs of the country are enormous and the financial resources and managerial capacity available to meet the need, even on the most optimistic projections, fall somewhat short. In this situation, NHP-2002 has had to make hard choices between various priorities and operational options. NHP-2002 does not claim to be a road map for meeting all the health needs of the populace of the country. Further, it has to be cognized that such health needs are also dynamic, as threats in the area of public health keep changing over time. The Policy, while being holistic, offers the necessary risk of recommending differing emphasis on different policy components. Broadly speaking, NHP-2002 focuses on the need for enhanced funding and an organizational restructuring of the national public health initiatives in order to facilitate more equitable access to the health facilities. Also, the Policy is focused on those diseases which are principally contributing to the disease burden – TB, malaria and blindness from the category of historical diseases; and HIV/AIDS from the category of 'newly emerging diseases'. This is not to say that other items contributing to the disease burden of the country will be ignored; but only that the resources, as also the principal focus of the public health administration, will recognize certain relative priorities. It is unnecessary to labour the point that under the umbrella of the macro-policy prescriptions in this document, governments and private sector programme planners will have to design separate schemes, tailor-made to the health needs of women, children, geriatrics, tribal and other socio-economically underserved sections. An adequately robust disaster management plan has to be in place to effectively cope with situations arising from natural and man-made calamities.

One nagging imperative, which has influenced every aspect of this Policy, is the need to ensure that 'equity' in the health sector stands as an independent goal. In any future evaluation of its success or failure, NHP-2002 would wish to be measured against this equity norm, rather than any other aggregated financial norm for the health sector. Consistent with the primacy given to 'equity', a marked emphasis has been provided in the policy for expanding and improving the primary health facilities, including the new concept of the provisioning of essential drugs through Central funding. The Policy also commits the Central Government to an increased underwriting of the resources for meeting the minimum health needs of the people. Thus, the Policy attempts to provide guidance for prioritizing expenditure, thereby facilitating rational resource allocation.

This Policy broadly envisages a greater contribution from the Central Budget for the delivery of Public Health services at the State level. Adequate appropriations, steadily rising over the years, would need to be ensured. The possibility of ensuring this by imposing an earmarked health cess has been carefully examined. While it is recognized that the annual budget must accommodate the increasing resource needs of the social sectors, particularly in the health sector, this Policy does not specifically recommend an earmarked health cess, as that would have a tendency of reducing the space available to Parliament in making appropriations looking to the circumstances prevailing from time to time.

The policy highlights the expected roles of different participating groups in the health sector. Further, it recognizes the fact that, despite all that may be guaranteed by the Central Government for assisting public health programmes, public health services would actually need to be delivered by the State administration, NGOs and other institutions of civil society. The attainment of improved health levels would be significantly dependent on population stabilization, as also on complementary efforts from other areas of the social sectors – like improved drinking water supply, basic sanitation, minimum nutrition, etc. to ensure that the exposure of the populace to health risk is minimized.

Any expectation of a significant improvement in the quality of health services, and the consequential improved health status of the citizenry, would depend not only on increased financial and material inputs, but also on a more empathetic and committed attitude in the service providers, whether in the private or public sectors. In some measure, this optimistic policy document is based on the understanding that the citizenry is increasingly demanding more by way of quality in health services and the health delivery system, particularly in the public sector, is being pressed to respond. In this backdrop, it needs to be recognized that any policy in the social sector is critically dependent on the service providers treating their responsibility not as a commercial activity but as a service, albeit a paid one. In the area of public health, an improved standard of governance is a prerequisite for the success of any health policy.

## Trends in Policy Development

Although the National Health Policy (NHP) in India was not framed until 1983, India has built up a vast health infrastructure and initiated several national health programmes over last five decades in government, voluntary and private sectors under the guidance and direction of various committees (Bre, Mudaliar, Kartar Singh, Srivastava), the Constitution, the Planning Commission, the Central Council of Health and Family Welfare and Consultative Committees attached to the Ministry of Health and Family Welfare. The period after 1983 witnessed several major developments in the polices impacting the health sector – adoption of National Health Policy in 1983, 73rd and 74th Constitutional Amendments in 1992, National Policy in 1993, National Health Policy in 2002, National Policy on Indian System of Medicine and Homeopathy in 2002, Drug Policy in 2002, introduction of Universal Health Insurance schemes for the poor in 2002, Drug Policy in 2002, introduction of Universal Health Insurance schemes for the poor in 2003, and inclusion of health in Common Minimum Programme of the UPA Government in 2004.

The first National Health Policy in 1983 aimed to achieve the goal of 'Health for All' by 2000 AD, through the provision of comprehensive primary health care services. It stressed the creation of an infrastructure for primary health care; close coordination with health-related services and activities (like nutrition, drinking water supply and sanitation); the active involvement and participation of voluntary organizations; the provision of essential drugs and vaccines; qualitative improvement in health and family planning services; the provision of adequate training; and medical research aimed at the common health problems of the people.

The main objective of the revised National Health Policy, 2002 is to achieve an acceptable standard of good health among the general population of the country and has set goals to be achieved by the year 2015. The major policy prescriptions are as follows:

- Increase public expenditure from 0.9 per cent to 2 per cent by 2010.
- Increase allocation of public health investment in the order of 55 per cent for the primary health sector; 35 per cent and 10 per cent to secondary and tertiary sectors respectively.
- Gradual convergence of all health programmes, except the ones (such as TB, malaria, HIV/AIDS, RCH), which need to be continued till moderate levels of prevalence are reached.
- Need to levy user charges for certain secondary and tertiary public health services, for those who can afford to pay.
- Mandatory two-year rural posting before awarding the graduate medical degree.

- Decentralizing the implementation of health programmes to local self-governing bodies by 2005.
- Setting up of Medical Grants Commission for funding new Government Medical and Dental colleges.
- Promoting public health discipline.
- Establishing two-tier urban health care system – Primary Health Centre for a population of one lakh and Government General Hospital.
- Increase in government funded health research to a level of 2 per cent of the total health spending by 2010.
- Appreciation of the role of private sector in health and enactment of legislation by 2003 for regulating private clinical establishments.
- Formulation of procedures for accreditation of public and private health facilities.
- Cooption of NGOs in national disease control programmes.
- Promotion of tele medicine in tertiary health care sector.
- Full operationalization of National Disease Surveillance Network by 2005.
- Notification of contemporary code of medical ethics by Medical Council of India.
- Encouraging setting up of private insurance instruments to bring secondary and tertiary sectors into its purview.
- Promotion of medical service for overseas users.
- Encouragement and promotion of Indian System of Medicine.

The first National Health Policy, in 1983, aimed to achieve the goal of 'Health for All' by 2000 AD through the provision of comprehensive primary health care services. It stressed the creation of an infra-structure for primary health care; close coordination with health-related services and activities (like nutrition, drinking water supply and sanitation); active involvement and participation of voluntary organizations; provision of essential drugs and vaccines; qualitative improvement in health and family planning services; provision of adequate training; and medical research aimed at the common health problems of the people.

Through the 73rd and 74th Constitutional Amendment Acts (1992), the local bodies (Municipalities and Panchayats) have been assigned 29 development activities, which have a direct and indirect bearing on health. These include health and sanitation (covering hospitals, PHCs and dispensaries), family welfare, drinking water, women and child development, the public distribution system and poverty alleviation programmes.

The Common Minimum Programme announced by the UPA government in 2004 has proposed to raise public spending on health to at least 2–3 per cent of the Gross Domestic Product (GDP) over the next five years, with focus on primary health care. The present government has proposed to take all steps to ensure availability of life saving drugs at reasonable prices through revival of Public Sector Units in the manufacture of critical bulk drugs.

The budget 2004–05 has proposed three major initiatives in the health sector. They are: (i) redesigning the Universal Health Insurance scheme introduced in 2003 to make it exclusive for below poverty level people with a reduced premium, (ii) introduction of Group Health Insurance scheme for members of Self Help Groups and Credit Link Groups at a premium of ₹ 120 per person for an insurance cover of ₹ 10,000, and (iii) exemption of income tax for the hospitals working in rural areas.

# 14

# Ministry of Health and Family Welfare

## A Catalyst for Promoting Reproductive Health

India is rapidly gaining ground in the international scenario as a popular destination for foreign international students and even for some others who opt to migrate to this mystical land for the tourism. The country, which had been reeling under the onslaught of British colonial rule, managed odds and has successfully created a niche for itself. It has metamorphosed into one of the most favoured destinations for travel, much due to the presence of several renowned world heritage sites and spiritualistic forces, which pulls enthusiastic travellers towards it.

Ministry of Health and Family Welfare comprise the following divisions:

- Ministry
  - — Ministry of Health and Family Welfare
- Departments
  - — Department of Ayurveda, Yoga and Naturopathy, Unani, Siddha and Homoeopathy (AYUSH)
  - — Department of Family Welfare
  - — Department of Health
  - — Pharmacopoeia Laboratory for Indian Medicine (PLIM)
- Attached Offices
  - — Directorate General of Health Services (DGHS)
- Subordinate Offices
  - — Central Institute of Psychiatry (CIP)
  - — Homoeopathic Pharmacopoeia Laboratory (HPL)
  - — National Institute of Communicable Disease (NICD)

- Autonomous Bodies
  - — All India Institute of Medical Sciences (AIIMS)
  - — International Institute for Population Sciences (IIPS)
  - — Jawaharlal Institute of Postgraduate Medical Education and Research (JIPMER) Lala Ram Swarup Institute of Tuberculosis and Respiratory Diseases
  - — Morarji Desai National Institute of Yoga (MDNIY)
  - — National Institute of Ayurveda
  - — National Institute of Homoeopathy (NIH)
  - — National Institute of Mental Health and Neuro Sciences (NIMHANS)
  - — National Institute of Naturopathy (NIN)
  - — National Tuberculosis Institute (NTI)
  - — North Eastern Indira Gandhi Regional Institute of Health and Medical Sciences (NEIGRIHMS) Post Graduate Institute of Medical Education and Research, Chandigarh
  - — Rashtriya Ayurveda Vidyapeeth
- Boards
  - — National Board of Examinations
  - — National Medicinal Plants Board (NMPB)
- Councils
  - — Central Council for Research in Ayurveda and Siddha (CCRAS)
  - — Central Council for Research in Homoeopathy (CCRH)
  - — Central Council for Research in Unani Medicine (CCRUM)
  - — Indian Council of Medical Research (ICMR)
  - — Medical Council of India (MCI)
- PSUs and Joint Ventures
  - — Hindustan Latex Limited (HLL)
  - — Hospital Services Consultancy Corporation (I) Limited (HSCC)
  - — Indian Medicines Pharmaceutical Corporation Limited (IMPCL)
- Divisions/Units/Wings/Branches ...
  - — Indian Society for Medical Statistics (ISMS)
  - — Institute of Immunohaematology
  - — Malaria Research Centre (MRC)

  - National Institute of Cholera and Enteric Diseases (NICED) Reproductive and Child Health (RCH)
  - Tuberculosis Research Centre, Chennai
- Others
  - Central Government Health Scheme (CGHS), Allahabad
  - Central Government Health Scheme (CGHS), Kolkata
  - Central Government Health Scheme (CGHS), Mumbai
  - CODEX India
  - Food Safety, India
  - National AIDS Control Organization (NACO)
  - National Family Health Survey (NFHS)
  - National Vector Borne Disease Control Programme (NVBDCP)

### Central Government Health Schemes (CGHS)

The Central Government Health Schemes was started in 1954 with the objective of providing comprehensive medical care to the Central Government employees, both serving and retired and is also providing service to members and former members of parliaments, judges of Supreme Court and High Court, freedom fighters, former Governors and former Vice-Presidents of India.

#### *Schemes and Programmes*

- Central Government Health Schemes
- National AIDS Control Programme
- National Leprosy Eradication Programme
- Vector Borne Disease Control Programme
- National TB Control Programme
- National Programme for Control of Blindness
- National Cancer Control Programme
- National Iodine Deficiency Disorder Control Programme
- Mental Health Programme
- Drugs
- Rashtriya Arogya Nidhi (RAN)
- Prevention of Food Adulteration Programme

The Central Government Health Scheme in India is a comprehensive health care to the CGHS beneficiaries.

The Central Government Health Scheme is applicable to the following categories of people residing in CGHS covered cities:

1. All Central Government Servants paid from Civil Estimates (other than those employed in Railway Services and those employed under Delhi Administration except members of Delhi Police Force).
2. Pensioners drawing pension from Civil Estimates and their family members (Pensioner residing in non-CGHS areas also may obtain CGHS Card from nearest CGHS covered city)
3. Hon'ble Members of Parliament
4. Hon'ble Judges of Supreme Court of India
5. Ex-Members of Parliament
6. Employees and Pensioners of Autonomous Bodies covered under CGHS (Delhi)
7. Ex-Governors and Ex-Vice Presidents
8. Former Prime Ministers
9. Former Judges of Hon'ble Supreme Court of India and Hon'ble High Courts
10. Freedom Fighters

It provides service through following categories of systems:

1. Allopathic
2. Homeopathic
3. Indian System of Medicines e.g.
   (i) Ayurveda
   (ii) Unani
   (iii) Yoga
   (iv) Sidha System

The main components of the Scheme are:

1. The dispensary services including domiciliary care
2. FW and MCH Services
3. Specialist consultation facilities both at dispensary, polyclinic and hospital level including X-Ray, ECG and Laboratory Examinations.
4. Hospitalization
5. Organization for the purchase, storage, distribution and supply of medicines and other requirements
6. Health Education to beneficiaries

The dispensary is the backbone of the Scheme. Instructions on these various matters have been issued from time to time for the guidance of the specialists and medical officers. With the rapid and continuous expansion of the Scheme, however, not only situation has changed and problems arisen but also the rapidly expanding staff have not approved practices, procedures and instructions in regard to their various duties and responsibilities. In the paragraphs is set out the gist of provisions of the Scheme, various instructions and order issued form time to serve as a Compendium for the guidance of the CGHS staff.

## CGHS Cards

### *Definition of Family*

In accordance with the initial instructions, the term of 'Family' for the purposes of the Scheme shall consist of the government servant's wife or husband, as the case may be, children and stepchildren and parents who are mainly dependent on and residing with the Government servant concerned. Subsequently, in pursuance of the recommendations of the Fourth Central Pay Commission, it has been decided that for availing the medical facilities under the scheme, parents, sisters, widowed sisters, widowed daughters, minor brothers and children will be deemed dependent on the government employee if they are residing with him and their income from all sources including pension and pension equivalent of DCRG benefit is less than ₹ 1,500 per month.

### *Entitlement of the Scheme*

All Central Government Servants paid from Civil Estimates (other than those employed in Railway Services and those employed under Delhi Administration except members of Delhi Police Force) having their headquarters in cities where the Scheme is functioning and members of their families, are entitled for the CGHS medical facilities.

### *Transfer*

In case the Central Government employee is transferred to uncovered city leaving behind his family, the government employee is not entitled for the medical benefits either for himself or for his family under the Scheme but will be governed under CS(MA) Rule.

### *Family Welfare Activities*

The beginning of family welfare activities in Central Government Health Scheme was made in 1955 when Family Welfare Centres in six dispensaries were established under a full time Lady Medical Officer. In the year 1976, each allopathic dispensary of Central Government Health Scheme, Delhi was given one Family Welfare worker for Family Welfare and MCH services. IUD programme was introduced under CGHS in 1965 in three centres and it was subsequently extended to all allopathic dispensaries of CGHS, Delhi in December, 1976.

In other CGHS Centres the Family Welfare Programme depends upon the State Government Hospitals and other recognized hospitals, where Central Government Health Scheme beneficiaries avail facilities.

### Family Welfare Activities of CGHS, Delhi

In CGHS Delhi at present 87 allopathic dispensaries, two maternity centres and one gynae and maternity hospital are functioning to provide ante-natal, post-natal family welfare and MCH services to the CGHS beneficiaries. In addition to these services Lodi Road, II and Chitra Gupta Road dispensaries have a separate set-up of MSW to distribute conventional contraceptives. Distribution centres have also been set up in some of the larger offices and industrial establishments.

Besides giving advice and guidance to the married couples, the centres also supply family planning materials. Family Welfare Cell, CGHS, Delhi arranged to impart training in IUCD insertion to a number of lady medical officers as well as Family Planning para-medical staff with a view to enable them to conduct the programme more effectively with enhanced skill.

### Family Welfare Activities

*(a) Family Learning Methods*

1. Sterilization
2. IUD
3. Nirodh
4. Oral pills

*(b) Maternal and Child Health*

1. Ante-natal/Perinatal/Post-natal check ups

*(c) Immunization*

1. DPT
2. Polio
3. TT

4. DT
5. Measles and MMR
6. BCG. (Given by public Hospital/Local Bodies)

*(d) Information, Education and Communication Activities*

1. Documentaries/Film Shows
2. Orientation Training camp
3. Seminars
4. Composite programmes
5. Group Meetings
6. Well baby shows
7. Exhibitions

### *Family Welfare Services Under CGHS, Delhi*

The Central Government Health Scheme provides free of cost a package of Family Welfare services to the CGHS beneficiaries and to those who are not. Certain benefits, however, are available to Government employees only. It provides consultation and guidance at the dispensary level to all eligible couples along with specialized services in the CGHS hospitals. It supplies conventional contraceptives (such as Nirodh) to the beneficiaries, free of cost.

### *Copper-T (IUCD)*

The facility for insertion of Copper-T is available at CGHS dispensaries. The insertion is performed by trained lady medical officers.

### *Antenatal and Postnatal Checkup*

Each dispensary provides facilities for regular antenatal and postnatal checkups of female beneficiaries.

### *Well Baby Clinic*

The health of small babies and children is well cared for at the dispensaries and necessary expertise, consultation, immunization and treatment are provided to the beneficiaries.

### *Immunization Programme*

The entire range of essential immunization programme is carried out in dispensaries to protect children against polio, diphtheria, whooping cough and tetanus.

### *Medical Termination of Pregnancy*

The facilities for medical termination of pregnancy can be availed of, in the CGHS: approved hospitals and CGHS Maternity Centres (e.g. Srinivaspuri and Kalkaji in New Delhi) along with Maternity Hospital, Rama Krishna Puram.

### *Admission of Maternity Cases*

The beneficiaries are advised to get the names registered in the CGHS approved hospitals well in time so that the patient can get all medical facilities in time.

If the beneficiaries intend to go for confinement in a recognized private hospital, they can obtain permission from the concerned department, once pregnancy is confirmed by Medical Officer of CGHS Dispensary/Government Specialist. However, antenatal check up is to be obtained through dispensary/Government Hospitals.

### *Vasectomy and Tubectomy*

These terminal methods of sterilization can be availed of, at the CGHS approved hospitals/centres, as approved institution by Directorate of Family Welfare, Delhi Administration.

Duties of Chief, Medical/Sr Medical Officer/MO:

1. The medical officer will provide comprehensive medical care including preventive and curative, family welfare and MCH and health education to the beneficiaries.
2. He will also scrutinize the CGHS 'token number' before providing treatment. As per rules, production of card is necessary at the time of each visit, whether it be a new case or old.
3. He will restrict himself to general list of the formulary. But in case he has to prescribe any specialist item he should take prior concurrence from Chief Medical Officer, in charge. He will not write of his own any medicine meant for consultants/Specialist.
4. *Issue of Chit:* All Medical Officers must issue chits for restricted medicines in his/her own handwriting. The chits must show the name and quantity (in words and figures) clearly and must be signed and properly dated. No cutting/overwriting will be allowed on chits.
5. *Domiciliary Visit:* He/she should undertake domiciliary visit as per instructions issued from time to time and should not avoid the same. Even by implication, beneficiaries must not be asked to provide transport.

6. *Family Welfare Programme MCH and. Health Education:* All Medical Officers must take active interest to promote the Family Welfare programme, MCH and Health Education.
7. He/she should help Chief Medical Officer/Medical Officer in charge in maintaining cleanliness of the dispensary, supervision of the work at dressing room, injection room, checking of various dispensary accounts and general administration, as desired by the Medical Officer-in-charge/CMO I/C.
8. *Specialist Consultation:* The Medical Officer may refer a case to a specialist according to the instructions already laid down.
9. *Emergency Duty:* The Medical Officer is required to perform emergency duty by turn during non-working hours and on Sundays and Gazetted holidays in the functioning of the dispensary as per instructions issued from time to time.

The Medical Officer will keep the medical certificate, fitness certificate books and chit books and authority slips under his safe custody and under no circumstances will this be handled by any other staff.

The Medical Officer will perform such other duties as may be assigned to him by the Medical Officer-in-charge/Zonal Headquarters or Directorate from time to time.

## Reproductive Health

In recent years, levels of mortality in India have been declining and gender differentials in mortality narrowing. This, however, should not be interpreted to mean that reproductive health does not continue to be a matter of critical importance. This review of India's reproductive health situation underscores this note of caution. The review focuses on the fertility-related aspects of reproductive health in India, its levels, determinants and interventions designed to improve it; it touches on such issues as sterility and sexually transmitted diseases. Recognizing that reproductive health goes beyond the medical, we attempt here to synthesize the evidence available from a variety of sources: social science, public health and medical.

There is a tendency to equate reproductive health with maternal mortality, so at the outset we must note that reproductive health encompasses both mortality and health (WHO, 1991; Sai and Nassim, 1989). Such measures as maternal, foetal, prenatal and neonatal mortality are undoubtedly the most critical manifestations of poor reproductive health, but this should not detract from other important quality-of-life concerns such as anaemia, morbidity, obstetric conditions, birth weight, abortion and related complications, closely-spaced pregnancies, unmet need for contraception, infertility and incidence of STDs. Together, these mortality and morbidity indicators, are a true reflection of reproductive health. Equally important are factors underlying reproductive health. Reproductive health in India is largely influenced by poverty-related and socio-cultural factors on the one hand, and programme interventions on the other. Socio-cultural factors which impinge on reproductive health include women's lack of awareness of health practices, strong seclusion norms which inhibit health-seeking, adolescent marriage, large family size norms which in turn encourage frequent and closely spaced pregnancies, and a general devaluation of women which makes them the last to obtain food or health care and which requires of them long periods of physical activity. Interventions directed towards reproductive health include the Maternal and Child Health, Integrated Child Development Services and Family Planning Programmes. This review considers each of these underlying sets of factors and the ways in which they affect reproductive health at various stages of the life cycle.

### Level of Maternal, Perinatal and Neonatal Mortality

Currently the main indicator of women's health, maternal mortality, is recognized as the tip of the iceberg of the problems caused by sexuality and reproduction (Sai and Nassim, 1989). Unfortunately, maternal deaths are notoriously under-reported even in the more developed world, since often when the cause of death is a non-obstetric condition, precipitated by an obstetric condition, the latter is not reported; underestimates in the range of 33–50 per cent have thus been observed even in the USA (Royston and Armstrong, 1989). In India, misclassification is compounded by sparse and unreliable civil registration data and few community level studies. Results from hospital studies are more numerous and point to high rates but are misleading since they are not representative of the population at large.

India's maternal mortality ratio (MMR) is estimated at 400–500 per 1,00,000 live births – about fifty times higher than that of many industrialized nations and six times as high as that of neighbouring Sri Lanka (UNICEF, 1991; Acsadi and Johnson-Acsadi, 1990). This appears to be an underestimate and a more realistic estimate is probably 555 as estimated by Mari Bhat et al. (1992), though higher estimates in the range of 700–900 (Mathai, 1989) have also been made.

Even so, using the estimated MMR of 400–500, in the global perspective, it is estimated that India accounted for 19 per cent of all live births worldwide, and for as much as 27 per cent of all deaths.

Not only is the risk of dying from maternal causes high, but also, women in India are repeatedly exposed to these risks as a result of high and closely-spaced fertility stretching from adolescence to menopause. Maternal deaths in India account for about one per cent of all deaths and two per cent of all female deaths annually, but this translates into over ten per cent of all deaths among women in the reproductive ages and 13.2 per cent among rural women in 1987 (UNICEF, 1991). The lifetime risk of dying from pregnancy-related causes in India – with a total fertility rate of 4–5 and a maternal mortality ratio of around 500 per 1,00,000 live births – is as high as one in 27 (Royston and Armstrong, 1989).

More intensive investigations of maternal mortality come from small field studies. There are few community or household level studies of maternal mortality. Notable among these is a 1985–86 village level study in Anantapur, Andhra Pradesh, which found a ratio of 830 and 545 in rural and urban areas respectively (Bhatia, 1988). Maternal deaths accounted for 38 per cent of all deaths to women in the reproductive ages in rural areas and 28 per cent in urban. Maternal mortality ranges from 2,166 per 1,00,000 live births in the least developed villages (as measured by location, communication and transport facilities, educational and other amenities), to 1,523 and 803 respectively among somewhat and adequately developed villages, to 516 in highly developed villages. As many as 66 per cent of maternal deaths had not been recorded by health workers; reasons could range from inability in attributing cause of death to simply a vested interest in minimizing reported maternal deaths.

Hospital-based studies of maternal mortality are more widely available. Ratios observed among these are expected to be higher than those for the community in general, because given that no more than 20 per cent of all deliveries occur in hospitals, it is the high risk cases who are more likely to be observed. A look at hospital-based studies indicates wide variation in maternal mortality ratio – ranging from 224 in a study in Madras to over 2000 in certain years in studies in Haryana and West Bengal, with the majority reporting ratios around 1,000–1,500.

Data on maternal mortality from vital registration systems, health service statistics and the few sample surveys that exist are unreliable, incomplete and of limited coverage. Indirect techniques to estimate maternal mortality seem promising in these circumstances; one example is the 'sisterhood' method (Graham et al., 1989), which derives estimates of maternal mortality from faulty data.

Aside from maternal mortality, high rates of miscarriage and stillbirth as well as of prenatal and neonatal mortality are a direct consequence of poor reproductive health and antenatal, natal and neonatal care. For example 1.5 million prenatal deaths occur annually; the prenatal mortality rate is 66 per 1,000 live births as compared to 10–20 in many developed countries. In limited prospective studies, prenatal mortality rates ranging from 46–80 in rural areas, and 39 to 47 in urban, have been observed (Singh and Paul, 1988).

Over this eleven-year period 1976–87, there has been a modest decline of roughly 25 per cent, that is, about 2.2 per cent annually in each measure of mortality: infant mortality fell from 129 to 94, post-neonatal mortality from 52 to 38; neonatal and prenatal mortality from 77 to 58 and from 67 to 50 respectively; and stillbirths from 18 to 13. Over the 1980–85 period, it has been post-neonatal rather than neonatal or prenatal mortality which has recorded major declines, suggesting that the exogenous causes of death have been more effectively controlled than the endogenous: while the infant mortality rate fell by 17 per cent, post-neonatal mortality recorded an 18 per cent decline compared to a decline of 13 per cent in neonatal and 14.2 per cent in prenatal mortality, and 10 per cent in the stillbirth rate. On the whole, neonatal deaths account for about 60 per cent of all infant deaths and 50 per cent of neonatal deaths occur in the first week of life; nearly 25 per cent of all neonatal deaths (i.e. 15% of all infant deaths) occur in the first 24 hours of life (Holla, 1985). In short, the evidence reiterates the importance of endogenous factors which are a reflection of poor reproductive health.

## Causes of Maternal, Perinatal and Neonatal Deaths

### *Maternal Deaths*

India is typical of a high mortality setting. Sepsis, abortions, haemorrhage, toxaemia and anaemia account for the large majority of all maternal deaths over the decade of the 1980s (Registrar General, 1987; Bhatia, 1988). In 1981, for example, these five conditions accounted for three-quarters (75%) of all maternal deaths, and 72 per cent in 1986. Anaemia accounts for 17–25 per cent of all deaths; haemorrhage for 16–22 per cent; sepsis for 8–13 per cent of all deaths; and, despite legislation, roughly 10 per cent of all maternal deaths are attributed to abortion. Toxaemia accounts for another 10–12 per cent. That infective diseases become exacerbated and life-threatening in pregnancy is evident from both hospital and local level sample surveys (Bhatia, 1988); Bhatia in fact observes that 10 per cent of after maternal deaths resulted from infective hepatitis and 7 per cent from gastro-enteric diseases.

This cause of death distribution suggests that a large number of maternal deaths are preventable, if attention is paid to three principal underlying conditions among women in India: poor health care, poor nutrition and high and closely spaced fertility stretching from adolescence to menopause. A number of medical studies report on preventable maternal deaths: by and large, well over two-thirds of all maternal deaths are held to be preventable (Agarwal et al., 1982; Bhaskar Rao, 1980; Panat and Mehendale, 1987; Roy Chowdhury and Sikdar, 1982; Mitra and Khara, 1983; Sinha, 1986). A multicentric study from some eleven states and union territories in the late 1970s suggests that 70 per cent of all deaths were preventable; a more recent study of deaths in New Delhi suggests that about 90 per cent were (Raichowdhuri et al., 1990). The Anantapur study of maternal mortality suggests that 41 per cent of the deaths could have definitely been prevented and 37 per cent could have possibly been prevented (Bhatia, 1988).

### *Perinatal and Neonatal Deaths*

Between 1980 and 1986, diseases peculiar to infancy accounted for a steady three-fifths or more of all infant deaths. More specifically, over one-quarter of all infant deaths in 1986 were attributed to prematurely (27%), almost one-tenth to respiratory infection (9%), and 7 per cent to diarrhoea of the newborn. Another 8 per cent resulted from other causes including cord infection.

Local level studies reiterate that perinatal and neonatal mortality are overwhelmingly due to maternal factors, notably poor nutrition and inadequate ante-and infra-natal care. Various studies report that prematurity and low birth weight are directly responsible for about one-quarter of all infant deaths and are associated factors in about 50 per cent of all neonatal deaths (Roy Choudhary and Jayaswal, 1989; Agarwal and Agarwal, 1987; Singh and Paul, 1988). Bacterial infection (mostly tetanus) is responsible for about one-tenth of all early infant deaths (Singh and Paul, 1988).

Study after study reports the links between maternal education, age and parity and early infant mortality (Roy Choudhary and Jayaswal, 1989; Agarwal and Agarwal, 1987). A multicentric hospital study (Mehta, 1983) reports a prenatal mortality rate of 58 per 1000 live births among uneducated women, compared to 41 among women with any education. A study in Bihar and Uttar Pradesh (Agarwal and Agarwal, 1987) observes that neonatal mortality is even more sensitive to maternal factors than is infant mortality. Neonatal mortality was about three times as high among illiterate women (99 in Bihar and 78 in Uttar Pradesh) as among women with more than a primary school education (36 and 29 respectively); corresponding disparities in infant and in post-neonatal mortality are less dramatic.

### *Childhood and Adolescence*

This pattern of high maternal and early infant mortality in India is a reflection of a series of social, cultural and economic circumstances which can be traced to the low status women occupy relative to men, and its seeds are sown long before the occurrence of pregnancy. Here we examine childhood and adolescence factors which impinge subsequently on reproductive health.

### *Nutrition and Health Care*

The poor nutritional and growth status of the mother is a reflection of her own growth as a foetus, newborn, child and adolescent. Nutritional status is recognized as a major risk factor for maternal and peri/neonatal mortality as well as the incidence of low birth weight and preterm infants. Follow-ups of cohorts of girls (Ramachandran, 1989) confirm that growth levels in childhood are an important determinant of age at menarche, nutritional status and weight in adulthood.

Under conditions of wide gender disparities which exist in India, malnourishment and limited access to health care are considerably more evident among females than among males from birth onwards (Das Gupta, 1987; Acsadi and Johnson-Acsadi, 1990). Boys are fed better (Das Gupta, 1987; Khan et al., 1988) and are much more likely to receive early access to health care in case of illness. Studies which have monitored growth and nutritional status among children (Srikantia, 1989; Government of Maharashtra and UNICEF–WIO, 1991) confirm gender disparities in growth and severe malnutrition from an early age. One consequence of this is poor adolescent weight and height: it is estimated (Gopalan, 1989) that 47 per cent of 15-year olds in India have body weights less than 38 kg and 39 per cent have heights less than 145 cm.

### *Early Marriage and Adolescent Childbearing*

The early onset of childbearing has disturbing consequences for reproductive health. As many as 6.2 per cent and 43.4 per cent of girls aged 10–14 and 15–19 respectively are already married at this age. In some northern states, in fact, a number of household surveys suggest that between 20 and 40 per cent of all girls are married by age 15. Following marriage, there are socio-cultural pressures on the young woman to conceive as soon as possible – this is one means whereby she can attain both prestige and security in her new home. Hence, adolescent marriage is synonymous with adolescent childbearing. And while most adolescent fertility occurs within marriage, there is some evidence of sexual activity among unmarried girls, not only in urban but also in rural areas.

It is estimated that as many as 10–15 per cent of all births annually occur to women in their early teens, before they are physically fully developed (Mathai, 1989; Kapil, 1990). The extra nutritional demands of pregnancy come at the heels of the adolescent growth spurt, which itself requires additional nutritional inputs, and results in the poor nutritional status of the pregnant adolescent (Ramachandran, 1989). As a result of the combined effects of shorter average maternal height, competition for nutrients between the mother's growth needs and the growth needs of her foetus, and also due to poorer placental functions of adolescent mothers, the risks of maternal mortality and peri- and neonatal-mortality are exceptionally high among adolescents (Leslie, 1991).

Hence, it is not surprising to note that maternal deaths are concentrated in the youngest ages: 1986 data from rural India suggest that as many as 45 per cent of all maternal deaths took place among women aged under 24 (Registrar General, 1987; rates for adolescents are not separately available). Evidence of differentials in age-specific maternal mortality levels come from both small-scale surveys and hospital studies. Estimates derived from Bhatia's village level study in Andhra Pradesh (Acsadi and Johnson-Acsadi, 1990) suggest that adolescent maternal mortality ratios are almost twice as high as those reported for women aged 25–39: 1,484 per 1,00,000 live births among women aged 15–19 compared to 735, 708 and 736 for women aged 25–29, 30–34 and 35–39 respectively. A hospital study in a relatively low mortality setting in Bombay (now Mumbai) (Pachauri and Jamshedji, 1983) indicates that compared to women aged 20–29, adolescents experienced (a) a higher mortality rate (206 and 138 respectively); (b) higher spontaneous abortion (158 and 77) and stillbirth (35 and 29) rates; and (c) more difficulties in the ante-(29 and 28%) and infra-(12 and 9%) natal periods.

Not only are adolescent mothers more likely to die or suffer from morbidity, but the children they bear are also exposed to considerable risk. Neonatal mortality rates among adolescents are reported to be six times those of older women in a high mortality setting in rural Bihar and Uttar Pradesh (203 and 34 respectively; Agarwal and Agarwal, 1987) and 1.4 times that of older women in a low mortality hospital setting in Mumbai (Pachauri and Jamshedji, 1983). Adolescent mothers are also more likely to give birth to low-birth-weight and pre-term babies and experience other pregnancy-related complications (Aras et al., 1990; Pachauri and Jamshedji, 1983), even when exposed to identical levels of antenatal care and immunization and despite virtually identical levels of weight and hemoglobin at 20 weeks of pregnancy (Aras et al., 1989).

## Pregnancy and Antenatal Care

### *Pregnancy and Antenatal Factors*

The concept of special care during the antenatal period is not unknown traditionally in India. Pregnancy is associated with a number of cultural practices, ranging from those concerning diet to special rites. By and large, however, existing traditional practices concerning diet, combined with traditional omissions, notably the reluctance to seek antenatal care, do little to enhance reproductive health.

### *Antenatal Care (ANC): Registration, Visits*

Traditionally, little attention has been paid to women in the antenatal period, even traditional *dais* (midwife) coming into the picture only at delivery. The maternal and child health programme seeks to address this period of neglect. Under this programme, all pregnant women are to be routinely followed up either in the health centre or at home, and provided immunization, iron supplementation and regular check-ups to monitor the pregnancy. The available evidence on this programme, however, suggests that while antenatal care undoubtedly improves maternal and infant well-being, this service reaches few pregnant women. Few women are even aware of these services. On the national level, it is estimated that no more than 40–50 per cent of all pregnant women in India receive any antenatal care at all (Singh and Paul, 1988; Starrs and Measham, 1990; Acsadi and Johnson-Acsadi, 1990). And fewer women are actually registered for antenatal care: only 21 per cent of all pregnant women in the rural sector and 47 per cent in the urban (UNICEF, 1991; quoting NSS, 1986–87).

Local level sample surveys give a more disturbing picture of ANC service utilization and programme awareness (see also Gopalan, 1989; Mathai, 1989). A study of antenatal care services in Bihar, Rajasthan, Orissa (now Odisha), Maharashtra and Gujarat finds that maternal and child health (MCH) services hardly reached pregnant women: only between 5 and 22 per cent of all pregnant women in rural areas and between 20 and 50 per cent in urban areas (Kanitkar and Sinha, 1989). These findings are reiterated by other studies in these and other states, including Uttar Pradesh, Bihar, Rajasthan (Khan and Prasad, 1983; Mehta et al., 1983; Khan et al., 1988) and Punjab (Bhatinda district, Singh et al., 1988). It is only in Kerala where antenatal services are reported to have reached a large proportion of women (Khan and Prasad, 1983; Mehta et al., 1983).

Where visits do occur, they occur infrequently and their content is unclear (Jain and Agarwal, 1986; Murthy et al., 1990). Whereas at least five antenatal check-ups are considered ideal, pregnant women who received antenatal care have rarely had more than one or two contacts and that, too, only when halfway through the pregnancy (Gopalan, 1989).

The reasons for this poor utilization of services are cultural and socio-economic on the one hand but also a result of poor quality of services on the other. Kanitkar and Sinha (1989) observe that the large majority of women who did not utilize antenatal services considered it unnecessary. This could reflect the traditional notion that childbearing is not an event worthy of medical attention. It could also reflect dissatisfaction with the accessibility, quality and effect of services; a disturbing minority cited such reasons as lack of knowledge and economic and transportation problems. All these factors underscore the need for concentrated mass education efforts, a stepped-up domiciliary visit schedule and a general improvement in the quality of services.

Women who have received antenatal care experience lower maternal and early infant mortality, fewer complications and higher birth weight. As far as maternal mortality is concerned, the study in Anantapur, Andhra Pradesh, observes significant differences in visits for antenatal care between women who had died and those who had survived childbearing. Of women who had died, only 16 per cent had at least one antenatal visit to the health centre, compared to 27 per cent among women who survived (Bhatia, 1988). As far as prenatal mortality is concerned, a multicentric hospital study (Mehta and Jayant, 1981) found that two–thirds of all women who suffered a perinatal death had not received a single antenatal check-up; 30 per cent of all prenatal deaths (and half of all identifiable causes) are attributed to insufficient antenatal attention (Mehta, 1983). Antenatal care also affects birth weight: a study in Mumbai (Arcs et al., 1990) reports that 59 per cent and 69 per cent of women whose infants weighed less than 2.0 and 2.5 kilogrammes respectively had received antenatal care, compared to 86 per cent of those whose infants weighed 2.5 kilogrammes or more.

### *Identification and Referral of High-Risk Cases*

As a result of limited antenatal contacts, high-risk cases escape identification. In Anantapur for example, 49 per cent of the women who had died suffered anaemia, hepatitis and hypertension, which should have been identified as high-risk factors. Other risk factors which are to be identified by grassroots workers include age, weight, height, birth interval, parity (one, or more than 4), previous history of difficult pregnancy or infant loss, evidence of antenatal haemorrhage, poor weight gain (under 5 kilogrammes), excessive weight gain (to detect toxaemia), diarrhoea, dysentery or fever during pregnancy (Singh and Paul, 1988). However, frequently this is not done. And even if a high-risk case is identified, mothers frequently do not get satisfactory treatment at referral institutions (the PHC for example) because of lack of competent staff, equipment and even facilities for transporting the woman to the referral facility (Kapil, 1990).

### *Immunization*

Service statistics suggest that 16.18 million pregnant women were immunized against tetanus during 1988–89 (Ministry of Health and Family Welfare, 1990). We estimate (from 1988 population figures and 1986–89 crude birth rates) that this represents no more than 62.4 per cent of all pregnant women, with wide statewise variation. Community and survey-based assessments of antenatal immunization suggest that the situation may be far worse. In contrast to estimates from service statistics, surveys in rural Bihar, Gujarat and Odisha report rates fewer than 15 per cent; and in rural Maharashtra, about 28 per cent (Kanitkar and Sinha, 1989). A village-level study in Uttar Pradesh (Khan and Prasad, 1983) observed that of the 1,800 women who were pregnant in the year preceding the survey, only ten per cent received tetanus immunization (compared to an estimated 46 per cent from service statistics).

As a result of poor antenatal immunization, neonatal tetanus persists. Tetanus is estimated to account for some 2,30,000 to 2,80,000 infant deaths each year, well over half of which occur in Bihar and Uttar Pradesh (Sokhey, 1988; Singh and Paul, 1988; UNICEF, 1991). Tetanus is held to account for anywhere between one-and two-thirds of all neonatal deaths (Sokhey, 1988; Singh and Paul, 1988; UNICEF, 1984; Kapil, 1980; Agarwal and Agarwal, 1987).

### *Nutrition in the Antenatal Period*

There exists in India a wide range of cultural practices regarding diet during pregnancy, both on how much and on what to eat. Unfortunately, these are unlikely to foster improvements in antenatal nutrition since they tend to discourage increases in women's already meagre average daily food intake (Ramachandran, 1989) and in such nutritional items as leafy vegetables during pregnancy. A village level study in Uttar Pradesh (Khan et al., 1988) suggests that even when women are aware of the importance of diet during pregnancy, cultural and economic priorities deny them access to better nutrition: one pregnant woman's daily food intake was four chapatis, two dishes of vegetables and two cups of tea only. Another study in rural Uttar Pradesh (Tripathi et al., 1987) observes that weight gain during pregnancy was of the order of only 6.0–6.5 kg among poorly nourished women and 8.1–8.3 kg among better nourished women.

As a result, anaemia is widespread among pregnant women (haemoglobin levels below 11.0 g/dl); it is estimated to range from 40–50 per cent in urban areas to 50–70 per cent in rural areas (UNICEF, 1991; Kapil, 1990; Bhardwaj et al., 1990; Mathai, 1989), higher in such states as Bihar and Uttar Pradesh (Agarwal and Agarwal, 1987) and almost 90 per cent in rural areas where hookworm infestation is endemic (Ramachandran, 1989). Haemoglobin levels tend to deteriorate in the course of pregnancy; compared to a mean level of 10.8 g/dl among non-pregnant women, haemoglobin levels fell steadily to 10.4 g/dl, 9.7 g/dl and 9.4 g/dl respectively in the first, second and third trimesters of pregnancy (Srikantia, 1989a). Parity also affects haemoglobin levels: while 24 per cent of women with two or fewer pregnancies had haemoglobin levels below 9 g/dl, the corresponding proportion among women with three or more pregnancies was over 42 per cent.

Thus, not only is anaemia a leading direct cause of maternal deaths, but it also contributes indirectly by aggravating other complications of pregnancy such as eclampsia, antepartum haemorrhage, sepsis and genito-urinary tract infections. And not only does it affect mortality, but it impairs the health of many more women; puerperal morbidity tends to be 3–4 times higher in women with haemoglobin levels below 6.5 g/dl compared to normal women (Kapil, 1990). Consequences of maternal anaemia for infants are equally acute. For example, three-fifths of all infants born to women with haemoglobin levels less than 5.0 g/dl were low birth weight, compared to one-quarter of those born to women with normal haemoglobin levels (Ramachandran, 1989); prenatal mortality rates are ten times higher among severely anaemic women compared to normal women. A study in Uttar Pradesh shows that 62 per cent of infants born to women who gained less than 5 kg during pregnancy were low birth weight compared to 38 per cent among women who gained 7–9 kg (Mathai, 1989). Links between low birth weight and early infant death are well known: low-birth-weight infants account for over 70 per cent of all prenatal deaths, 90 per cent of all early neonatal deaths and half of all infant deaths (Ramalingaswami, 1985; Singh, 1986).

### *Food and Iron Supplementation*

Food and iron supplementation have been found to improve such maternal health attributes as weight gain, incidence of anaemia, complications during pregnancy and childbirth and birth weight (Dawn and Mitra, 1990; Iyengar, 1975). These findings have prompted a variety of strategies for supplementing the diets of pregnant women. The most ambitious of these is the Integrated Child Development Services (ICDS) programme, in which pregnant and lactating women are provided supplementary nutrition (500 kilocalories and 25 gramme of protein) daily Unfortunately, though this programme has been implemented for over a decade now, there is little information available on changes in reproductive health indicators in areas served by the programme. The little that is available from service statistics suggests that little more than half (51%) of all pregnant and lactating women eligible for this supplementary nutrition actually receive it (Ministry of Welfare, Department of Women and Child Development, 1991). In some states, the situation is worse: for example, both ICDS reports and an assessment of the utilization of ICDS services in Rajasthan (Jain and Agarwal, 1986) put this figure at 40 per cent.

The national anaemia prophylaxis programme of iron and folic acid distribution, in which pregnant women are provided with 100 iron and folic acid tablets during pregnancy, was initiated as early as the 1950s. However, both service statistics and sample surveys confirm that this programme has not been very successful. From service statistics, we find that no more than an estimated one-third of all pregnant and lactating women (as estimated from population and birth rate figures for 1988–89) have received iron and folic acid supplementation. Even more discouraging are the results of the few sample surveys on antenatal care, particularly in the four large northern states. A village level study in Uttar Pradesh (Khan et al., 1988) observed that only seven per cent of all pregnant women received iron and folic acid supplementation (compared to 26% for the state as a whole as estimated from service statistics). A micro-level evaluation by the Indian Council of Medical Research has shown that the programme has had little effect on the prevalence of anaemia among pregnant women (UNICEF, 1991); worse, there was little difference in the prevalence of anaemia between those who were supplied the tablets (88.1%) and those who were not (87.6%). Reasons underlying this ranges from inadequate supplementation to low acceptance, to poor quality of tablets.

### *Work in the Antenatal Period*

In India, the average rural woman neither increases her nutritional intake nor reduces her physical activity through her pregnancy (Ramachandran, 1989). The combination of poor pre-existing nutritional levels, inadequate diet during pregnancy, heavy physical activity and frequent childbearing results in further deterioration of maternal nutritional status and poor growth of the foetus (Tripathi et al., 1987). A village level study in Uttar Pradesh (Khan et al., 1988) observed that pregnant women work for as long as 13–14 hours a day, and throughout the pregnancy; time use data of five pregnant women suggests an average of 13 hours of physical labour, including both wage and domestic work and no more than 6–7 hours of rest. Reports of similarly long average work days among pregnant women come from Andhra Pradesh, too (Mathai, 1989). Walking long distances to collect fuel and water results in high calorie expenditure, which is rarely offset by additional food intake. Even when pregnant women are aware of the need for additional rest during pregnancy, economic and domestic demands on their time take precedence and few women can afford to reduce physical labour during pregnancy (Khan et al., 1986).

### *During the Birth*

Contact with the health care network at the intranatal stage is even poorer than at the antenatal stage. At the time of delivery, no more than twenty per cent of all women have some contact with medical or paramedical personnel. Deliveries are largely conducted by untrained personnel and in unhygienic conditions, both of which contribute significantly to poor maternal health.

### *Attendance at Birth*

A decade ago, in 1984, no more than 15 per cent of all rural births were performed in an institution and as many as two-thirds were delivered by untrained workers and others. And in such states as Bihar, Jammu & Kashmir, Madhya Pradesh, Odisha, Rajasthan and Uttar Pradesh, more than three out of four births are delivered by an untrained attendant. And what is disturbing is the evidence that over the 1971 to 1987 period, the picture has hardly changed. The proportion of births conducted institutionally increased from 8 to 15 per cent in rural areas and from 32 to 47 per cent in urban. The proportion of births delivered by untrained attendants fell from 81 per cent in 1971 to 68 per cent in 1987 in rural areas and from 43 per cent to 39 per cent in urban areas. Even so, there are rural areas of the country where nine out of ten births are delivered by an untrained attendant (Khan et al., 1986 for Uttar Pradesh; Kanitkar and Sinha, 1989 for Bihar, Rajasthan and Gujarat).

In these circumstances, the role of the estimated 5,00,000 traditional birth attendants in India – about one per 1,000 population – becomes especially important (Singh and Paul, 1988; Planning Commission, 1985). Collaboration between the health sector and the traditional birth attendant is an important way of bridging two very different cultures concerning reproductive health but this link has not yet been effectively exploited. And the little evidence which is available (for example, Kumar and Walia, 1983) suggests that trained attendants do in fact have significantly better health care knowledge and can better recognize high-risk conditions, suggesting the importance of training of traditional birth attendants. But we have little evidence on reproductive health outcomes in areas served by trained *dais* (midwife), and this is a topic worthy of further investigation.

### *Birth Hygiene*

For the most part, delivery continues to be conducted under unhygienic conditions. A 1984–85 study of traditional birth attendants (Sharma and Bali, 1989) in slums in Delhi reveals that, among intranatal practices, as many as 80 per cent did not wash their hands before delivery (119/141) and two-thirds used an unsterilized (but fresh) blade to cut the cord. This is quite consistent with a hospital based study of neonates with tetanus which reports that in all cases, unsterilized blades, knives or broken glass were used to cut the cord (Kumar et al., 1988). We would do well to be reminded that China's success in reducing the number of deaths from sepsis and neonatal tetanus is attributed largely to the teaching of simple hygienic principles of clean hands, clean perineum and clean cord care.

## Other Factors Affecting Reproductive Health

Other factors concerning reproductive health range from conditions in the immediate postnatal period (morbidity, breast-feeding and nutrition, and birth spacing) to more general concerns such as contraception and abortion on the one hand, and infertility and exposure to sexually transmitted diseases on the other.

### *Morbidity*

For every maternal death in India, there are at least 20 mothers suffering from impaired health (Kapil, 1990), suggesting an additional 2.4 million mothers with impaired health and efficiency as a result of pregnancy-related causes. Complications in pregnancy and childbirth can result in poor maternal health: incontinence, uterine prolapse and infertility are commonly associated with pregnancy-related complications. Pelvic inflammatory disease is commonly associated with unclean hands or instruments during delivery and can lead to infertility. Infectious diseases are more common and more serious in pregnancy.

Despite the fact that most maternal and neonatal deaths occur in the immediate postnatal period, few women are visited by health workers during this period. In Anantpur, for example, as many as 60 per cent of maternal deaths took place within five days of delivery (Bhatia, 1988) and yet we have evidence that no more than one-third of all who have just given birth are visited by health workers in the first week after delivery (Mathai, 1989). Given the cultural setting in which neither mother nor child is allowed out of the house in the first 40 days, this lack of contact during the early postnatal period could have serious implications for reproductive health.

Maternal morbidity has serious implications in terms of the chronic suffering and poor quality of life it brings. Yet universally, indicators of maternal morbidity remain undeveloped and no systematic attempt at classifying them has been made. The little evidence available from India suggests a high incidence of gynecological diseases. A village level investigation of rural women in Maharashtra (Bang et al., 1989) observed on physical examination that some 92 per cent were found to have one or more gynecological diseases; infections of the genital tract, including pelvic inflammatory disease, vaginitis and cervicitis, contributed half of this morbidity. Despite this high prevalence, only 8 per cent had undergone gynecological examination and treatment in the past.

### *Breast-feeding and Lactational Amenorrhoea*

Breast-feeding continues to be fairly universal and prolonged in India, up to about 24 months in rural areas. During lactation, women continue to subsist on average on 1,200–1,600 kilocalories daily, out of which 450–500 are required to meet the demands of milk production (Ramachandran, 1989a), leaving 800 calories to meet the woman's requirements; this ratio is suggestive of considerable daily weight loss and maternal depletion. At the same time, however, prolonged breast-feeding has tremendous advantages for the infant. Even so, unhealthy traditional breast-feeding practices continue which have a negative effect on early infant survival: even in the metropolis of Mumbai (UNICEF–WIO, 1991), colostrums is discarded, prelacteal feeds are given and the introduction of supplementary foods is delayed to well beyond six months. As a result of this, compounded by poor hygiene and sanitation, growth faltering is commonly observed after six months among low income households (Ramachandran, 1989a).

### *Frequent Childbearing*

Women in South Asia have more pregnancies than in any other region of the world other than Sub-Saharan Africa. Women in India remain largely valued for their reproductive performance, and large numbers of children and sons in particular (at least two) are widely desired. With a total fertility rate of 4.3, the average woman spends a large proportion – about one-third – of her reproductive years in pregnancy and lactation. Early, frequent and rapid childbearing is then the norm, reinforcing, in turn, women's already poor reproductive health and enhancing their chances of pregnancy-related complications. Unfortunately there are few studies in India on the relationship between birth intervals and maternal depletion, health or mortality. An analysis of all maternal deaths occurring in three hospitals in Bangkok, however, confirms that women with a previous birth interval of less than two years had a 250 per cent higher risk of dying than women with a longer birth interval (Royston and Armstrong, 1989). Studies in India (Ramachandran, 1989) indicate that morbidity among women who conceive during lactation is considerably higher than in other women; the mean birth weight of infants born within a twelve-month interval from a previous birth was significantly lower than those born after a twelve-month interval.

Finally, there is the familiar link between the length of the birth interval and infant mortality: a study in Punjab in the 1970s reports infant mortality rates of 206 for those born after an interval of less than one year, compared to 132 and 108 for births occurring after intervals of 2–3 and more than 4 years respectively (Sadik, 1980). Another study (Chatterjee, 1989) indicates that births occurring within 12 months of a previous one are exposed to a mortality rate of 200 compared to 100 in cases where the birth interval exceeds 12 months. Apart from higher mortality, short birth intervals are associated with growth faltering of the immediately older sibling.

### *Contraception*

Though contraceptive prevalence rates have been increasing, more births in India continue to be averted by the practice of prolonged breast-feeding than by contraception. Where contraception is practiced, it is usually for limiting rather than spacing fertility and, indeed, knowledge of non-terminal methods is poor. While 42 per cent of all currently married women in the reproductive ages practise some form of contraception, few (only 12%) use a non-terminal method, reflecting the unbalanced focus of the family planning programme on terminal rather than reversible methods. As a result, the current pattern of contraception offers women little relief from closely spaced pregnancies. Rather, it compresses childbearing into fewer years, usually terminating childbearing by the early thirties, by which time over three children have already been born.

Morbidity (and even mortality) arising from contraception is not unknown. In particular, the camp approach to sterilization and the increasing focus on IUDs have been associated with a variety of side-effects and more serious conditions ranging from excessive bleeding to pelvic inflammatory disease-pointing once more to a need for more hygienic service delivery conditions in general.

There continues to be considerable unmet need for family planning (currently married women who want no more children but are not using a method of contraception). Estimates of unmet need for India are of the order of 20 per cent: if women who wanted no more children were able to avoid another pregnancy, it is estimated that maternal mortality ratios would fall by up to 40 per cent (see Acsadi and Johnson-Acsadi, 1990).

### *Induced Abortion*

A sad reflection of the extent of unmet need is the fact that roughly five million abortions are performed annually in India, most of them illegally. In 1987–88, only about half a million abortions were performed under the health services network, while another estimated 4.5 million abortions occurred illegally (UNICEF, 1991). About two out of five legal abortions occur because of contraceptive failure (Ministry of Health and Family Welfare, 1989). There has also been a tendency in India to misuse amniocentesis to detect the sex of the foetus, and resort to abortion (usually of the female foetus) to arrive at the desired sex composition of children; this suggests the disturbing possibility of increased abortions and repeat abortions. Women resort to illegal abortions in large numbers for many reasons. Registered practitioners are unavailable: in 1984 for example, only about 1,000 physicians of a total of roughly 15,000 trained to perform abortions were in rural areas. Abortion can involve a cost to the patient, for saline and drugs, and this can be prohibitive for the average rural woman. Information about legal termination services is inadequate; there is limited publicity about the law and there is a widely held perception that abortion is illegal. And abortion services at approved centres tend to be impersonal and unattractive.

Mortality and morbidity arising from abortion continue to be high. We have seen that about 10 per cent of all maternal deaths are due to abortions: largely from sepsis and haemorrhage (84% from sepsis and 10 per cent from haemorrhage in one study (Kamalajayaram and Parameswari, 1988). Even so, the actual number of deaths due to abortion may be as high as 15–25 per cent (Starrs and Measham, 1990) since the majority of deaths from abortion are unreported as such, and most illegal abortions are conducted by untrained practitioners under unhygienic conditions. This is corroborated by evidence from hospital based studies (Bansal and Sharma, 1985; Mather and Rohatgi, 1981; Kamalajayararn and Parameswari, 1988) suggesting a high incidence of abortion-related mortality and morbidity.

### *Infertility and Sexually Transmitted Diseases*

Far less evidence is available on the levels and patterns of infertility. Evidence from the 1981 Census (Ministry of Health and Family Welfare, 1989) and a village level study in Maharashtra (Bang et al., 1989) puts the level of infertility at 6–7 per cent, compared to 2–3 per cent in other developing countries (Sai and Nassim, 1989). Infertility poses a serious threat to female well-being in a culture which prizes reproduction – preventing her from achieving the family size which she desires and exposing her to various kinds of emotional harassment or marital disharmony. Factors underlying infertility include, among other things, women's poor health and nutrition status which can lead to repeated miscarriages and foetal waste, unhygienic obstetric and abortion procedures and even such debilitating diseases as tuberculosis.

Even less is known of the levels and patterns of sexually transmitted diseases which have severe implications for the reproductive health of both women and men. The available evidence suggests a relatively high prevalence of STDs. For example, an intensive village-level investigation of 650 women in Maharashtra (Bang et al., 1989) suggests that a disturbingly large proportion of women were suffering from syphilis (10.5%) and gonorrhoea (0.3%). Finally, about a million men and women are estimated to be suffering from HIV/AIDS with dangerous potential for its wider spread.

## Prospects for Improvements in Reproductive Health

Reproductive health features prominently in the government's stated goals for 'Health For All' by 2,000. Targets have been set for a variety of reproductive health components ranging from mortality rates to such health-related measures as levels of antenatal care, trained attendance at delivery, immunization and birth weight. Unfortunately, despite these programmes and these goals, the situation today remains discouraging: the chances of achieving these goals seem remote.

Rather than simply a medical problem, poor reproductive health is, of course, ultimately a reflection of the series of social, cultural and economic circumstances, which are not responsive to short-term strategies and go beyond the health sector. The most basic long-term solutions are of course poverty- and gender-related and here changes in female status in general are the key, and the expansion of educational and economic opportunities for women, improvement in nutrition and prevention of adolescent marriage are of particular importance.

Short-term benefits to reproductive health can accrue through well-implemented interventions which reduce not only mortality but also morbidity. Such interventions do, of course, exist but the thrust of their services has been so skewed that health benefits have been limited. While an impressive array of programmes exist in India to improve reproductive health, in practice the focus has been on sterilization, so that maternal and child health care, health and nutrition education, birth spacing and safe abortion have been relatively neglected. Programmes suffer from poor outreach, quality of services and care, and an inability to adapt services and messages to the cultural milieu of their beneficiaries. First, improvements in the quality of services and care are an important means by which to encourage service utilization and dispel the cynicism with which services are currently viewed. Second, in a culture where few women seek health services and seclusion practices inhibit health centre visits, outreach is critical; domiciliary visits by health personnel have to be not only frequent but of good quality and must cover a range of services, from antenatal care to nutrition, immunization, birth spacing and health education. Third, and equally important in a society in which the large majority of women are uneducated and unexposed to new ideas, information needs of rural women must be satisfied through culturally acceptable messages.

The assessment of reproductive health levels is handicapped by a scarcity of good data on most reproductive health outcomes, including both mortality and especially quality of life indicators. Most of the work currently available is clinic based and medically oriented but this is inadequate when it comes to assessing reproductive health and its underlying causes. Rigorous indirect estimates of maternal mortality, at the state and district levels are essential. Micro-level analyses of the links between reproductive health outcomes and their socio-economic and cultural antecedents in different settings would go a long way in tailoring services in a locally relevant way. So would studies on the impact of interventions designed to redress reproductive health deficiencies.

Finally a word of caution, it is tempting to infer from the fact that mortality levels have declined and gender differentials narrowed that the *reproductive health* of women is not a matter of serious concern. Evidence presented in this review offers strong support countering this inference. There is no denying that reproductive health in India continues to be unacceptably poor, and that national commitment to and investment in its improvement have been inadequate.

## Reproductive Health and Rights

In general, reproductive health issues are addressed through a variety of complementary, and sometimes contradictory, laws and policies. The manner in which these issues are addressed reflects a government's commitment to advancing reproductive health. The following section presents key legal and policy provisions that together determine women's reproductive rights and choices in India.

### *General Health Laws and Policies*

The Constitution enjoins the state to make the 'improvement of public health' a primary responsibility. The National Health Policy, adopted in 2002, and the Tenth Five-Year Plan create the primary framework for the delivery of public health services, and both aim to raise the health status of the population through ensuring equal access to primary health care for all citizens. The policy prescriptions of the National Health Policy are largely reflected in the Tenth Five-Year Plan.

The emphasis on primary health care in India's contemporary health and development policies is rooted in the thinking of the 1946

Bhore Commission Report, which declared that primary health care is a basic right of all individuals, regardless of their ability to pay for services or other socio-economic factors. The commission established primary health care as the foundation for the public health care system in India and developed the blueprint for the delivery of primary health care services in the public sector. India further manifested its commitment to these principles in 1978, at the International Conference on Primary Health Care held in Alma-Ata, USSR, at which it pledged to attain the Alma-Ata Declaration's goal of 'Health for All' by the year 2000 by striving to ensure all individuals' equal access to primary health care services.

### *Objectives*

The primary objective of the National Health Policy is to realize an 'acceptable standard of good health' among the general population. To achieve this goal, the policy points to the need to improve access to health services among all social groups and in all areas of the country. It proposes to improve access by establishing new facilities in areas where they are lacking and improving and upgrading existing facilities. The policy sets forth several time-bound objectives, which include the following:

- a reduction in maternal mortality and infant mortality rates to 100 in 1,00,000 and 30 in 1,000, respectively, by 2010;
- zero level of growth of HIV/AIDS by 2007;
- a 50 per cent reduction in mortality due to tuberculosis, malaria and other vector and water-borne diseases by 2010;
- an increase in the utilization of public health facilities;
- From less than 20 per cent to more than 75 per cent by 2010.

The policy also recognizes that women and other 'underprivileged' groups disproportionately experience poor access to health services, and it aims to facilitate such groups' access to basic health care services. Under the policy, the Central Government is to give top funding priority to programmes targeting women's health.

Some of the broad objectives of the Tenth Five-Year Plan also address health issues. The plan recognizes that 'economic growth cannot be the only objective of national planning ... over the years, development objectives are being defined not just in terms of increases in GDP or per capita income but more broadly in terms of enhancement of human well-being'. In view of the importance of citizens' health to national development, the plan commits to providing services such as essential primary health care, emergency life saving services, and services, under national programmes for disease control and family welfare free of cost to all, and further commits to providing essential health care services to people living below the poverty line. The plan specifically recognizes the failings of the Ninth Five-Year Plan with regard to quality of care objectives and commits to introducing quality control concepts and tools ... into every aspect of health care in order to ensure that the population and the system benefit from defined and institutionalized norms, accountability and responsibility. The plan also proposes to address deficiencies in the government's provision of health care services to low-income populations in urban slums and remote rural and tribal areas. Strategies and programmes for the prevention, control and treatment of communicable diseases comprise continued areas of focus.

## Infrastructure of Health Care Services

### *Government Facilities*

Health is a shared responsibility of the Central and State governments, although it is effectively a state responsibility in terms of execution of policies and services. The Ministry of Health and Family Welfare is the main governmental body in charge of developing national health policies and broad-based public health initiatives and coordinating implementation efforts of states. The ministry's divisions include the Department of Health, the Department of Family Welfare and the Department of Indian Systems of Medicine and Homeopathy.

India has a massive and largely under-funded public health infrastructure through which it primarily finances and delivers curative health care services and implements centrally sponsored family welfare and disease control programmes, including those relating to tuberculosis, HIV/AIDS, malaria, and leprosy.

In urban areas, primary health care services are delivered through a large network of health facilities, including postpartum centres, urban health posts and urban family welfare centres. There are 550 postpartum centres at the district level and 1,012 centres at the sub-district level.

These facilities provide the following services:

- essential obstetric care;
- early detection of complications arising from anaemia, bleeding, toxemia, obstructed labour, and sepsis;

- emergency maternity services, including vacuum extraction, delivery by caesarian section, blood transfusion and manual removal of placenta;
- all public health interventions for baby's well-being;
- family planning services for permanent and spacing methods of contraception; and
- satellite outreach services for the population and referral services for subdistrict centres and primary health centres.

There are presently 871 urban health posts, which provide primary health care, family welfare and maternity services. There are 1,083 urban family welfare centres, which also provide family welfare services.

In rural areas, a three-tiered infrastructure of sub centres, primary health centres and community health centres deliver primary health-care services to the rural population. The network of subcentres consists of 1,37,292 functioning facilities, which serve as the first contact point between the primary health care system and the community subcentres provide basic drugs for women and children's minor ailments and essential health needs. They are staffed by one male multipurpose worker and one female multipurpose worker/auxiliary nurse & midwife. One female health assistant oversees the work of a group of six subcentres and provides technical guidance and supervision to auxiliary midwife nurses. More than 97,000 of functioning subcentres are funded by the Department of Family Welfare; the remaining facilities are funded by state governments.

Primary health centres are established and funded by states and generally serve as the first contact point between the village community and a medical officer. There are currently 22,807 functioning primary health centres. These facilities provide 'curative, preventive, promotive' health care and family planning services. Each is staffed by a medical officer and 14 paramedical and other workers, and serves as a referral unit for a group of six subcentres.

Community health centres are similarly established and maintained by states and serve as a referral unit for a group of four primary health centres. Community health centres also provide obstetric care and specialist consultations. There are presently 3,027 functioning community health centres in India. Each is staffed by four medical specialists – a surgeon, physician, gynecologist, and pediatrician – and 21 paramedical and other workers.

A network of government hospitals also delivers primary, secondary and more specialized health care services to both the urban and rural population. These include district, subdistrict and rural hospitals. The majority of hospitals are located in urban areas.

### *Private Run Facilities*

The private health sector is composed largely of for-profit medically trained providers who operate their own clinics or work in facilities ranging from nursing homes with inpatient facilities that have generally fewer than 30 beds to large corporate hospitals. There are approximately 67,000 private hospitals, accounting for 93 per cent of all hospitals in India, a dramatic increase from an estimated 3,000 private hospitals in 1981. Qualified and registered private doctors and institutions are not readily available in remote rural and tribal areas, both because of a lack of social infrastructure and the inability of people to pay.

The private sector also includes a broad range of non-governmental actors. More than 7,000 voluntary agencies are involved in health-related activities, although their services are unevenly distributed among states and generally limited in scope. In addition to providing health services independent of the government, some NGOs help implement government health programmes sponsored by the Ministry of Health and Family Welfare. The government also has given funding to some NGOs to establish health care facilities in rural and marginalized urban areas in an effort to improve the quality and availability of their health services.

## Financing and Costs of Health Care Services

### *Government Financing*

Since independence, successive five-year plans have provided the framework for policy and funding decisions related to the development of India's health care infrastructure. Aggregate expenditure for health is about 5.2 per cent of GDP. In contrast, public health investment is about 0.9 per cent of GDP, which the National Health Policy aims to increase to 2.0 per cent by 2010. Spending on health is more often for curative than preventive care. State spending on health accounts for 75 per cent – 90 per cent of total public expenditure on health and is largely tied up in salary expenditures.

The central and state governments equally share spending on most national health programmes. The central government fully funds national programmes relating to disease control, including HIV/AIDS, and family planning. Central government funds also support medical education, training for nurses, emergency relief measures, and pilot projects to develop disease control or other health care strategies. States are responsible for most spending on primary, secondary and tertiary health institutions.

Health financing in India is predominantly private. Private health spending accounts for more than 80 per cent of total health spending, one of the highest proportions of private spendings in the world. Almost all such spending is out-of-pocket at the point of service. The private sector accounts for most curative care services in the country, although quality and distribution of services varies widely across states. The distribution of private services is heavily skewed towards the highest income groups. Although low-income individuals rely on public services for most of their health care needs, 79 per cent of outpatient care for those below the poverty line is provided by the private sector. However, this care is generally of low quality and provided by untrained practitioners.

Various international organizations and United Nations agencies provide significant technical and material assistance for many health and family welfare programmes in India. The World Bank, European Commission, United Nations Population Fund (UNFPA), United Nations Children's Fund (UNICEF), and other bilateral donors contribute funding to the Reproductive and Child Health Programme, the country's primary national programme focused on reproductive health. The World Bank contributed USD 248.3 million to the first phase of the programme, which spanned 1997–2002, and an equal amount for the second phase. The European Commission approved assistance of ECU 200 million while UNFPA provided USD 100 million for the programme.

From 2001–2002, the World Health Organization (WHO) contributed funding and technical assistance to the implementation of more than 33 projects. Its funding amounted to approximately USD 13.7 million during this period. Some important WHO activities in India include supplying essential medicines, drugs and kits to primary health centres; helping control the spread of communicable diseases; and providing and promoting health education to low-income individuals and adolescents.

### Costs

The Tenth Five-Year Plan articulates a 'continued commitment' to providing essential primary health care, emergency life saving services, and services under government disease control and family welfare programmes, free of cost to all individuals. However, user charges currently apply for some health care services at public facilities, including public hospitals. Hospitalization due to major illness is a cause of debt among all income groups. Individuals receiving inpatient hospital treatment spend 58 per cent of their total annual expenditure on health care.

Less than 10 per cent of the total population is covered by health insurance in the governmental and private sectors, and those covered are primarily from upper-income groups, or government or industrial employees.

Central government employees and their families living in the capital and 18 other major cities are entitled to health care coverage through Central Government Health Schemes. Covered services include: outpatient care in all systems of medicine; emergency services in the Allopathic system (Western, curative medical system); free supply of necessary drugs; home visits to patients with serious illnesses; family welfare services; treatment in specialized hospitals in both the public and private sector; and a 90 per cent advance for necessary specialized hospital procedures.

In 1948, the Employees' State Insurance Act introduced a national health insurance programme for industrial employees. The act provides for compulsory state insurance for sickness, pregnancy and employment-related injury in all but seasonal factories. Under the act, employees and employers contribute to a fund held and administered by a corporation constituted under the Act.

In June 2000, the government launched a new group insurance scheme called Janashree Bima Yojana. The programme covers all families below the poverty line in urban and rural areas. In urban areas, coverage extends to people slightly above the poverty line as well. Families receive ₹ 20,000 on natural death, ₹ 50,000 on death or total permanent disability caused by accident, and ₹ 25,000 on partial permanent disability due to an accident.

The Health Ministers Discretionary Grant is a little known source assistance distributed by health ministers to help low-income individuals defray the costs of hospitalization and medical treatment, where free health services are unavailable. Low-income individuals qualify for such funds, but there are otherwise no fixed guidelines for determining eligibility. In 1999–2000, a total of ₹ 44,89,000 in assistance was distributed to 270 patients.

Public sector insurance companies are designing an insurance scheme called *Janraksha* targeted to needy populations. The programme would require subscribers to pay a premium of ₹ 1 per day to entitle them to receive inpatient treatment costing up to ₹ 30,000 per year at designated hospitals. Covered services also would include outpatient treatment at a cost of up to ₹ 2,000 per year at designated clinics such as those in public hospitals, medical colleges, private trust hospitals, and NGO-operated institutions.

Life Insurance Corporation of India launched *Jeevan Bharati* in March 2003, an insurance plan exclusively for women aged 18–50, the benefits of which include coverage for critical illnesses such as cancers of the breast, ovary and fallopian tubes and for congenital defects of newborn babies.

## Regulation of Health Care Providers

India has established statutory regulatory councils to monitor the standards of medical education, promote medical training and research activities, and oversee the qualifications, registration and professional conduct of doctors, dentists, nurses, pharmacists, and practitioners of non-traditional medical treatments such as Ayurveda, Siddha, Unani, yoga, and Naturopathy.

The Medical Council of India, established under the 1933 Indian Medical Council Act as repealed by the 1956 Indian Medical Council Act, oversees the licensing, educational standards, training and research activities of doctors, and maintains a register of all qualified medical practitioners in India. The council is also empowered to establish ethical and professional standards for medical practitioners. Violations of prescribed standards may result in the removal of a practitioner's name from a state medical register.

Similarly, the Dental Council of India, the Indian Nursing Council and the Pharmacy Council of India are statutory bodies that regulate the professions they oversee. The Central Council of Indian Medicine and the Central Council of Homeopathy regulate the educational and clinical programmes of the Indian Systems of Medicine and Homoeopathy, which include Ayurveda, Siddha, Unani, yoga, and Naturopathy treatments.

### *State Medical Councils have also been Established with Similar Overall Objectives*

The Indian Council of Medical Research is the primary governmental body that formulates, coordinates and promotes biomedical research. The Union Health Minister presides over the council's governing body. The council's research priorities, in line with those of the National Health Policy, include control and management of communicable diseases; fertility control; maternal and child health; and the development of alternative strategies for health care delivery. The council issued the Ethical Guidelines for Biomedical Research on Human Subjects in 2000. The guidelines provide for the establishment of institutional ethics committees to review all ethical aspects of proposed research protocols and monitor ethical compliance of approved projects. (See 'Regulation of Reproductive Technologies and Patients' Rights' sections for more information on the guidelines.)

## Regulation of Reproductive Health Technologies

### *Assisted Reproductive Technologies*

There is currently no law that regulates assisted reproductive technologies despite the emergence of a considerable number of specialized hospitals and infertility clinics in India.

The Delhi Artificial Insemination (Human) Act, enacted by the Delhi Legislative Assembly in 1995, legalizes the donation of semen and ova. The act calls for the registration of all sperm banks that store, sell, donate, and supply semen. It also requires that all semen be tested for HIV infection and prohibits the segregation of sperm according to gender markers for the X or Y chromosome. It mandates the confidentiality of donors and recipients and requires the written consent of both the woman who is receiving the sperm and her husband. Non-compliance with the Act results in strict punishment.

The Ethical Guidelines for Biomedical Research on Human Subjects also address ethical issues involved in assisted reproductive technologies. The guidelines address issues such as informed consent, donor selection protocol, the legitimacy of a child born through assisted reproductive technologies, surrogacy and the right of children born from such procedures and their adoptive parents to access relevant health information about a child's genetic parents. The guidelines also mandate minimal screening of all relevant parties for sexually transmissible infections (STIs), HIV/AIDS and hepatitis.

The Indian Council of Medical Research and the Draft National Academy of Medical Sciences have formulated the Draft National Guidelines for Accreditation, Supervision and Regulation of Assisted Reproductive Technology clinics in India, which were released for public debate in September 2002. The guidelines address the issues of surrogacy and the rights of the child born through various assisted reproductive technologies. They also express concern about the affordability and feasibility of related services.

The guidelines include the following provisions:

- Assisted reproductive technology clinics must not be a party to any chimerical dement in donor programmes or in gestational surrogacy;
- No assisted reproductive technology procedure shall be done without the spouse's consent;
- Sex selection at any stage – either before or after the fertilization or abortion of embryos of any particular sex – should not be permitted except to avoid the risk of transmission of a genetic abnormality linked to the biological parents or associated with pre-implantation genetic diagnosis;
- Use of sperm donated by a relative or a known friend of either the wife or the husband should not be permitted. It will be the responsibility of the assisted reproductive technology clinic to obtain sperm from appropriate banks;
- No relative or person known to the couple may act as a surrogate;
- Surrogacy by assisted conception should only be considered for patients who are physically or medically unable to carry a pregnancy to term;
- Sperm or egg donors may consent to have their embryos stored for up to five years for use by another couple or for research purposes;
- The sale or transfer of human embryos or any part thereof, or of gametes in any form and in any way, to parties outside of the country must be prohibited;
- A child born through assisted reproductive technologies is presumed to be the legitimate child of a surrogate couple, born within wedlock and with all the attendant rights of parentage, support and inheritance;
- Although there is no legal bar on an unmarried or single woman receiving artificial insemination, it is universally recommended that this procedure be performed only on married women who have the written consent of their husbands;
- There is an urgent need to treat infertility like any other disease and to require the government, an employer or an insurance carrier to cover all attendant expenses for one child.

### *Sex Determination Techniques*

In response to the proliferation and misuse of prenatal diagnostic centres for the purpose of among others, sex determination, leading to female feticide, the national legislature enacted the Pre-Conception and Pre-Natal Diagnostic Techniques (Prohibition of Sex Selection) Act in 1994, which has been amended twice, most recently in 2003. The Act prohibits the use of prenatal diagnostic tests for the purpose of determining foetal sex and the practice of 'sex selection'. Such tests may only be conducted at registered facilities and for limited purposes, including the detection of chromosomal abnormalities, genetic metabolic diseases, sex-linked genetic disorders and congenital anomalies.

For a prenatal diagnostic test to be authorized, one or more of the following conditions must be present:

- the pregnant woman is above age 35;
- the pregnant woman has undergone two or more spontaneous abortions or foetal losses;
- the pregnant woman has been exposed to potentially teratogenic agents such as drugs, radiation, infection, or chemicals;
- the pregnant woman or her spouse has a family history of 'mental retardation' or 'physical deformities'; or
- Any other condition specified by a supervisory board constituted under the Act.

Where authorized prenatal diagnostic tests are conducted, the Act prohibits medical providers from disclosing the foetus's sex to the pregnant woman or her relatives The advertisement of foetal sex determination services is also prohibited under the Act.

Contravention of the Act's provisions by those performing or seeking prohibited services is punishable with imprisonment and a fine. Medical practitioners also may have their licenses suspended for a first offense and revoked upon a second offense. A woman who is 'compelled' to undergo prenatal testing for the purpose of determining the sex of the foetus or to practise sex selection may not be punished under the Act. The Act provides a rebuttable presumption that any pregnant woman who undergoes such a test was 'compelled' by her husband or other relative.

The Act provides for the creation of supervisory boards at the central, state and union territory levels to monitor implementation of the Act, advise the government on related policy matters and conduct awareness-raising activities about the practice of sex selection and female foeticide.

The 2002 Indian Medical Council (Professional Conduct, Etiquette and Ethics) Regulations specifically prohibit medical practitioners from performing sex determination tests for the purpose of female foeticide. Violations of this provision constitute professional misconduct rendering the physician subject to criminal penalties and disciplinary action from the council.

The Ethical Guidelines for Biomedical Research on Human Subjects addresses the issue of prenatal diagnosis. 'The guidelines state that' [prenatal diagnosis] should be performed only for reasons relevant to the health of the fetus or the mother. [It] should not be performed solely to select the sex of a child (in the absence of an X-linked disorder). They urge medical practitioners to 'recognize the human and economic costs involved ... and limit its use to situations where there is a dear benefit'.

In September 2003, the Supreme Court directed the central and state governments to enforce laws banning ultrasound scans for the purposes of determining the sex of the foetus.

## Patients' Rights

There is no single national law that governs patients rights. Patients can seek remedial measures against doctors for medical negligence under the 1872 Indian Contract Act, Indian Penal Code, Law of Torts, the 1986 Consumer Protection Act, and the Indian Medical Council Act. Under the Indian Contract Act, a doctor is required to use 'reasonable professional skill and care'. A patient may sue under the Act for breach of contract in civil court for his or her doctor's failure to apply this level of skill and care.

Under the Indian Penal Code, medical practitioners can be held criminally liable for causing the death of a patient by negligence. Acts performed without criminal intent and in good faith to prevent other harm, or in good faith with the patient's express or implied consent or without consent when obtaining consent is impossible, are protected. A patient may also seek damages for medical negligence under the Law of Torts.

Under the Consumer Protection Act, patients may seek compensation for suffering loss or injury due to their medical practitioner's negligence. Although the Act does not expressly protect harm caused by medical services, judgments under the Act have held that paid, but not free, medical services are covered by the Act. Compensation has been granted in a number of medical negligence cases. Courts have also articulated the duty of medical practitioners to act with a reasonable degree of skill, care and knowledge.

A patient may also file a complaint with the appropriate State Medical Council for an act of professional misconduct by a medical provider. The council would then conduct an inquiry. The council may issue a warning, or suspend or terminate the provider's medical license, but is not empowered to award monetary damages to the patient.

The Ethical Guidelines for Biomedical Research on Human Subjects set forth the duties and rights of medical researchers and human research subjects with respect to issues including informed consent, non-exploitation, privacy, confidentiality, professional competence, accountability, and transparency.

In the 2000 Supreme Court case, *State of Haryana and Others v. Smt Santra,* the court held the state liable for a doctor's negligence in unsuccessfully performing a sterilization procedure after the patient became pregnant as a result of the failed procedure. The court awarded the patient monetary damages.

## Reproductive Health Laws and Policies

There is no comprehensive national health law or policy on reproductive health. However, several aspects of reproductive health are addressed in the Reproductive and Child Health Programme, a national programme aimed at providing integrated health and family welfare services for women and children. The Ministry of Health and Family Welfare reoriented and renamed its former Family Welfare Programme as the Reproductive and Child Health Programme in 1997, to improve the quality, distribution and accessibility of services and to meet the health care needs of women and children more effectively. The programme's key components include the following:

- prevention and management of unwanted pregnancy;
- services to promote safe motherhood;
- services to promote child survival; and
- prevention and treatment of reproductive tract infections and STIs.

The programme marked an important shift in the government's provision of reproductive health services 'from a focus on achieving method-specific contraceptive targets to providing client-centred quality services'. It abolished demographic targets and provider incentives that were identified by the central government for contraceptive use, and replaced them with a decentralized participatory approach to planning and monitoring reproductive and child health services, involving panchayats, women and community groups. Pursuant to this new approach, health plans are formulated at the primary health centre and subcentre levels, not at the national or state level as they were under the Family Welfare Programme. The decentralized participatory approach seeks to adapt the concepts for reproductive health and rights that emerged from the International Conference on Population and Development (ICPD).

## Family Planning

The Reproductive and Child Health Programme and National Population Policy, adopted in 2000, establish the framework for the government's delivery of family planning services.

A key objective of the Reproductive and Child Health Programme is to promote contraceptive use and provide a full range of contraceptive methods, including condoms, oral pills, IUDs, and male and female sterilization.

The National Population Policy aims to address the unmet need for contraception in order to meet the medium-term objective of reducing the national fertility rate to replacement levels by 2010 and the long-term objective of stabilizing the population growth rate by 2045. One of the 14 national socio-demographic goals identified in the policy is to achieve universal access to family planning information, counselling and services, including a wide range of contraceptives.

### *Contraception*

Almost half of married women of reproductive age currently use modern contraceptive methods.[285] There are wide differences between states in the levels of unmet need, with the highest levels in Bihar and Uttar Pradesh.[286] Female sterilization is the most widely known and used method in all states although, again, there are substantial differences between states and districts.[287] Thirty-four per cent of currently married women who have undergone sterilization, 3 per cent use condoms, 2 per cent use the pill, 2 per cent use IUDs, 2 per cent rely on male sterilization, and 5 per cent use traditional or other methods. Prevalence rates for almost all methods are higher in urban than in rural areas, with condom use more than four times higher in urban than in rural areas. Current contraceptive use peaks at 67 per cent among women aged 35–39. The variation in contraceptive use by age is similar across urban and rural areas.

### *Contraception: Legal Status*

There is no specific statute that exclusively governs or controls the manufacture, advertisement, sale or standards of contraceptives. Guidelines about contraception relate primarily to the approval of contraceptives as drugs. The key central statutes are the 1940 Drugs and Cosmetics Act and the 1945 Drugs and Cosmetics Rules. Testing and trials of contraceptives are conducted by the Indian Council of Medical Research.

Emergency contraception pills are available by prescription in family planning clinics, pharmacies and, more recently, in all urban government dispensaries and most rural primary health care centres. Dedicated Levonorgestral-only products were officially registered in India in January 2002. In April 2003, the Federation of Obstetrics and Gynecological Society of India established an emergency contraceptive hotline.

In the 1998 Supreme Court case *All India Democratic Women Association v. Union of India,* petitioners challenged the use of the drug quinacrine as a method of female sterilization and contraception. The court disposed of the petition based on the government's assurances that it intended to ban the use of the drug as a method of contraception. A few months later, the government issued a notification banning the import, manufacture, sale and distribution of quinacrine for use as a contraceptive and established penalties for violators of the ban.

At the direction of the Supreme Court, the Drugs Technical Advisory Board, a statutory body constituted under the Drugs and Cosmetics Act, issued a statement in 1995 recommending that Depo-Provera not be included in India's family planning programmes. In January 2002, the government abandoned its plan to offer injection through the Reproductive and Child Health Programme. Ministry of Health officials have stated that although injection will not be offered through government programmes, they may be made available in the private sector.

### *Regulation of Information on Contraception*

No specific statute regulates the dissemination of information regarding advertisement, promotion or packaging of contraceptives. Media and penal laws determine the legality of publicizing contraceptives. Previously, obscenity laws within the Indian Penal Code prohibited advertising a drug for the prevention of conception. These rules have since been liberalized to provide prima facie protection for 'ideas having social importance ... unless obscenity is so gross ... that the interest of the public dictates the other way'.

### *Sterilization*

Female sterilization is the most commonly used form of contraception in India. About 29 per cent of the approximately 74.22 million couples who use a government-approved family planning method are 'protected' against conception by sterilization. Female sterilization accounts for 95 per cent of all reported sterilizations. The median age for female sterilization is 25.7. Acceptance of sterilization increased in all major states from 1997 to 1999, specifically, by 15.9 per cent in Andhra Pradesh; 17.6 per cent in Assam; 3.3 per cent in Gujarat; 4.9 per cent in Punjab; 2.2 per cent in Rajasthan; 0.9 per cent in Tamil Nadu; and 12.5 per cent in Uttar Pradesh.

### *Sterilization: Legal Status*

No specific central statute regulates the provision of sterilization services. The Standards for Female and Male Sterilization issued by the Ministry of Health and Family Welfare set forth the eligibility criteria for sterilization. Applicants for sterilization must be married. Male applicants should 'ideally' be below the age of 60, while female applicants must be between the ages of 22–45. Couples must have at least one child above the age of one. The standards also require that applicants be given counselling prior to undergoing the procedure; applicants should be informed about all available methods of family planning, the permanent nature of the procedure, the risk of complications and the inability of sterilization to protect against reproductive tract infections, STIs or HIV/AIDS. Applicants should be informed specifically of their option to decide against sterilization without sacrificing their right to receive other reproductive health services. All counselling should be provided in a language the client can understand. Sterilization may only be performed with the applicant's informed written consent, which should be given free of 'coercion' or 'physical or mental stress. In the case of pregnant women, the standards prohibit health providers from obtaining a woman's consent when she is 'sedated or ... experiencing stress associated with some pregnancy-related events/problems'. A spouse's written consent is not required for sterilization.

### *Sterilization Policies*

Although the Reproductive and Child Health Programme abolished centrally determined targets for method-specific contraceptives, including sterilization, certain government incentives for sterilization still exist. In order to further the goals of the National Population

Policy, a government health insurance plan was proposed to provide insurance incentives to couples below the poverty line who are undergoing sterilization. Such couples with no more than two children would be eligible for family health insurance, including hospitalization, of up to ₹ 5,000 and personal accident insurance for the spouse undergoing the sterilization procedure. In certain states, such as Andhra Pradesh, low-income individuals who are sterilized after one or two children receive priority for anti-poverty benefits, including housing, land, wells and loans.

### *Government Delivery of Family Planning Services*

In urban areas in India, a network of government hospitals and urban family welfare centres is primarily responsible for providing family planning methods and services. In rural areas, primary health centres and subcentres provide these services.

The public health sector is the source of contraception for 76 per cent of current users of modern methods. Government facilities provide condoms, oral contraceptives and IUDs free of charge. The government launched a Social Marketing Programme for condoms in 1968 and for oral contraceptives in 1987, through which condoms and oral pills are made available by marketing companies or NGOs at highly subsidized rates and through diverse outlets.

Sterilization and IUD insertions are mostly performed in government hospitals and primary health centres. On occasions, sterilization camps are organized in rural or urban areas throughout the country. In 1987, a joint NGO–go eminent programme established Centres of Excellence in Medical Colleges in different parts of the country to provide training in government standards for male and female sterilization. A UNFPA-funded non-scalpel vasectomy project is also being implemented by the Ministry of Health and Family Welfare. The project, which will train 1,500 medical personnel throughout the country to perform non-scalpel vasectomies, aims to promote male sterilization and male involvement in furthering family welfare.

To encourage grassroots participation in the formulation of family planning services, the government allows medical personnel at the local and district levels to submit annual action plans and monthly activity reports to district family welfare officers, who then inform state and national officials. The government also instituted an Empowered Action Group in the Ministry of Health and Family Welfare to facilitate the planning of area-specific programmes with the involvement of voluntary associations, community organizations and Panchayat Raj (local government) institutions. Part of the group's mandate is to explore the possibility of socially marketing contraceptives in order to make them more accessible.

By promoting a participatory approach to family planning services, the National Population Policy stresses the importance of panchayat institutions in furthering decentralized planning and programme implementation in the context of the policy's goals of meeting unmet need and achieving population stabilization. It urges panchayats to form representative committees to prepare 'need-based, demand-driven, socio-demographic plans at the village level.'

### *Family Planning Services Provided by NGOs and the Private Sector*

Family planning services are provided by private hospitals and clinics as well as NGOs. Despite its provision of more than three-fourths of the country's curative health-care services, the private health sector provides less than one-third of all maternal and child health and family planning services. Seventeen per cent of modern contraceptive users rely on the private sector for their supply. The major factors limiting the private sector's participation in family planning services include: the focus until now on curative services; the variable quality of services; and the inability of low-income people to pay for these service. One of the aims of the Tenth Five-Year Plan is to more closely involve the private sector in the provision of family planning services.

About one per cent of current users of modern contraceptive methods obtain their method from NGOs. The Department of Family Welfare funds roughly 97 large NGOs and more than 800 smaller NGOs in ten states. However, a large number of districts in states with high fertility and mortality rates have no NGO presence. The National Population Policy aims to increase the role of NGOs and voluntary organizations in raising awareness about reproductive and child health interventions and improving community participation. To increase NGO participation, the Department of Family Welfare reached out to several well-established NGOs, such as the Family Planning Association of India and the Voluntary Health Association of India, to help select, train, assist and monitor smaller NGOs working at the village level.

## Maternal Health

Recent government estimates of India's maternal mortality ratio range from 407 to 540 maternal deaths per 1,00,000 live births. Maternal deaths account for an estimated 15 per cent of all deaths of women of reproductive age. Most maternal deaths are caused by haemorrhage (29.7%), anaemia (19%) and sepsis (16.1%). Over half of all deliveries take place in private homes, while one-third take place in health facilities. Forty-two per cent of deliveries are attended by a health professional. Older women as well as women from scheduled tribes, illiterate women and low-income women generally do not receive prenatal check-ups.

### *Policies*

One of the primary goals of the National Health Policy and National Population Policy is to reduce the maternal mortality rate to less than 100 maternal deaths per 1,00,000 live births by 2010. In support of this goal, the Tenth Five-Year Plan gives emphasis to maternal health services including the following:

- essential obstetric care through early registration of pregnancy and screening of pregnant women to detect risk factors;
- identification and management of high-risk mothers;
- appropriate management of anaemia and hypertension disorders; and
- Referral care for at risk mothers.

Priority areas also include services for the prevention, detection and management of reproductive tract infections and STIs, and special efforts to promote institutional deliveries and safe home deliveries. The government also commits to making special efforts to promote access to health care during pregnancy at primary health centres.

On the occasion of International Women's Day on 8 March 2003, the Ministry of Health and Family Welfare initiated a programme that compensates pregnant women for their travel costs to health centres. The programme additionally provides a sum of ₹ 1,000 for the birth of a daughter and ₹ 500 for the birth of a son.

Several initiatives undertaken in previous five-year plans and health policies have been incorporated into the government's current policies. The Universal Immunization Programme, launched in 1985, became part of the Reproductive and Child Health Programme in 1997. As a result of this initiative, the number of pregnant women who were vaccinated against tetanus toxoid more than doubled between the start of the programme and 2001. The interventions of the Child Survival and Safe Motherhood Programme, which was launched in 1992 in 72 districts and had expanded to 466 districts by the end of the Eighth

Five-Year Plan, also became part of the Reproductive and Child Health Programme. During the Ninth Five-Year Plan, a training programme for *dais* (midwives) was initiated in 142 districts in 15 states. Around 358 Reproductive Child Health camps were also held to improve access in rural areas to primary-care services.

The government also has launched a nationwide scheme of women's health groups called *Mahila Swasthya Sanghs* in villages. These groups provide a forum for discussing women's health concerns and issues. Group participants also receive short-term training and counselling by local health care workers as well as educational and informational materials. More than 34,000 such groups have been formed in various states and union territories.

### *Nutrition*

Approximately one-third of newborn children are of low birth weight, indicating that many pregnant women suffer from nutritional deficiencies. The Constitution's Directive Principles of State Policy enjoin the state 'to regard raising the level of nutrition and standard of living of its people and the improvement of public health as among its primary duties'.

The 1993 National Nutrition Policy gives special priority to at-risk women, mothers and children. During the Ninth Five-Year Plan, several interventions were adopted as part of the policy, including the following:

- screening of all pregnant women and lactating mothers for chronic energy deficiency;
- identifying women who weigh less than 40 kg and providing them with adequate health care before, during and after pregnancy, as well as neonatal care, under the Reproductive and Child Health Programme; and
- ensuring that such women receive food supplementation through the Integrated Child Development Services Scheme.

The Integrated Child Development Services Scheme, launched in 1975, is a major intervention in combatting malnutrition and provides food supplementation to children below age six as well as to expectant and nursing mothers, with a special emphasis on the girl child. It has grown to be the world's largest child development programme, covering more than 17 million children and pregnant and lactating mothers.

# 15

# Abortion and Sexually Transmissible Infections (STIs) and HIV/AIDS

There is no precise estimate of the total number of induced abortions in India because government data only accounts for abortions performed in government-approved facilities, which are a fraction of the total number of abortions that occur every year. According to government data, an estimated 1.7 per cent of pregnancies end in induced abortion, although there are wide interstate differences ranging from 0.3 per cent in Bihar to 6 per cent in Manipur. The government also estimates that between 4 million and 6 million abortions are performed illegally and that unsafe abortion accounts for 9 per cent of maternal deaths. Non-governmental studies suggest that an estimated 6.7 million abortions occur annually and that 4.5 per cent to 16.9 per cent of all maternal deaths result from unsafe abortion.

## Abortion: Legal Status

The 1971 Medical Termination of Pregnancy Act sets forth the grounds for legal abortion, which include the following:

- risk to the woman's life;
- grave injury to the woman's physical or mental health; and
- substantial risk of foetal impairment.

In determining whether the continuation of a pregnancy would jeopardize a woman's health, the law permits consideration of socio-economic factors affecting the woman's 'actual or reasonable foreseeable environment'. Physical or mental injury to health may also be presumed when the pregnancy is the result of rape or contraceptive failure on the part of the man or woman.

Abortions may only be performed by registered medical practitioners and in government hospitals or facilities approved for abortion by the government or district level committees. For pregnancies of up to 12 weeks, an abortion is permitted upon the good faith opinion of one registered medical practitioner. For pregnancies between 12 and 20 weeks, the opinions of two practitioners are required. For pregnancies beyond 20 weeks, abortion is prohibited except when 'immediately necessary to save the life of the pregnant woman'. Registered medical practitioners must adhere to an elaborate procedure for reporting abortions performed.

The pregnant woman's consent, or that of a legal guardian where she is a minor or lacks mental capacity, is also required for legal abortion. The consent of the woman's husband is not required. The central government has issued regulations to safeguard the confidentiality of a woman seeking legal abortion.

The government approved the distribution of mifepristone and misoprostol, two drugs used in medical abortion, in March 2002. Medical abortion is available in government-approved hospitals and at all registered abortion clinics. Trials are underway to test the efficacy, dosage and safety of drugs for medical termination of pregnancy between 12 and 20 weeks. Early pilot studies report that medical abortion may be especially beneficial in rural settings and suggest that nurses trained to insert intrauterine devices could also administer the drugs for medical abortion.

The Medical Termination of Pregnancy Act imposes a fine of up to ₹ 1,000 for willful contravention of its provisions. Pursuant to amendments to the Act in 2002, penalties for unauthorized clinics and unregistered practitioners performing abortions were increased. The termination of a pregnancy by an unauthorized person or in an unauthorized facility is punishable with two to seven years imprisonment. The owner of an unauthorized facility performing abortion is also subject to the same punishment.

All other penalties are provided in the Indian Penal Code. Any individual, including the pregnant woman herself, who causes a miscarriage for reasons other than to save the life of the mother, is punishable by up to seven years imprisonment and/or fines. The severity of the punishment increases if the woman is at a late stage of pregnancy, which the penal code defines only as 'quick with child'. The act of causing a miscarriage without the woman's consent is punishable by life imprisonment or a period of ten years and a fine.

### *Regulation of Information on Abortion*

A 2002 Supreme Court directive ordered state governments to enforce the ban on sex-selective abortion and punish clinics that advertise and promote sex-selective abortion.

### *Abortion Policies*

The Tenth Five-Year Plan identifies the improvement and expansion of, and women's access to, early and safe abortion services as continuing areas of government focus. Government strategies for reducing abortion-related morbidity include meeting unmet needs for contraception to reduce the number of pregnancies; improving access to safe abortion services; and 'ensuring that women do accept appropriate contraception at the time of [abortion] to prevent unwanted pregnancies requiring a repeat [abortion]'.

A major goal of the National Population Policy is the expansion of the availability of safe abortion services. In accordance with this policy and the Reproductive and Child Health Programme, actions have been initiated to improve and expand abortion facilities and women's access to them, particularly in rural areas. Specific strategies for improving women's access to safe abortion services include these:

- decentralizing the registration of abortion clinics from the state to the district level;
- simplifying the regulations for reporting of abortion;
- training physicians in the government, private and voluntary sector in abortion;
- providing manual vacuum aspiration syringes to recognized abortion centres where there is a trained physician but no vacuum aspiration machine;
- using manual vacuum aspiration for performing abortion in community health centres and primary health centres; and
- Exploring the feasibility and safety of introducing non-surgical methods of abortion in medical college hospitals and extending the service in a phased manner to district hospitals.

The National Population Policy also calls for the provision of post-abortion care, including services to manage complications and identify other health needs of post-abortion patients, and refer them to appropriate services. As part of post-abortion care, physicians may also be trained to provide family planning counselling and services such as insertion of IUDs, sterilization, oral contraceptives, and condoms.

### *Government Delivery of Abortion Services*

More than 8,500 hospitals and clinics are authorized to perform abortions. The United Nations Special Rapporteur on Violence Against Women has reported that 1,800 of India's 20,000 primary health centres have certified abortion facilities. Less developed but more populous states often have fewer abortion facilities than smaller and more developed states. For example, Maharashtra, a more developed state, has over one-fifth of the country's registered abortion facilities. The four large, less developed states of Bihar, Madhya Pradesh, Rajasthan and Uttar Pradesh contain 40 per cent of the country's population but only 16.7 per cent of its total registered facilities.

Not all registered abortion facilities are fully functional or have ever provided abortion services. According to an analysis of abortion facilities in Gujarat, Maharashtra, Uttar Pradesh and Tamil Nadu from 1995–1997, about one-fourth of the primary health centres in Maharashtra and Uttar Pradesh, one-third of those in Gujarat and one-half of those in Tamil Nadu were providing abortion services. Up to half of surveyed primary health centres had never offered abortion services, even though they were approved as abortion facilities. In contrast, the majority of community health centres, rural hospitals and subdistrict hospitals surveyed were equipped to provide abortion services. According to national regulations, all community health centres, postpartum centres and other higher-level health facilities are expected to provide abortion services. In each of the four states that were surveyed, the main reason why abortion services were not offered was the lack of trained providers. Some clinics cited lack of adequate equipment as the primary reason.

To alleviate the shortage of trained providers in primary health centres, community health centres and subdistrict hospitals, the government is assisting states and union territories in hiring doctors trained in abortion techniques to pay weekly or bimonthly visits to these facilities to perform abortions and other reproductive health services.

Abortion services provided by NGOs and the private sector: Several NGOs play an important role in providing safe abortion services in India. Parivar Seva Sanstha, one of the country's largest NGOs working in the field of reproductive health, operates abortion care centres in urban areas throughout the country. The Family Planning Association of India provides counselling as well as abortion services at the district level.

To support NGOs in providing abortion services, the government has proposed a plan to provide equipment and free training to authorized abortion facilities in the NGO sector.

## Sexually Transmissible Infections (STIs) and HIV/AIDS

There are approximately forty million new reported cases of STIs every year. In rural areas, STI treatment facilities are not usually available.

The incidence of HIV/AIDS has been on the rise for more than a decade and has reached alarming proportions in recent years. With nearly four million people infected with HIV, India has the world's second largest population of HIV-infected people. At the end of 2001, there were 1.5 million women living with HIV/AIDS. Studies indicate that a growing number of women attending prenatal clinics are testing HIV-positive.

### *Relevant Laws*

There is no separate national legislation on STIs or HIV/AIDS. However, there area number of legal provisions and court decisions that apply to persons living with STIs and HIV/AIDS. Under the Indian Penal Code, negligently or malignantly engaging in any act that one knows is likely to spread the infection of any disease dangerous to life is a crime punishable by imprisonment ranging from six months to two years and possibly a fine. To date, this provision has been applied to STIs such as syphilis and gonorrhea, but it has not been applied to HIV/AIDS.

Under most matrimonial laws, a spouse's infection with a communicable venereal disease is a ground for divorce. To date, there are no reported cases where divorce has been sought on the basis of a spouse's infection with HIV/AIDS.

As stated above, there are no national laws specific to HIV/AIDS. However, the state of Goa has introduced the 1985 Goa, Daman and Diu Public Health Act, as amended by the 1987 Goa Public Health Act, which contains provisions specific to persons affected by HIV/AIDS. This Act contains provisions for the isolation of persons found to be sera positive, under certain prescribed conditions. Attempts have been made to introduce HIV/AIDS specific legislation in the legislative assemblies of two more states.

Although there are no laws per se that prohibit discrimination against persons living with STIs or HIV/AIDS, some court decisions have upheld such persons' right to nondiscrimination, primarily in the health-are, employment and armed forces contexts. In *MX v. ZY,* the Bombay High Court held that the constitutional right to nondiscrimination requires that people living with HIV/AIDS not be refused treatment at public hospitals or terminated from their place of employment in the public sector on the basis of their HIV status. In *Parmanand v. the Union of India,* the Supreme Court held that private health care providers may not refuse to treat HIV-infected individuals in emergency situations.

Other court decisions have undermined the rights of persons living with HIV/AIDS. In *Mr X v. Hospital Z,* the Supreme Court ruled that health care workers are liable under the Indian Penal Code for failing to disclose a patient's HIV status to his or her partner(s). The original ruling also suspended the right of HIV-positive individuals to marry, though this right was later restored in an order issued by the court in December 2002. However, HIV-positive individuals who know their status must still obtain informed consent from their prospective spouses prior to marriage.

There are also several legal standards that address blood safety and transfusion services. In 1993, amendments to the Drugs and Cosmetics Act and accompanying rules required the screening of blood for five transmissible infections, including HIV/AIDS. Blood banks must obtain a license from the relevant authority, and these licenses must be renewed at regular intervals. A 1996 Supreme Court decision also generated key changes in the regulation of the country's blood supply. In *Common Cause v. Union of India and others,* the court set forth mandatory licensing of blood banks, a ban on professional blood donations and strict guidelines for holding blood donation camps.

### *Policies for the Prevention and Treatment of STIs and HIV/AIDS*

One year after the first HIV case was identified in 1986, the government formulated the National AIDS Control Programme under the Ministry of Health and Family Welfare. In 1992, the Ministry established the National AIDS Control Organization as the focal governmental body for the formulation and implementation of HIV/AIDS-related policies and programmatic initiatives.

In 2002, the government announced the National AIDS Prevention and Control Policy and National Blood Policy. The general objective of the National AIDS Prevention and Control Policy is to contain HIV/AIDS transmission and reduce the impact of the disease on infected persons and on the health and socio-economic well-being of the general population. One specific target is to achieve a zero growth rate of new HIV infections by 2007. Other objectives include the following:

- creating a socio-economic environment that helps prevent HIV/AIDS;
- providing care and support to people living with HIV/AIDS and ensuring the protection and promotion of their human rights, including their rights to access the health care system, education, employment, and privacy;
- mobilizing the support of NGOs and community-based organizations in initiatives for the prevention and alleviation of HIV/AIDS;
- decentralizing the National AIDS Control Programme to the field level with adequate financial and administrative delegation of responsibilities;
- strengthening programme management capabilities in state governments, municipal corporations, panchayat institutions and leading NGOs participating in the National AIDS Control Programme;
- integrating the National AIDS Control Programme with other national programmes such as Reproductive and Child Health, tuberculosis control, and the Integrated Child Development Scheme, and with the primary health care system;
- preventing women, children and other socially marginalized groups from becoming vulnerable to HIV infection by improving their health education, legal status and economic prospects;
- providing adequate and equitable health care to HIV-infected individuals and drawing attention to the public health rationale for overcoming stigmatization, discrimination and seclusion in society;
- maintaining constant interaction with international and bilateral agencies for support and cooperation in the field of research in vaccines, drugs and emerging systems of health care;
- ensuring the availability of adequate and safe blood and blood products for the general population through promotion of voluntary blood donation; and
- promoting a better understanding of HIV/AIDS among young people, especially students, youth and other sexually active groups.

The National AIDS Prevention and Control Policy also gives special priority to the prevention and control of STIs as a strategy for controlling the spread of HIV/AIDS. The policy provides for the integration of services for treatment of STIs as well as reproductive tract infections at all levels of health care, including:

- strengthening STI clinics in all district hospitals, medical colleges and other facilities by providing technical support, equipment and drugs;
- undertaking a massive training programme for all medical and paramedical workers involved in providing services for reproductive tract infections and STIs;
- ensuring that all STI clinics provide counselling services and good quality condoms for STI patients; and
- utilizing NGOs to provide such counselling services at STI clinics.

The National Blood Policy aims to ensure accessibility and adequate supply of safe and quality blood and blood components collected from voluntary and non-remunerated blood donors. The objectives of this policy include the following:

- making available adequate resources to develop and reorganize blood transfusion services in the entire country;
- making the latest technology available for operating blood transfusion services;
- launching extensive awareness programmes for donor information, education, motivation, recruitment and retention in order to ensure a safe blood supply;
- encouraging the appropriate clinical use of blood and blood products;
- encouraging research and development in the field of transfusion medicine and related technology; and
- taking adequate regulatory and legislative steps for the monitoring and evaluation of blood transfusion services and eliminating profiteering in blood banks.

The Action Plan for Blood Safety was developed in 2003 to implement the objectives set forth in the National Blood Policy. The action plan provides for the following:

- accreditation of blood banks;
- disclosure of the status of all infections transmitted through blood transfusions;
- multiage response through partnerships between government, private sector, the Red Cross Society of India, the Indian Council of Medical Research, Medical Council of India, NGOs, community-based organizations, and others;

- rational use of blood and blood products among clinicians; and
- external quality control mechanisms for public sector blood banks.

In an effort to expand the range of preventive methods available to women against HIV transmission, the government is considering introducing microbicides-creams or gels that can prevent transmission of STIs and HIV when applied at the mouth or female genitals – in its HIV/AIDS prevention programmes.

### *Regulation of Information on STIs and HIV/AIDS*

Restrictions on the right to freedom of expression and information on STIs and HIV/AIDS are traditionally covered by laws governing obscenity, censorship and the public interest. The Indian Penal Code criminalizes the sale, publication, distribution and advertisement of 'obscene' materials, but does not specifically define 'obscene'. The code does not prohibit materials if they are 'for the public good'. In May 2000, the authors of a controversial pamphlet entitled 'AIDS and Us' were arrested under the 1980 National Security Act for circulating the pamphlet.

## Health Care Programmes

### *Health and Health Care*

Health and health care need to be distinguished from each other for no better reason than that the former is often incorrectly seen as a direct function of the latter. Heath is clearly not the mere absence of disease. Good health confers on a person or groups freedom from illness and the ability to realize one's potential. Health is, therefore, best understood as the indispensable basis for defining a person's sense of well-being. The health of populations is a distinct key issue in public policy discourse in every mature society often determining the deployment of huge society. They include its cultural understanding of ill health and well-being, extent of socio-economic disparities, reach of health services and quality and costs of care and current biomedical understanding about health and illness.

Health care covers not merely medical care but also all aspects of preventive care too. Nor can it be limited to care rendered by or financed out of public expenditure within the government sector alone but must include incentives and disincentives for self-care and care paid for by private citizens to get over ill health. Whereas in India, private out-of-pocket expenditure dominates the cost financing health care, the effects are bound to be regressive. Heath care at its essential core is widely recognized to be a public good. Its demand and supply cannot, therefore, be left to be regulated solely by the invisible head of the market. Nor can it be established on considerations of utility maximizing conduct alone.

What makes for a just health care system even as an ideal? Four criteria could be suggested: First, universal access and access to an adequate level, and access without excessive burden. Second, fair distribution of financial costs for access and fair distribution of burden in rationing care and capacity and a constant search for improvement to a more just system. Third, training providers for competence empathy and accountability, pursuit of quality care adds cost-effective use of the results of relevant research. Last, special attention to vulnerable groups such as children, women, disabled and the aged.

## Major Disease Control Efforts

A careful analysis of the Global Burden of Disease (GBD) study focusing on age-specific morbidity during 2000 in ten most common diseases (excluding injuries) shows that sixty per cent of morbidity is due to infectious diseases and common tropical diseases, a quarter due to lifestyle disorders and 13 per cent due to potentially preventable prenatal conditions. Further domestic R&D has been so far muted in its efforts against estimated annual aggregate health expenditure in India of ₹ 80,000 crores. R&D expenditure in India for public and private sector combined was ₹ 1,150 crores only. India must play a larger part in its own efforts at indigenous R&D as very little worldwide expenditure on R&D is likely to be devoted to infectious diseases. For instance, out of the 1,233 new drugs that came into the market between 1975 and 1997, only 11 were indicated specifically for tropical country diseases.

We have already the distinction of elimination or control acceptable to public health standards of small pox and guinea worm diseases. In the draft National Health Policy-21, it has now been proposed to eliminate or control the following diseases within limits acceptable to public health practice: (A good deal of the effort would be feasible.)

- Polio, Yaws and leprosy by 2005 which seems distinctly feasible though the removal of social stigma and reconstructive surgery and other rehabilitation arrangements in regard to leprosy would remain inadequate for a decade or more.
- Kalaazar by 2010 and Filalriasis by 2010, which also seems feasible due to its localized prevalence and the possibility of greater

community based work involving primary health care institutions in the simple but time-limited tasks or public health programmes.

- Blindness prevalence to 0.5 per cent by 2010 seems less feasible due to a greying population. At present the programme is massively supported by foreign aid as there are many other legitimate demands on domestic health budgets:
- AIDS reaching zero growth by 2007 appears to be problematic as there are disputes even about base data on infected population. On most reckonings, affordable vaccines are not likely to be available soon nor anti-retro viral drugs appear likely at affordable prices in the near future. Further the prevalence curve of AIDS in India is yet to show its shape. There is also larger unresolved question of where HIV/AIDS should be fitted in our priorities of public health, especially in this massively foreign aided programme, what happen if aid does not become available at some point.

### *Unfinished Burden of Communicable Diseases*

Apart from the above, there remains a vast unfinished burden in preventing controlling or eliminating other major communicable diseases and in bringing down the risk of deaths in maternal and prenatal conditions. Endemic diseases arising from infection or lack of nutrition continue to account for almost two-thirds of mortality and morbidity in India. Indeed, eleven out of thirteen diseases recommended by the Bhore Committee were infectious diseases and at least three of them may well continue to be with us for the next two decades barring leprosy which is almost on the path to total control by 2005, the other key communicable diseases will be TB, malaria and AIDS – to which diarrhea in children and complicated and high risk maternity should be added in view of their pervasive incidence and avoidable mortality among the poorer and underserved sectors,

#### *Tuberculosis*

Tuberculosis has had a worldwide resurgence including in India. It is estimated about 14 million persons are infected, i.e. 1.55 of total population suffer from radiologically active tuberculosis. About 1.5 million cases are identified and more than 3,00,000 deaths occur every year. Between NFHS 1 and NFHS 2 the prevalence has increased from 4,678 per lakh population to 544. Unfortunately, prevalence among working age adults (15–59) is even as higher as 675. All these may well be underestimates in so far as patients are traced only through hospital visits. Only about half reach the hospital. Often wrong diagnosis by insufficiently trained doctors or misunderstood protocols is another key problem in both public and private sectors. TB is a widespread disease of poverty among women living and working in poorly ventilated places and with other undernourished persons in urban slums it is increasingly affecting the younger adults also in the economically productive segments. No universal screening is possible. Sputum positive test does not precede diagnosis but drugs are prescribed on the basis of fever and shadows, as a result incomplete cure becomes common and delayed tests only prove the wrong diagnosis too late. Improved diagnosis through better training and clear protocols and elimination of drug resistance through incomplete cure should be priority. Treatment costs in case of drug resistance can soar close to ten times the normal level of ₹ 3,000 to 4,000 per person treated. Similarly, even though the resistant strain may cover only 8 per cent at present, it could suddenly rise and as it approaches 20 per cent or so, there is a danger that TB may get out of control. The directly observed therapy (DOTS) programme trying for full compliance after proper diagnosis is settling down but already has some claims of success. More tan 3,000 laboratories have been set up for diagnosis and about 1.5 lakh workers trained and with total population coverage by 2007, cure rates (already claimed to have doubled) may rise substantially. There is reason to hope that DOTS programmes would prove a greater success over time with increased community awareness generation. The key issue is how soon and how well can it be integrated into the PHC system and made subject to routines of local accountability, without which no low cost regime of total compliance is feasible in a country as large as India.

An optimistic assessment could be that with commitment and full use of infrastructure, it will be possible to arrest further growth in absolute numbers of TB cases keeping it below 1.5 million till 2010 even though the population will be growing. Once that is done TB can be brought down to less than a million, it would lie within internationally accepted limits and disappear as a major communicable disease in India by 2020.

*Malaria*

As regards malaria, we have had a long record of success and failure and each intervention has been thwarted by new problems and plagued by recrudescence. At present, India has a large manpower fully aware of all aspects of malaria but often low in motivation. It can be transformed into a large-scale work force for awareness generation, tests and distribution of medicine. In spite of past successes, there is evidence of re-emergence with focal attacks of malaria with the virulent falciparum variety especially in tribal areas. Priority tribal area malaria stands fully funded by the Centre. About 2 million cases of malaria are recorded all over India every year with seasonal high incidence of local failures of control. Drug resistance in humans and insecticide resistant strains of mosquitoes present a significant problem. But there is a window of opportunity in respect of DDT sensitive areas in eastern India where even now malaria incidence can be brought down by about 50 per cent within a decade and be beneficial for control of kalazaar and JE. There is growing interest and community awareness of biological methods of control of mosquito growth. Unfortunately, diligent ground level public health work is in grave disarray in these areas but can be improved by better supervision, greater use of panchayat raj institutions and building on modest demonstrated successes. As regards a vaccine, there seems to be no sufficient incentive for international R&D to focus on a relatively lower priority or research. Roll back malaria programmes of the WHO are more likely to concentrate on Africa whose profile of malaria is not similar to ours. The search for a vaccine continues but has little likelihood of immediate success.

In spite of various difficulties, if the restructuring of the malaria workforce and the strengthening of health infrastructure takes place, one can expect that the incidence can be reduced by a third or even up to half in the next decade or so. For this, it is necessary that routine tasks like timely spraying and logistics for taking blood slides testing and their analysis and organic methods of reducing mosquito spread, etc. are downstaged to community level and preformed under supervision through panchayat participation, public education and local monitoring. Malaria can certainly be reduced by a third even up to a half in ten years, and there is a prospect of near freedom from malaria for most of the country by 2020.

### *AIDS*

There is finally the case of HIV/AIDS. The magnitude in the numbers of HIV infected and of AIDS patients by 2025 can be known only as trends emerge over a decade from now, when better epidemiological estimates are available, but at present these figures are hotly contested. We can start with the number infected with HIV as per NACO sentinel surveillance in 2000 a cumulative total 3.86 million, a figure disputed in recent public health debate. We can then assume that about 10 per cent will turn into full-blown cases of severe and intractable stage of AIDS. There is as yet no basis to know how many of those infected will become

AIDS patients; preventive efforts focused on behaviour change will show up firmly only after a decade or so. During this period one can assume an additional 10 per cent growth to account for new cases every year. The Draft NHP 2001 seeks to stop further infection by educating and counselling, and condom supplies to level it off around 2007, which seems somewhat ambitious. We have yet to make a decisive dent into the problem of awareness with the broader population and so far we have been at work only on high risk groups. National Family Health Survey (NFHS-2) shows only a third of woman reporting that they even knew about the HIV/AIDS. Further such awareness efforts must be followed by multipronged and culturally compatible techniques of public education that go beyond segments easier to be convinced or their behaviour changed. There are voices already raised about the appropriate lateness of IEC mass media content and of the underemphasis of face-to-face counselling, calling for innovative mobilization strategies rooted in indigenous belief systems.

What it implies is that we may be carrying by 2015 close to 5 million infected and unto a tenth of them could turn into full-blown cases We may not be able to level off infection by 2007 – further, these magnitudes may turn out in actual fact to be wildly off the mark. On any account it is clear that AIDS can lead to high mortality among the productive groups in society affecting economic functioning as also public health. Even if 10 per cent of them, say 50 to 60,000 cases, become full-blown cases, the state has the onerous and grim choice to look at competing equities and decide on a policy for free treatment of AIDS patients with expensive anti-retroviral drugs. And if it decides not to, the issue remains as to how to evolve humane balanced and affordable policies that do not lead to a social breakdown. In about a decade, vaccine development may possibly be successful and drugs may by more effective but they may not always be affordable nor can be given free.

There would hopefully be wider consultation with persons with caring sensibilities including AIDS patients on how to counsel in different eventualities and to get the balance right between hospital and home care, and how to develop a humane affordable policy for anti-retroviral drugs for AIDS patients. Is there a case for providing them with drug free of cost merely to extend their lives for few years? The matter involves a true dilemma, for public health priorities themselves certainly argue for more funds should address diseases constituting bigger population-based hazards. Investments made in such expensive interventions can instead be made in supporting hospice efforts in the voluntary and private sectors.

Whatever position may emerge in research or spread of infection of case fatalities, a multipronged attempt for awareness, must continue and tough choices must get discussed openly without articulating special, often urban middle class, interests denying other views and especially public health priorities of the poor. The promotion of barrier protection must increase but has to be related to a system of values, which would be acceptable to the people's beliefs. We need to strengthen sentinel surveillance systems and awareness effort. We also need sensitive feed back on the effects they leave on younger minds for a balanced culturally acceptable strategy. All this is feasible and can be accomplished if we are not swept away by the power of funding, and advocacy and fear of being accused to be out of line with dominant world opinion.

In any case, many of the ill cannot afford the high prices or have access to it from public agencies. The strict patent regimen under Trade-Related Aspects of Intellectual Property Rights (TRIPS) is bound to prevail, notwithstanding the ambivalently worded Doha decision of WTO that public health emergencies provide sufficient cause of countries to use the flexibility available from various provisions of TRIPS. A recent analysis reveals that the three drug regimen recommended will cost $ 10,000 per person per year from Western companies and the treatment will be lifelong. Three Indian companies are offering to Central Government anti-retroviral drugs at $600/₹ 30,000/per person per year and to an international charity at an even lower price $ 350/₹ 13,000/per year, provided it was distributed for humanitarian relief free in S. Africa. It has been public policy in Brazil that the drug is supplied free to all AIDS victims should be no exception. If drugs are supplied acting on a public health emergency basis and prices can stabilize at ₹ 1,000 or so per year the public health budget should be able to accommodate the cost weighed against true public criteria. But the aim of levelling off infection of 2007 still seems unlikely.

### Maternal and Prenatal Deaths

Maternal and prenatal deaths are sizeable but the advantage here is that they can be prevented merely by more intensive utilization of existing rural health infrastructure. Policy and implementation must keep steady focus on key items such as improved institutional deliveries, better trained birth attendants and timely antenatal screening to eliminate anaemia, and at the same time isolate cases needing referral or other targeted attention. After all, Tamil Nadu has by such methods ensured close to 90 per cent institutional deliveries backed by a functional referral. Firm administrative will and concurrent supervision of specified screening tasks included in Maternal and Child Health (MCH) services can give us a window of opportunity to dramatically bring down within a few years alarming maternal mortality currently one of the highest in the world. From NFHS I data, it was estimated at 424 per lac births it has risen to 540 per lac births in NFHS II, but the WHO estimate puts it higher at 570. There can be a systematic campaign over five years to increase institutional deliveries as near as possible to the Tamil Nadu level, also taking into account assisted, home deliveries by trained staff with doctors at call. For the interim Traditional Birth Attendant (TBAs) should be relied on through a mass awareness campaign involving Gram Panchayats too. Over a period of time there is no reason why ANMs entitled benefits of children to help in their growth and not remain as welfare measure. Using the infrastructures fully and with community participation and extensive social mobilization, many tasks in nutrition are feasible and can be in position to make impact by 2010.

### *Child Health and Nutrition*

Associated with this is the issue of infant and child mortality, (70 out of 1,000 dying in the first year and 98 before five years) and low birth weight (22% UW at birth ands 47% EJW at below 3 years). Most mortality occurs from diarrhoea and the stagnation in IMR in the last few years is bound to have a negative effect on population stabilization goals. A recent review of the Ninth Plan indicated that even with accelerated efforts we may reach at best IMR/50 by 3002, but more likely IMR/56, since the easier part of the problem is taking child mortality is over every part gain hereafter will deal with districts at greater risk and needing better organizational efficiencies in immunization. At the same time, more streamlined registered care home (RCH) services are getting established as part of public systems and through private partnerships Therefore, there is every reason to hope that the National Population Policy (NPP) 2000 target of 30 per thousand live births by 2010 will be met, barring a few pockets of inaccessible and resource lean areas with stubborn persistence of poverty and dominantly composed of weaker sections (e.g. in part of Odisha as seen from NFHS II).

As regards childhood diarrhea, deaths are totally preventable by simple community action and public education by targeting children of low birth weights and detecting early those children at risk from malnutrition through proper low cost screening procedure; the present arrangement has got too burdened with attempting total population coverage getting all children weighed even once in three months and making ANMs depots for Oral Rehydration Salts (ORS) and for simple drugs for fever and motivating the community to take pride in healthy children are the lessons of the success of the Tamil Nadu Nutrition Project, If this is done there is a reasonable chance of two-thirds decline in moderate malnutrition and abolition of serious grades completely by 2015. The success can be built upon till 2025 for reaching levels comparable to China.

Concentration on preventive measures of maternal and child health, and in particular, improved nutrition services will be particularly useful because it will help that generation to have a head start in good health and are going to be a part of the demographic bonus. The bonus is a young adult bulge of about 340 million (with not less than 250 million from rural population and about 100 million born in this century). The bonus will appear in a sequence with South Indian States completing the transition before North Indian States, spread over the next three decades. To ensure best results at this stage the present nutritional services must be converted into targeted (and entitled) benefits of children to help in their growth and not remain only as a welfare measure. Using the infrastructures fully with community participation and extensive social mobilization many tasks in nutrition are feasible, and can be in position to make impact by 2010.

Mild and moderate malnutrition still prevalent in over half of our young population can be halved if food as the supplemental pathway to better nutrition becomes a priority, both for self-reliance and lower costs. There has been a tendency for micro-nutrient supplementation to overwhelm food derived nourishment. This trend is assisted by foreign aid but over a long run may prove unsustainable. By engaging the adolescents into proper nutrition education and reproductive health awareness we can seamlessly weave into the nutritional security system of our country a corps of informed interconnected and imaginative ideas that can be tried out. Such social mobilization at low cost can be the best preventive strategy as has been advocated for long, by the Nutrition Foundation of India (Gopalan, 2001) and can be a priority in this decade over the next two plan periods.

# 16

# Primary Health Care

## Primary Health Care in India

In 1977, the Government of India launched a Rural Health Scheme, based on the principle of 'placing people's health in people's hands'. It is a three-tier system of health care delivery in rural areas based on the recommendation of the Shrivastav Committee in 1975. Close on the heels of these recommendations an international conference at Alma-Ata in 1978, set the goal of an acceptable level of 'Health for All' the people of the world by the year 2000 through primary health care approach. As a signatory to the Alma-Ata Declaration, the Government of India is committed to achieving the goal of Health for All, through primary health care approach which seeks to provide universal comprehensive health care at a cost which is affordable.

Keeping in view the WHO goal of 'Health for All' by 2000 AD, the Government of India evolved a National Health Policy based on primary health care approach. It was approved by Parliament in 1983. The National Health Policy has laid down a plan of action for reorienting and shaping the existing rural health infrastructure with specific goals to be achieved by 1985, 1990 and 1995 within the framework of the Sixth (1980–85) and Seventh (1985–90) Five-Year Plans and the new 20-point Programme. Steps are already under way to implement the National health Policy objectives towards achieving health for all by the year 2000, these are described below:

## Village Level

One of the basic tenets of primary health care is universal coverage and equitable distribution of health resources. That is, health care must penetrate into the farthest reaches of rural areas and that everyone should have access to it. To implement this policy at the village level, the following schemes are in operation:

### *Village Health Guides Scheme*

A Village Health Guide is a person with an aptitude for social service and is not a full time government functionary. The Village Health Guides Scheme was introduced on 2 October 1977 with the idea of securing people's participation in the care of their own health. The scheme was launched in all States except Kerala, Karnataka, Tamil Nadu, Arunachal Pradesh and Jammu & Kashmir which had alternative systems (e.g. Mini-health Centres in Tamil Nadu) of providing health services at the village level.

The health guides are now mostly women. A circular was issued by Government of India in May 1986 that male health guides would be replaced by female health guides. The health guides come from and are chosen by the community in which they work. They serve as links between the community and the governmental infrastructure. They provide the first contact between the individual and the health system.

The guidelines for their selection are:

1. they should be permanent residents of the local community, preferably women,
2. they should be able to read and write, having minimum formal education at least up to the VI standard,
3. they should be acceptable to all sections of the community and
4. they should be able to spare at least 2 to 3 hours every day for community health work.

After selection, the health guides undergo a short training in primary health care. The training is arranged in the nearest, primary health centre, subcentre or any other suitable place for the duration of 200 hours, spread over a period of 3 months. During the training period they receive a stipend of ₹ 200 per month.

On completion of training, they receive a working manual and a kit of simple medicines belonging to the modern and traditional systems of medicine in vogue in that part of the country to which they belong. Broadly, the duties assigned to health guides include treatment of simple ailments and activities in first aid, mother and child health including family planning, health education and sanitation. The manual or guidebook gives them detailed information about medical care of common illnesses and of what they can and cannot do. In practical terms, they know exactly what should be done when confronted with a situation, when they can begin treatment by themselves and when they should refer the patient immediately to the nearest health centre.

The health guides are free to attend to their normal vocation. They are expected to do community health work in their spare time of about 2 to 3 hours daily for which they are paid an honorarium of ₹ 50 per month and drugs worth ₹ 600 per annum. As the training involves expenditure, the Government will not train another health guide from the same village before three years. As of date, there are 3.23 lakh village health guides functioning in the country. The training programme is being continued during the (Ninth Plan Period, 1997–2002) to achieve the national target of one health guide for each village or 1,000 rural population.

### *Local Dais*

Most deliveries in rural areas are still handled by untrained *dais* (midwife) who are often the only people immediately available to women during the perinatal period. An extensive programme has been undertaken, under the Rural Health Scheme, to train all categories of local *dais* (traditional birth attendants) in the country to improve their knowledge in the elementary concepts of maternal and child health and sterilization, besides obstetric skills. The training is for 30 working days. Each *dai* is paid a stipend of ₹ 300 during her training period. Training is given at the PHC, subcentre or MCH centre for 2 days in a week, and on the remaining four days of the week they accompany the health worker (female) to the villages preferably a day' in their own area. During her training she is required to conduct at least 2 deliveries under the guidance and supervision of the HW (F), ANM or HA (F). The emphasis during training is on asepsis so that home deliveries are conducted under safe hygienic conditions, thereby reducing the maternal and infant mortality.

After successful completion of training, each *dai* is provided with a delivery kit and a certificate. She is entitled to receive an amount of ₹ 10 per delivery provided the case is registered with the subcentre/PHC. To each infant registered by her, she will receive ₹ 3. These *dais* are also expected to play a vital role in propagating small-family norms since they are more acceptable to the community. Although the national target is to train one local *dai* in each village, the Eighth Five-Year Plan objective was to train all untrained *dais* practising in the rural areas.

### *Anganwadi Worker*

Angan literally means a courtyard. Under the ICDS (Integrated Child Development Services) Scheme, there is an anganwadi worker for a population of 1,000. There are about 100 such workers in each ICDS Project. As of date over 532 ICDS blocks are functioning in the country. The anganwadi worker is selected from the community she is expected to serve. She undergoes training in various aspects of health nutrition, and child development for 4 months. She is a part-time worker and is paid an honorarium of ₹ 200–250 per month for the services rendered, which include health check-up, immunization, supplementary nutrition, health education, non-formal pre-school education and referral services. The beneficiaries are especially nursing mothers, other women (15–45 years) and children below the age of 6 years. Along with Village Health Guides, the anganwadi workers are the community's primary link with the health services and all other services for young children.

## Subcentre Level

The subcentre is the peripheral outpost of the existing health delivery system in rural areas. They are being established on the basis of one subcentre for every 5,000 population in general and one for every 3,000 population in hilly, tribal and backward areas. As on 31 March 2003, 1,38,368 subcentres were established in the country – the total requirement is estimated to be 1.34 lakh.

Each subcentre is manned by one male and one female multipurpose health worker. At present the functions of a subcentre are limited to mother and child health care, family planning and immunization. It is proposed to extend the facilities to all subcentres for IUD insertion, and simple laboratory investigations like routine examination of urine for albumin and sugar. Creation of these facilities would go a long way in securing greater acceptance of IUD and early detection of complications of pregnancy. The work at subcentres is supervised by male and female health assistants. According to the revised norm, one female HA will supervise the work of 6 female HWs. The job descriptions of these workers have been published as Manuals by the Rural Health Division of the Ministry of Health and Family Welfare.

## Primary Health Centre Level

The concept of primary health centre is not new to India. The Bhore Committee in 1946, gave the concept of a primary health centre as a basic health unit, to provide, as close to the people as possible, an integrated curative and preventive health care to the rural population with emphasis on preventive and promotive aspects of health care. The Bhore Committee aimed at having a health centre to serve a population of 10,000 to 20,000 with 6 medical officers, 6 public health nurses and other supporting staff. But in view of the limited resources, the Bhore Committee's recommendations could not be fully implemented, even after a lapse of 50 years.

The health planners in India have visualized the primary health centre and its subcentres as the proper infrastructure to provide health services to the rural population. The Central Council of Health at its first meeting held in January 1953, had recommended the establishment of primary health centres in community development blocks to provide comprehensive health care to the rural population. The number of primary health centres established since then had increased from 725 during the First Five-Year Plan to 5,484 by the end of the Fifth Plan (1975–1980) – each PHC covering a population of 1,00,000 or more spread over some 100 villages in each community development block. These centres were functioning as peripheral health service institutions with little or no community involvement. Increasingly, these centres came under criticism as they were not able to provide adequate health coverage, partly because they were poorly staffed and equipped, and partly because they had to cover a large population of one lakh or more. The Mudaliar Committee in 1962 had recommended that the existing primary health centres should be strengthened and the population to be served by them to be scaled down to 40,000.

### *Community Health Centres*

As on 31 March 2003, 3,076 community health centres were established by upgrading the primary health centres, each community health centre covering a population of 80,000 to 120 lakh (one in each community development block) with 30 beds and specialists in surgery, medicine, obstetrics and gynaecology, and paediatrics with X-ray and laboratory facilities. For strengthening preventive and promotive aspects of health care, a new non-medical post called community health officer has been created at each community health centre. The community health officer is selected from amongst the supervisory category of staff at the PHC and district level with minimum of 7 years experience in rural health programmes. Some states have not accepted this scheme and have opted for a second medical officer.

The specialists at the community health centre may refer a patient directly to the State level hospital or to the nearest/appropriate Medical College Hospital, as may be necessary, without the patient having to go first to the sub-divisional or District Hospital.

### *Defining Primary Health Care*

A new approach to health care came into existence in 1978, following an international conference at Alma-Ata (USSR). This is known as 'primary health care'. It has all the hallmarks of a primary health care delivery, first proposed by the Bhore Committee in 1946 and now espoused worldwide by international agencies and national governments.

Before Alma-Ata, primary health care was regarded as synonymous with 'basic health services', 'first contact care', 'easily accessible care', 'services provided by generalists', etc. The Alma-Ata international conference gave primary health care a wider meaning. The Alma-Ata conference defined primary health care as follows:

> Primary health care is essential health care made universally accessible to individuals and acceptable to them, through their full participation and at a cost the community and country can afford.

The primary health care is equally valid for all countries from the most to the least developed, although it takes varying forms in each of them. The concept of primary health care has been accepted by all countries as the key to the attainment of Health for All by 2000 AD. It has also been accepted as an integral part of the country's health system.

### *Elements of Primary Health Care*

Although specific services provided will vary in different countries and communities, the Alma-Ata Declaration has outlined eight essential components of primary health care.

1. education concerning prevailing health problems and the methods of preventing and controlling them;
2. promotion of food supply and proper nutrition;
3. an adequate supply of safe water and basic sanitation;
4. maternal and child health care, including family planning;
5. immunization against major infectious diseases;
6. prevention and control of locally endemic diseases;
7. appropriate treatment of common diseases and injuries; and
8. provision of essential drugs.

### *Principles of Primary Health Care Equitable Distribution*

The first key principle in the primary health care strategy is equity or equitable distribution of health services, i.e. health services must be shared equally by all people irrespective of their ability to pay, and all (rich or poor, urban or rural) must have access to health services. At present, health services are mainly concentrated in the major towns and cities resulting in inequality of care to the people in rural areas. The worst hits are the needy and vulnerable groups of the population in rural areas and urban slums. This has been termed as social injustice. The failure to reach the majority of the people is usually due to inaccessibility. Primary health care aims to redress this imbalance by shifting the centre of gravity of the health care system from cities (where three-quarters of the health budget is spent) to the rural areas (where three-quarters of the people live), and bring these services as near people's homes as possible.

### *Community Participation*

Notwithstanding the overall responsibility of the Central and State Governments, the involvement of individuals, families, and communities in promotion of their own health and welfare, is an essential ingredient of primary health care. Countries are conscious of the fact that universal coverage by primary health care cannot be achieved without the involvement of the local community. There must be a continuing effort to secure leaning full involvement of the community in the planning, implementation and maintenance of health services, besides maximum reliance on local resources such as manpower, money and materials. In short, primary health care must be built on the principle of community participation (or involvement).

One approach that has been tried successfully in India is the use of village health guides and trained *dais*. They are selected by the local community and trained locally in the delivery of primary health care to the community they belong, free of charge. By overcoming cultural and communication barriers, they provide primary health care in ways that are acceptable to the community. It is now considered that 'health guides' and trained *dais* are an essential feature of primary health care in India. These concepts are revolutionary. They have been greatly influenced by experience in China where community participation in the form of barefoot doctors took place on an unprecedented scale.

### *Intersectional Coordination*

There is an increasing realization of the fact that the components of primary health care cannot be provided by the health sector alone. The

Declaration of Alma-Ata states that 'primary health care involves, in addition to the health sector, all related sectors and aspects of national and community development, in particular agriculture, animal husbandry, food, industry, education, housing, public works, communication and others sectors'. To achieve such cooperation, countries may have to review their administrative system, reallocate their resources and introduce suitable legislation to ensure that coordination can take place. This requires strong political will to translate values into action. An important element of intersectional approach is planning – planning with other sectors to avoid unnecessary duplication of activities.

### *Appropriate Technology*

Appropriate technology has been defined as 'technology that is scientifically sound, adaptable to local needs, and acceptable to those who apply it and those for whom it is used, and that can be maintained by the people themselves in keeping with the principle of self-reliance with the resources the community and country can afford'. The term 'appropriate' is emphasized because in some countries, large, luxurious hospitals that are totally inappropriate to the local needs, are built, which absorb a major part of the national health budget, effectively blocking any improvement in general health services. This also applies to using costly equipment, procedures and techniques when cheaper, scientifically valid and acceptable ones are available, viz. oral rehydration fluid, standpipes which are socially acceptable, and financially more feasible than house-to-house connections, etc.

It will be seen from the above discussion that primary care is qualitatively a different approach to deal with the health problems of a community. Unlike the previous approaches (e.g. basic health services, and integrated health care, vertical health services) which depended upon taking health services to the doors of the people, primary health care approach starts with the people themselves. This approach signifies a new dynamism in health care and has been described as health by the people, placing people's health in people's hands. The ends of the primary health care approach are the same as those of earlier approaches (i.e. attainment of an acceptable level of health by every individual), but the means adopted are different, that is, more equitable distribution and nationwide coverage, more intersectional coordination and more community involvement in health related matters. In short, primary health care goes beyond the conventional health services. It forms part of the larger concept of Human Resources and Development,

### Food Supply, Infectious Diseases, Nutrition, Immunization

Roughly 3 million children die each year of vaccine preventable diseases (VPDs) with a disproportionate number of these children residing in developing countries. 'Vaccines remain one of the most cost-effective public health initiatives', yet the cover against VPDs remains far from complete; recent estimates suggest that approximately 34 million children are not completely immunized with almost 98 per cent of them residing in developing countries. Vaccination coverage in India is also far from complete despite a longstanding commitment to universal coverage. A recent evaluation of VPD coverage in India found that 18 million children did not receive any coverage in 2001–2002.

In India, immunization has been a central goal of the health care system from the 1970s, first through the Expanded Programme on Immunization (EPI) in 1978, and later with the universal immunization programme (UIP) since 1985. Constitutionally, health care is on the State's list of responsibilities and is financed by the State. The UIP is an exception; it is one of the few 100 per cent centrally sponsored family welfare programmes and provides support for vaccine storage, training of medical and paramedical staff, and all infrastructure needs specific to delivering immunization to infants at the village level.

Throughout the 1980s, gains in immunization coverage proved to be rapid for all VPDs; some VPDs showed gains from below 20 per cent coverage to over 60 per cent coverage by the early 1990s. Pulse polio immunization (PPI) campaign initiated in 1995, was successful in significantly increasing first-dose polio immunization coverage; however, there were limited gains in complete coverage for polio vaccines. Moreover, coverage of non-polio vaccines seemed to have remained unaffected by the PPI campaign. This limited success in expanding full coverage for VPDs has renewed the search of ways to expand coverage effectively. A natural place to start was by studying the strengths and weakness of the current vaccine delivery system through the rural health infrastructure in India.

India's rural health care system has a strong dependence on community health infrastructure and outreach, particularly in remote villages. Community health infrastructure has been shown to be an important correlate of health outcomes in other developing countries. In the Indian context, two studies have examined the role of health infrastructure on the utilization of maternal health care using national data, while others have examined the relationship between health infrastructure and child and maternal health at the State level. These studies have mixed findings. For example, one study used multivariate regressions to control for individual and household characteristics and found that distance to a health facility did not predict health services utilization. Others have used a similar analytic strategy, but different data, and the results indicated that presence of a health facility in the village significantly increased the likelihood of maternity care utilization. In this study, we examined the role of rural health infrastructure and community health workers in expanding immunization coverage in rural India.

We built on this prior research in four important ways. First, by characterizing the availability of rural health infrastructure in more detail than prior studies, we were able to discuss the effectiveness of different levels of health infrastructure in expanding coverage. Important differences in both the nature of services provided and the staffing at different levels of care are likely to have different effects on immunization coverage. We constructed a hierarchical measure of health infrastructure that captured the highest level of health facility available in the village, and thus we were able to examine whether it matters if the best available health facility in the village is a hospital or a less equipped, smaller facility.

Second, we also examined whether the availability of community health workers (CHWs) such as village health guides (VHG), Anganwadi workers (AWW), and trained birth attendants (TBA) affects immunization coverage.

Third, we classified the set of vaccines under the Universal Immunization Programme (UIP) into polio and non-polio vaccines to identify the effect of different mechanisms of immunization delivery. Since the Pulse Polio Immunization (PPI) campaign was initiated between the two National Family Health Survey (NFHS) waves, it is important to examine changes in coverage for polio and non-polio immunizations separately.

Finally, in addition to the usual household and individual covariates we included village-level variables as well as indicator variables for each State (state fixed effects) in our regression models to control for variations across areas in unobserved factors such as policy environment and governance that are correlated with health infrastructure as well as immunization coverage. Given that States differ markedly in terms of development and health related measures, it was important to adequately control for these differences.

## Rural Health Care System

The health care delivery system in rural India relies on a combination of primary health care infrastructure and community outreach. Table 1 and 2 provides details about various levels of government funded rural health infrastructure, the intended and actual populations that each level serves, the medical staff available at each level and the shortfall for each level. Community health centres (CHC) are the largest facility and are the most endowed in terms of medical staff and equipment, followed by primary health centres (PHC), and subsequently, subcentres (SC). CHCs are designed to serve a much larger population, followed by PHCs, and then SCs. However, there are substantial shortfalls at each level of health infrastructure; as of 2005, there were 10 per cent fewer PHCs and SCs than needed and 50 per cent fewer CHCs than needed.

From an immunization delivery perspective, one key problem in expanding coverage is the demanding, temperature-controlled environment needed to store vaccines before they are administered. Most CHCs and many PHCs, though not all, are currently a part of the 'cold chain' and are technically able to maintain a stock of vaccines at recommended temperature zones. While stock-outs at these levels have been reported, they are rare. Thus, the key area of concern is how effectively the immunization delivery system administers vaccines to infants in villages away from these cold chain facilities.

## Health Services Research

A comparison of interstate variations in expenditure on health suggests that Rajasthan spent 5.75 per cent of its budget on health, whereas it was only 3.63 per cent in case of Gujarat in 2003–2004. The State-wise expenditure on health also reveals that the share of health sector in the overall budget has been declining over time. For example, all the States spent 7.02 per cent of their budget on health in 1985–86, which declined to 5.72 per cent in 1991–92 and further to 4.97 per cent in 2003–04.

Low public sector spending on health services results in overdependence on private sector for getting health services. In India, the share of private sector on health care expenditure constitutes around 72 per cent and household sector being the major constituent of the private sector claims 68.8 per cent of expenditure on health care (Table 1). In other words out-of-pocket expenditure comprises major share of expenditure on health care. All the three layers of governments (federal, state and local) spend only 23.8 per cent of the total expenditure on health services. NGO sector is almost non-existent in terms of spending on health services. Its share is only 0.3 per cent.

**Table 1**

*Health Care Expenditure*

| | Private | | Government | | | Public | | NGOs | External Funds |
|---|---|---|---|---|---|---|---|---|---|
| | House-holds | Private Firms | Central | State | Local | Firms | Sector Banks | | |
| Health spending | 68.8% | 3% | 7.2% | 14.4% | 2.2% | 3% | 0.2% | 0.3% | 2% |
| Total | 71.8% | | 23.8% | | | 3.2% | | 0.3% | 2.% |

*Source:* Rao, et al., 2005.

The results of a recently concluded study in Muktsar District of Punjab State in India corroborate overdependence on private health service providers. Both in the rural and urban areas of Muktsar District majority of the people depend upon private health service providers. For example, out of 352 respondents, 276 respondents constituting 78.41 per cent of the total, use health services of the private sectors (see Table 2). In rural areas 75.7 per cent of the respondents and in urban areas 95.5 per cent respondents prefer to visit private health agency for treatment (Panjab University, 2008).

**Table 2**

*Choice of Health Agency by Ownership*

| Respondents | Private | Public | Total |
|---|---|---|---|
| Rural | 227 (75.66) | 73 (24.33) | 300 |
| Urban | 49 (94.23) | 03 (5.77) | 52 |
| Total | 276 (78.41) | 76 (21.59) | 352 |

*Source:* Field Survey, Panjab University, 2008.

Figures in Parentheses are Percentages.

Overdependence on private sector has resulted in glaring disparities in the distribution of health services between rich and poor. According to Rao, 'while taxation is considered the most equitable system of financing, as tax is a means of mobilizing resources from the richer sections to finance the health needs of the poor, out-of-pocket expenditures, the poor, who have the greater probability of falling ill due to poor nutrition, unhealthy living conditions, etc. pay proportionately more on health than the rich and access to health care is dependent on ability to pay' (Rao et al., 2005).

It is not only that distribution of health services are skewed across strata, skewness in their distribution is also found while studying Rural-urban access to health services in India. For example, in rural India there are 0.2 hospital beds per thousand population as against 3.0 in urban areas (see Table 3).

**Table 3**

*Rural-Urban Divide in Health Services in India*

| S. No. | Characteristics | Rural (per 1,000 population) | Urban (per 1,000 population) |
|---|---|---|---|
| 1. | Hospital Beds | 0.2 | 3.0 |
| 2. | Doctors | 0.6 | 3.4 |
| 3. | Public Expenditures | ₹ 80,000 | ₹ 5,60,000 |
| 4. | Out of Pocket | ₹ 7,50,000 | ₹ 11,50,000 |
| 5. | Infant Mortality Rate (IMR) | 74/1,000 Live Births | 44/1,000 Live Births |
| 6. | Under Five Mortality Rate (U5MR) | 133/1,000 Live Births | 87/1,000 Live Births |
| 7. | Births Attended | 33.5% | 73.3% |
| 8. | Full Immunization | 37% | 61% |

*Source:* Jhilam Rudra De (2008).

Similarly in rural areas there are only 0.6 doctors per 1,000 population, which is as high as 3.4 in urban areas. Rural-urban disparities are equally pronounced on account of outcome of health services. For instance Infant Mortality Rate (IMR) in rural areas in 74 per one thousand live births which is about 44 per thousand live births in urban areas. Similarly Under-Five Mortality Rate (UFMR) is 133 per thousand live births in rural areas and 87 per thousand live births in urban areas (De, 2008).

The Government of India has taken a new massive policy initiative known as National Rural Health Mission (NRHM) to reduce the divide between urban and rural areas in the field of health. The major objectives of NRHM are to improve the availability of and access to quality health care by people, especially for those residing in rural areas,

A government-funded review of NRHM also revealed its slow progress. The major problems in the implementation of the NRHM are: administrative constraints, governance issues, inadequacies in human resources as well as the poor investment in public health services in the recent past (Shrivastava, 2008).

Commercialization and privatization of health services and introduction of users' charges in pubic health institutions during post-globalization phase have excluded a sizeable number of populations, particularly belonging to socially disadvantaged groups and the poor from the coverage of health services provided by organized sector.

The unequal access to health services has succinctly been stated by the 11th Five-Year Plan of India (2007–2012), '... there is also a divide between those who have access to essential services such as health, education, drinking water, sanitation, etc. and those who do not. Groups which have hitherto been excluded from our society such as Scheduled Castes (SCs), Scheduled Tribes (STs) and some minorities and Other Backward Classes (OBCs), continue to lag behind the rest' (Planning Commission, 2006).

Gender disparities in health services are also very acute and deserve special attention of the policy makers. Gender disparities are found on account of utilization of health services both for in-patient and out-patient care. National Sample Survey Organization (NSSO) data reveal that in the rural areas the money spent per illness episode for out-patient care was ₹ 151 and ₹ 137 respectively for male and female. The respective amounts for urban areas were ₹ 187 and ₹ 164. Gender variation is expenditure spent for in-patient care is also reported (Saba and Ravindran, 2002). Glaring spatial disparities in health services and their outcomes are also found particularly in rural India (Kathuria and Sankar, 2005).

In addition to inequity in health services, the quality of health services and governance of public health organizations are also matter of concern. First, the infrastructural facilities are inadequate followed by their poor maintenance. Second, most of public health institutions are understaffed accompanied by a high absence rate among the personnel. Third, medicines are normally not available in the health institutions (Dreze, 2004).

## Health Care Delivery System

### *Introduction*

The health care services are divided under State list and Concurrent list in India. While some items such as public health and hospitals fall in the State list, others such as population control and family welfare, medical education and quality control of drugs are included in the Concurrent list. The Union Ministry of Health and Family Welfare (UMHFW) is the central authority responsible for implementation of various programmes and schemes in areas of family welfare, prevention and control of major diseases. In the case of health, the term infrastructure takes on a wider role than mere physical infrastructure. Health care centres, dispensaries or hospitals need to be manned by well-trained staff with a service perspective. In this chapter we include medical staff in our ambit of discussion on rural health infrastructure.

The current conditions of physical infrastructure, staff, access and usage are laid out here before identifying critical gaps, and requirements in infrastructure and services. Issues related to institutions, financing and policy are discussed in the context of these critical need gaps, and the potential role of the private sector in health care provisioning in villages is explored.

### *Physical Infrastructure*

The health care in rural areas has been developed as a three-tier structure based on predetermined population norms. The subcentre is the most peripheral institution and the first contact point between the primary health care system and the community. Each subcentre is manned by one Auxiliary Nurse Midwife (ANM) and one male Multipurpose Worker [MPW(M)]. A Lady Health Worker (LHV) is in charge of six subcentres, each of which are provided with basic drugs for minor ailments and are expected to provide services in relation to maternal and child health, family welfare, nutrition, immunization, diarrhoea control and control of communicable diseases. Subcentres are also expected to use various mediums of interpersonal communication in order to bring about behavioural change in reproductive and hygiene practices. The subcentres are needed for taking care of basic health, needs of men, women and children. As per the figures provided by the UMHFW there were 1,46,026 subcentres functioning in

September 2005 – about 12 per cent lower than the prescribed number as per government norms.

Primary Health Centres (PHCs) comprise the second tier in rural health care structure envisaged to provide integrated curative and preventive health care to the rural population with emphasis on preventive and promotive aspects. (Promotive activities include promotion of better health and hygiene practices, tetanus inoculation of pregnant women, intake of Iron, Folic Acid (IFA) tablets and institutional deliveries.) PHCs are established and maintained by State Governments under the Minimum Needs Programme (MNP)/Basic Minimum Services Programme (BMS). A medical officer is in charge of the PHC supported by fourteen paramedical and other staff. It acts as a referral unit for six subcentres. It has four to six beds for in patients. The activities of PHC involve curative, preventive and Family Welfare Services. There were 23,236 PHCs functioning in September 2005 compared to 23,109 a year earlier, according to the Ministry of Health. Though the numbers appear to be increasing there is still a shortfall of about 16 per cent when compared to the required norms for PHCs.

Community Health Centres (CHCs) forming the uppermost tier are established and maintained by the State Government under the MNP/BMS programme. Four medical specialists including Surgeon, Physician, Gynecologist, and Paediatrician supported by twenty-one paramedical and other staff are supposed to staff each CHC. Norms require a typical CHC to have thirty in-door beds with OT, X-ray, Labour Room, and Laboratory facilities. A CHC is a referral centre for four PHCs within its jurisdiction, providing facilities for obstetric care and specialist expertise. There were 3,346 CHCs in the country, almost a 50 per cent shortfall.

About 49.7 per cent of the subcentres, 78.0 per cent of the PHCs and 91.5 per cent of CHCs are located in the government buildings. The rest are located either in rented buildings or rent free Panchayat/Voluntary Society buildings. As on September 2005, overall 60,762 buildings are required to be constructed to house subcentres. Similarly, for PHCs 2,948 and for CHCs 205 additional buildings are still required.

Data on facilities within these centres are not available. Most reports and evaluation studies point to the lack of equipment, poor or absence of repairs, improper functioning, or lack of complementary facilities such as 24-hour running water, electricity back-ups, and so on. But conditions being what they are, unreliable electricity and water supplies also take their toll on the performance of these centres.

### *Human Resource*

Generally, rural public health facilities across the country are having a difficult time attracting, retaining and ensuring regular presence of highly trained medical professionals. The higher the level of training required for the position, the greater is this need gap.

There exists shortfall across all cadres in the posts of MPW(F)/ANM, MPW(M), Health Assistant (Female)/LHV, and that of Health Assistant (Male). The large shortfall in Male Health Workers, has resulted in poor male participation in Family Welfare and other health programmes and overburdening of the ANMs. This shortage is despite government efforts to train health workers through various training programmes throughout the country for more effective and systematic service delivery.

PHC is the first contact point between the village community and the Medical Officer. The dearth of trained doctors, lab technicians and pharmacists is acutely felt. What these data do not reveal is that even if the personnel are present, their level of participation in providing health services is lower than desired due to lack of supplies, inadequately functioning equipment, poor monitoring of the staff, and so on.

Overall, about 49.9 per cent of the sanctioned posts of specialists at CHCs were vacant in September 2005, which translates to a shortfall of 6,110 specialists at the CHCs as compared to the requirement for existing infrastructure on the basis of existing norms. Even though the government prescribes norms for health care infrastructure, it clearly lacks the capacity to implement them on the ground.

The paucity of skilled health workers is corroborated by results of a household survey based data. The round two of Reproductive Child Health Survey (RCHS), conducted by IIPS for Ministry of Health and Family Welfare sampled 15,794 villages from all states of the country in the period 2002–4. The results are quite revealing and, in fact, reinforce the administrative data available. Around 95 per cent of the villages have a health provider of some type. However, the majority are Anganwadi workers and can be categorized as health workers only under a very liberal definition of health care. The break-up by the type of health care provider is presented. The percentage of villages with trained birth attendants is alarmingly low (37%) and almost 64 per cent of the villages do not have any doctor.

### *Access to Infrastructure*

Even if a health care provider is not present in a village, he/she can be reached easily, some basic access issues would be taken care of. However, we find many limitations especially in the context of road connectivity and adequate transport services. Many of the health care facilities, public or private, are not accessible throughout the year to about a third of the villages. Private and government hospitals are relatively more accessible as they are typically located in areas well connected by metalled roads.

Administrative data of the above showed that (1) a well-defined system of public health care provision exists, (2) there is some shortfall in infrastructure, (3) there is a significant problem with the adequacy of working facilities (supplies and equipment) within these centres, (4) there is a significant lack of adequately trained staff, and (5) there continues to be a lack of adequate access to the facilities that exist.[2] This, of course, affects usage of the health care infrastructure and therefore, access to adequate health care, a concern we address in the detailed section on issues related to access, where we also introduce the important role being played by the private sector.

### *IT for Accessible Health Care Provisioning*

It is well known that many doctors are not willing to serve in the rural areas due to lack of facilities, even if they are paid high salaries. However, as telecom network is spreading swiftly and the government is keen to provide broadband connectivity to all parts of the country; information technology can be effectively harnessed to improve the delivery of health services.

Rural populations have been observed to typically report fewer ailments than those in urban areas. This could be due to many reasons including those related to perception, age, lack of appreciation of health care requirements and so on. It is important to note however, that the awareness level about ailments or health problems has increased both in rural and urban areas between 1995–6 and 2004 as revealed by the NSS 60th round 2004. While 52 per cent of rural untreated patients in 1995–6 did not consider their ailments as serious, this figure stood at only 32 per cent in 2004.

On the average, almost 9 per cent of the rural populations in 2004 report some ailment within the past fifteen days from the day of survey during NSS 60th Round. This figure was much lower in 1995–6 (only about 5.5%). It is not clear why this may have increased so dramatically, especially since NSS survey methodologies have not changed significantly between the two surveys. The incidence of treatment, however, does not appear to have changed significantly over the years and hovers around 82 per cent for rural areas and 90 per cent for urban in both 2004 and 1995–6 (NSSO, 2004).

Clearly an ailment reported may or may not be treated. We find that about 18 per cent of those with an ailment did not receive any treatment at all in rural areas (NSSO, 2004). Within this 18 per cent, there are subtler nuances hidden. For the poorest rural segments, this ratio stands at 24 per cent as opposed to about 10 per cent for the topmost rural economic groups. The reasons ascribed, range from lack of access (12 out of every 100 untreated in rural areas), to lack of finance (28 out of every 100 untreated). Incidence of untreated ailment considered serious enough by the patient to merit medical attention shows a distinct increase in 2004 at 68 per cent over 48 per cent in 1995–6. This should be viewed in the context of increased awareness among rural and urban populations about the seriousness of their health problems. When compared with urban areas, we find that early the accessibility issue is a serious one

### Health Care Delivery System

The challenge that exists today in many countries is to reach the whole population with adequate health care services and to ensure their utilization. The 'large hospital' which was chosen hitherto for the delivery of health services has failed in the sense that it serves only a small part of the population, that too, living within a small radius of the building and the services rendered are mostly curative in nature. Therefore, it has been aptly said that these large hospitals are more ivory towers of diseases than centres for the delivery of comprehensive health care services. Rising costs in the maintenance of these large hospitals and their failure to meet the total health needs of the community have led many countries to seek 'alternative' models of health care delivery with a view to provide health care services that are reasonably inexpensive, and have the basic essentials required by rural population.

### Social and Economic Inequalities of Health

The preset health care delivery system in India is highly selective, institutionalized, centralized and top-down. It has failed to address the need of the majority of rural poor and the marginalized. The main governance issues related to health sector in India are mobilization of physical infrastructure; access, accountability and transparency; issues related to human resource motivation and gender concerns. Access to health care is hindered not only by geographic, social and cost barriers, but also by inherent systemic and structural weaknesses of the public health care system, some of them are as follows:

- Compartmentalized structures and inadequate definition of roles at all levels of care; inefficient distribution, use and management of human resources so that people have to contend with lack of key personnel, unmotivated staff, absenteeism, long waiting time, inconvenient clinic hours/outreach, service times, unauthorized patient charging;
- Inadequate planning, management and monitoring of services/facilities; displaying insensitivity to local/community needs; ineffective or non-existent referral systems, resulting in underutilization of PHCs, overutilization of hospital services, duplication; of services and cost-ineffective provision of services; inadequate systems to enforce accountability and assure quality;
- Inadequate attention to health education and public disclosure. The mandate for contributing to universal access to quality health care services with accountability is a challenging task. Looking at the current national scenario of access and accountability of rural health care delivery system, it can be concluded that neither the public nor the private services come anywhere close to acceptable standards of quantity, quality and accountability.
- Under the circumstances, our search is for a model that makes for a just health care system as an ideal for rural India, the main criteria for this could be:
- Universal access, and access to an adequate level, and access without excessive burden;
- Fair distribution of financial costs for access and fair distribution of burden in rationing care and capacity and a constant search for improvement to a more just system;
- Training providers for competence, empathy and accountability, pursuit of equally care and cost-effective use of the results of relevant research; and
- Special attention to vulnerable groups such as children, women, disabled and the aged.

### *Private Sector in Health Care Reforms and Insurance*

In India, since the early 1990s, considerable work has been undertaken related to health sector reforms, which have involved various governments, international, multilateral agencies and other stakeholders. In fact, innovative experiments are also being done across the States with varying degrees of success. While support exists for supporting various reform initiatives, there is insufficient and inadequate systematic documentation and analysis on its various aspects. Such an overview and analysis of all related issues is necessary to provide evidence to policy makers and other stakeholders in terms of the various dimensions and impact of health sector reform. This analysis would also be useful in suggesting the preferred further activities under health sector reform in India.

While the nature and direction of health sector reforms are specific to each State, common themes and approaches, objectives and issues can be identified. There is a need for policy makers at the State and Central level to exchange experiences and information on health systems reform, sound warnings, disseminate successes and failures, to draw lessons from and draw on best practices from experiences of States, thereby leading to a better understanding of the concept of health sector reforms in India.

Recognizing the need for evidence-based information about and assessment of various initiatives undertaken as part of the health sector reform process in India, the Ministry of Health and Family Welfare, Government of India, in collaboration with the WHO Country Office, India has undertaken a review and documentation of health sector reform initiatives in India. The various methodologies employed included conducting a mailed survey to document reform initiatives underway in various states, compiling relevant information and data through secondary literature review, conducting an experience sharing at national level, in depth documentation of experiences in select States through state visits and interviews with state officials, representatives from bi-lateral and multi-lateral agencies, NGOs, etc. With a view to document, reform initiatives at the centre, interviews were held with select programme officials, key individuals and representatives from select bilateral and multilateral agencies.

As part of the first phase of this activity, reform initiatives underway in nine States, namely Gujarat, Himachal Pradesh, Karnataka, Madhya Pradesh, Odisha, Punjab, Rajasthan, Tripura and Uttaranchal have been compiled into a document. This document, primarily for policy makers at centre and state level, contains information related to genesis, content, process and outcome of health sector reforms across these states. Initiatives in areas such as financing (user fees, health insurance), changes in health system organization, delivery and management, decentralization, controlling out of select services, public-private partnerships), reorganization and restructuring of existing government health care system as well as reforms related to human resources have been outlined.

The government is supposed to create settings that will provide equal opportunity for an individual to fulfil these desires. There is an undisputed association between this social equality, social integration and health. The effect of social integration on health is conclusively documented in the theory of 'social support'.

The effect of social and economic inequality on health is profound too. Poverty, which is a result of social and economic inequality in a society, is detrimental to the health of population. The outcome indicators of health (mortality, morbidity and life expectancy) are all directly influenced by the standards of living of a given population. More so, it is not the absolute deprivation of income that matters, but the relative distribution of income (Wilkinson, 1992).

When applied to Indian context these social theories translate into millions of lives that perish due to a lack of socio-economic equality. Since the emergence of free India in 1947, economic egalitarianism dominated the economic policies. Socialism and government-centred economic policies were favoured over the profit-making private enterprise and capitalism. Though admirable for its motives, these policies led to overdependence on the bureaucracy and stifled the growth of free enterprise. Slow and unequal social mobilization in various parts of India led to an uneven economic growth. Caste and social polarization, literacy and educational levels, natural resources, levels of corruption and role of political leadership has resulted in some Indian states doing better than others on the economic front. This basic inequality was magnified by the rapid but unequal economic growth that India has witnessed in the last two decades. Amidst the rising standards of living, lie pockets of terrible poverty and deprivation.

### *Unequal Distribution of Health Care Resources in India*

Health care resources in India though not adequate, are ample. There has been a definite growth in the overall health care resources and health-related manpower in the last decade. The number of hospitals grew from 11,174 hospitals in 1991 (57% private) to 18,218 (75% private) in 2007. In 2000, the country had 1.25 million doctors and 0.8 million nurses. That translates into one doctor for every 1,800 people. If other systems including Indigenous System of Medicine (ISM) and homeopathic medicine are considered, there is one doctor per 800 people. It not only satisfies but also betters the required estimate of one doctor for 1,500 population. Approximately 15,000 new graduate doctors and 5,000 postgraduate doctors are trained every year. The country has an annual pharmaceutical production of about ₹ 260 billion (INR) and a large proportion of these medicines are exported.

To a casual observer this looks like a good proportion; however, on further study, unequal distribution of resources becomes apparent. The ratio of hospital beds to population in rural areas is fifteen times lower than that for urban areas. The ratio of doctors to population in rural areas is almost six times lower than that in the urban population. Per capita expenditure on public health is seven times lower in rural areas, compared to government health spending for urban areas. Though the spending on health care is 6% of gross domestic product (GDP), the state expenditure is only 0.9 per cent of the total spending. People using their own resources spend rest of it. Thus, only 17 per cent of all health expenditure in the country is borne by the state and 82 per cent comes as out of pocket payments by the people. This makes the Indian public health system grossly inadequate and underfunded. Only five other countries in the world are worse off than India regarding public health spending (Burundi, Myanmar, Pakistan, Sudan and Cambodia). As a result of this dismal and unequal spending on public health, the infrastructure of health system itself is becoming ineffective. The most peripheral and most vital unit of India's public health infrastructure is a primary health centre (PHC). In a recent survey it was noticed that only 38 per cent of all PHCs have all the essential manpower and only 31 per cent have all the essential supplies (defined as 60% of critical inputs), with only 3 per cent of PHCs having 80 per cent of all critical inputs.

The reduction on public health spending and the growing inequalities in health and health care are taking its toll on the marginalized and socially disadvantaged population. The Infant Mortality Rate in the poorest 20 per cent of the population is 2.5 times higher than that in the richest 20 per cent of the population. In other words, an infant born in a poor family is two and half times more likely to die in infancy, than an infant in a better off family. A child in the 'Low standard of living' economic group is almost four times more likely to die in childhood than a child in the 'High standard of living' group. Child born in the tribal belt is one and half times more likely to die before the fifth birthday than children of other groups. Female child is 1.5 times more likely to die before reaching her fifth birthday as compared to a male child. The female to male ratios for children are rapidly declining, from 945 girls per 1,000 boys in 1991, to just 927 girls per 1,000 boys in 2001.

Children below 3 years of age in scheduled tribes and scheduled castes are twice as likely to be malnourished than children in other groups. A person from the poorest quintile of the population, despite more health problems, is six times less likely to access hospitalization than a person from the richest quintile. This means that the poor are unable to afford and access hospitalization in a very large proportion of illness episodes, even when it is required. The delivery of a mother, from the poorest quintile of the population is over six times less likely to be attended by a medically trained person than the delivery of a well-off mother, from the richest quintile of the population. A tribal mother is over 12 times less likely to be delivered by a medically trained person. A tribal woman is one and a half times more likely to suffer the consequences of chronic malnutrition as compared to women from other social categories. These figures speak for themselves and bring to the fore unequal distribution of resources and the effect of it on public health parameters. This unequal distribution of resources is further complimented by inability of universal access to health care due to various access difficulties.

### *Access Difficulties to Health Care*

Universal access to health care is a norm in most of the developed countries and some developing countries (Cuba, Thailand and others). In India though, pre-existing inequality in the health care provisions is further enhanced by difficulties in accessing it. These access difficulties can be either due to:

1. Geographical distance.
2. Socio-economic distance.
3. Gender distance.

The issue of geographic distance is important in a large country like India with limited means of communication. Direct effect of distance of a given population from primary health care centre on the childhood mortality is well documented. It has been shown that the effect of difficult access to health centres is more pronounced for mothers with less education. The same study also states that distance from private hospitals does not affect the health parameters but the distance from public health centre does. Those who live in remote areas with poor transportation facilities are often removed from the reach of health systems. Incentives for doctors and nurses to move to rural locations are generally insufficient and ineffective. Equipping and resupply of remote health care facilities is difficult and inadequacies due to poor supply deter people from using the existent facilities. Maternal mortality is clearly much higher in rural areas as trained medical or paramedical staff attend fewer births, and transport in case of pregnancy complications is difficult. Geographical difficulties in accessing health care facilities thus is an important factor, along with gender discrimination – that contributes to higher maternal mortality in women who live in remote areas especially the tribal women in India.

A different aspect of health care access problem is noticed in cases of 'urban poor'. Data from urban slums show that infant and under-five mortality rates for the poorest 40 per cent of the urban population are as high as the rural areas. Urban residents are extremely vulnerable to macroeconomic shocks that undermine their earning capacity and lead to substitution towards less nutritious, cheaper foods. People in urban slums are particularly affected due to lack of good housing, proper sanitation and proper education. Economically they do not have back-up savings, large food stocks that they can draw down over time. Urban slums are also home to a wide array of infectious diseases (including HIV/AIDS, tuberculosis, hepatitis, dengue fever, pneumonia, cholera, and malaria) that easily spread in highly concentrated populations where water and sanitation services are nonexistent. Poor housing conditions, exposure to excessive heat or cold, diseases, air, soil and water pollution along with industrial and commercial occupational risks, exacerbate the already high environmental health risks for the urban poor. Lack of safety nets and social support systems, such as health insurance, as well as lack of property rights and tenure, further contribute to the health vulnerability of the urban poor. Though the health care facilities are overwhelmingly concentrated in urban areas, the 'socio-economic distance' prevents access for the urban poor. These socio-economic barriers include cost of health care, social factors, such as the lack of culturally appropriate services, language/ethnic barriers and prejudices on the part of providers. There is also significant lack of health education in slums. All these factors lead to an inability to identify symptoms and seek appropriate care on the part of the poor.

The third most important access difficulty is due to gender related distance. It is said that health of society is reflected from the health of its female population. That is completely disregarded in many of the South Asian countries including India. Gender discrimination makes women more vulnerable to various diseases and associated morbidity and mortality. From socio-cultural and economic perspectives women in India find themselves in subordinate positions to men. They are socially, culturally and economically dependent on men. Women are largely excluded from making decisions, have limited access to, and control over resources, are restricted in their mobility, and are often under threat of violence from male relatives. Sons are perceived to have economic, social or religious utility; daughters are often felt to be an economic liability because of the dowry system. In general, an Indian woman is less likely to seek appropriate and early care for disease, whatever the socio-economic status of family might be. This gender discrimination in health care access becomes more obvious when the women are illiterate, unemployed, widowed or dependent on others. The combination of perceived ill health and lack of support mechanisms contributes to a poor quality of life.

### *Effect on Health Outcome Indicators Due to Economic Inequality*

Health standards of a country reflect the social, economic, political and moral well-being of its ordinary citizen. Economic and social growth of a society and country is directly dependent on the health of its constituents. Healthy living conditions and access to good quality health care for all citizens are not only basic human rights, but also essential prerequisites for social and economic development. Any inequality in social, economical or political context between various population groups in a given society will affect the health indicators of that particular society. The most sensitive indicators of health of the society are infant and maternal mortality rates (IMR and MMR). IMR is still significantly high in India. Around 2.2 million infants die every year In fact, the National Health Policy 1983, target to reduce Infant Mortality Rate to less than 60 per 1,000 live births has still not been achieved. The National Health Policy had also set a target for 2,000 to reduce Maternal Mortality Rate to less than 200 per 1,00,000 live births. However, 407 mothers die due to pregnancy related causes, for every 1,00,000 live births even today. In fact, as per the National Family Health Survey (NFHS) in the last decade, Maternal Mortality Rate has increased from 424 maternal deaths per 1,00,000 live births to 540 maternal deaths per 1,00,000 live births. Apart from these avoidable deaths, India has seen persistence and resurgence of many infectious diseases. About 0.5 million people die from tuberculosis every year in India and this number has hardly changed in last five decades. Other communicable diseases like Malaria, Encephalitis, Kala Azar, Dengue and Leptospirosis to name a few, are far from being eradicated. The number of reported cases of malaria has remained at a high level of around 2 million cases annually since the mid-eighties. The outbreak of Dengue in India in 1996–97 saw 16,517 cases and claimed 545 lives. Simple curable diseases like diarrhoea, dysentery, acute respiratory infections and asthma also take their toll due to weak public health system and lack of awareness. Around 0.6 million children die each year from an ordinary illness like diarrhoea. While diarrhoea itself could be largely prevented by universal provision of safe drinking water and sanitary conditions, these deaths can be prevented by timely administration of Oral Rehydration Solution (ORS), which is presently administered in only 27 per cent of cases. Cancer claims over 0.3 million lives per year and tobacco related cancers contribute to 50 per cent of the overall cancer burden, which means that such deaths might be prevented by tobacco control measures. These health outcome indicators reflect a very disappointing state of public health care. The unfortunate fact is, these indicators have failed to improve in spite of various state-run programmes, mushrooming of private health care and a perceptible increase in the GDP. This underscores the importance of social and economic inequality as the stumbling block.

### Private Health Care and Economic Inequality

The growth of private health care sector has been largely seen as a boon; however, it adds to ever-increasing social dichotomy. The dominance of the private sector not only denies access to poorer sections of society, but also skews the balance towards urban-biased, tertiary-level health services with profitability overriding equality and rationality of care often taking a back seat. The increasing cost of health care that is paid by 'out of pocket' payments is making health care unaffordable for a growing number of people. The number of people who could not seek medical care because of lack of money has increased significantly between 1986 and 1995. The proportion of people unable to afford basic health care has doubled in the last decade. One in three people who need hospitalization and are paying out-of-pocket, are forced to borrow money or sell assets to cover expenses. Over 20 million Indians are pushed below the poverty line every year because of the effect of out-of-pocket spending on health care. In the absence of an effective regulatory authority over the private health care sector the quality of medical care is constantly deteriorating. Powerful medical lobbies prevent government from formulating effective legislation or enforcing the existing ones. A recent World Bank report acknowledges the facts that doctors overprescribe drugs, recommend unnecessary investigations and treatment and fail to provide appropriate information for patients, even in private health care sector. The same report also states the relation between quality and price that exists in the private health care system. The services offered at a very high price are excellent but are unaffordable for a common man. This re-emphasizes the role socio-economic inequality plays in health care delivery.

## Conclusion

Effects of social and economic inequality on health of a society are profound. In a large, overpopulated country like India with its complex social architecture and economic extremes, the effect on health system is multifold. Unequal distribution of resources is a reflection of this inequality and adversely affects the health of underprivileged population. The socially underprivileged are unable to access the health care due to geographical, social economic or gender related distances. Burgeoning but unregulated private health care sector makes the gap between rich and poor more apparent.

# 17

# Nutrition and Pregnancy

This chapter is on the nutrient intake and dietary planning that is undertaken before, during and after pregnancy. All dietary advice relating to pregnancy-related nutrition is noted by Mary E. Barasi as one of the major factors in determining the future well-being of a child conceived; some factors of a diet are even noted to reduce childhood morbidity and mortality due to helping the supply of nutrients to the mother.

In a precursory study into the link between nutrition and pregnancy in 1950, women who consumed minimal amounts over the eight-week period had a higher mortality or disorder rate concerning their offspring than women who ate regularly, because children born to well-fed mothers had less restriction within the womb.

Not only have physical disorders been linked with poor nutrition before and during pregnancy, but neurological disorders and handicaps are a risk that is run by mothers who are malnourished, a condition which can also lead to the child becoming more susceptible to later degenerative disease(s).

## Nutrition Before Pregnancy

### *Factors Mitigating Against Pre-pregnancy Nutrition*

It is known that good nutrition before pregnancy is important because of the amount of 'resources' childbirth requires. The process of pre-pregnancy nutrition is a process of 'building up' the immune system in preparation of pregnancy, and is known as being one of the major factors in determining the success rate of conceiving healthy children.

As with most situations, the most important factor in pre-pregnancy nutrition is ensuring that the mother is healthy and without any major factors which could worsen the chances of conceiving, factors such as anorexia or bulimia are thought to be direct links with infertility; the minimum body mass index (BMI) for conceiving mothers being 20.8.

This is also seen to be true with obese women with a BMI above 30 which is a direct result of decrementing amounts of insulin activity and sex hormones may reduce the viability of the ovum.

The ideal range of weight for women wishing to conceive children is thought to be optimal at body mass indexes between 20 and 26. If this, again, is used in conjunction with good nutrition and diet before pregnancy in terms of a normal balanced diet, then reserves of micronutrients, providing materials for pregnancy, would also be maximized.

- Magnesium and zinc supplementation for the binding of hormones at their receptor sites.
- Folic acid supplementation or dietary requirement of foods containing it for the regular growth of the follicle.
- Regular Vitamin D supplementation decreases the chances of deficiencies in adolescence. More importantly, it is known to reduce the likelihood of rickets with pelvic malformations which make normal delivery impossible.
- Regular Vitamin B12 supplementation again is known to reduce the chances of infertility and ill health.

## Nutrition During Pregnancy

### *Factors Mitigating Against Nutrition During Pregnancy*

As it is known, the embryo at conception, and in the subsequent weeks afterwards is the time when it is at its most vulnerable, as it is the time when the organs and systems develop within. The energy used to create these systems comes from the energy and nutrients in the mother's circulation and around the lining of the womb, such is the reason why correct nutrient intake during pregnancy is so important.

During the early stages of pregnancy, the placenta is not formed yet, so there is no mechanism to protect the embryo from the deficiencies which may be inherent in the mother's circulation, so it is critical that the correct amount of nutrients and energy are consumed.

One problem that was found in trials with pregnant women is that deficiencies in folic acid contributed towards neural tube defection; women who had 4 mg of folic acid in their systems due to supplementing 3 months before childbirth significantly reduced the risk of neural tube defect (NTD) within the foetus. This is now advocated by the UK department of health, recommending 400 micrograms per day of folic acid.

Intake of retinol, in extreme cases, has been linked to birth defects and abnormalities. However, regular intake of retinol is not seen as dangerous. It is noted that a 100 g serving of liver may contain a large amount of retinol, so it is best that it is not eaten daily during pregnancy, something which is also the same with alcohol intake in binge drinking.

Excessive amounts of alcohol have been proven to cause foetal alcohol syndrome. The World Health Organization recommends that alcohol should be avoided entirely during pregnancy, given the relatively unknown effects of even small amounts of alcohol during pregnancy.

### *Pregnancy Nutrition: Seafood, Meat and Herbal Tea*

You want what is best for your baby. That is why you add sliced fruit to your fortified breakfast cereal, sneak extra veggies into your favourite recipes and eat yogurt for dessert. But when it comes to pregnancy nutrition, did you know that what you do not eat and drink may be just as important as what you do? Start with the basics. Knowing what to avoid can help you make the healthiest choices for you and your baby.

#### *Seafood*

Seafood can be a great source of protein and iron, and the omega-3 fatty acids in many fish can help promote your baby's brain development. In fact, a British study suggests that skimping on seafood during pregnancy may contribute to poor verbal skills, behavioural problems and other developmental issues during childhood. However, some fish and shellfish contain potentially dangerous levels of mercury. An intake of too much of mercury may damage your baby's developing nervous system. Shrimp, lobster and scallops until they are milky white. Cook clams, mussels and oysters until their shells open. Discard any that do not open.

#### *Meat and Poultry*

During pregnancy, changes in your metabolism and circulation may increase the risk of bacterial food poisoning. Your reaction may be more severe than if you were not pregnant. Rarely, your baby may get sick, too.

To prevent food-borne illness, fully cook all meats and poultry before eating. Look for the juices to run clear, but use a meat thermometer to make sure. Skip medium or rare burgers and sausages. Be careful with hotdogs and deli meats, too. These are sources of a rare but potentially serious food-borne illness known as listeriosis. Cook hotdogs and heat deli meats until they are steaming hot – or avoid them completely.

*Dairy Products*

Dairy products such as skimmed milk, mozzarella cheese and cottage cheese can be a healthy part of your diet. But anything containing unpasteurized milk is a no-no. These products may lead to food-borne illness.

*Herbal Tea*

Although herbal tea may be soothing, avoid it unless your health care provider says it is OK – even the types of herbal tea marketed specifically to pregnant women. There is little data on the effects of specific herbs on developing babies. And large amounts of some herbal teas, such as red raspberry leaf, may cause contractions.

## Health Programmes for Women and Children

### *Programmes of Action*

The Indian government has initiated several measures to ensure that the problems of deprivation and discrimination faced by the poor women and children in India are overcome. These programmes of action aim at dealing with issues like health, education, rural development and better working conditions.

### *Health and Nutrition*

In the field of health, nutrition and family welfare, child survival, safe motherhood and nutritional anaemia have been receiving the highest priority. Apart from the extensive network of primary health care infrastructure, India has also the world's largest Integrated Child Development Services (ICDS) programme which offers a package of supplementary nutrition, immunization, health care, growth monitoring, pre-school education and health and nutrition education. Along with special initiatives like the Universal Immunization Programmes (UIP) these interventions have helped India substantially reduce the infant mortality rate and also bring malnourishment under control.

### *Education for All*

The Indian Constitution states that free and compulsory education for all children would be provided until they complete the age of fourteen years. While it has not been possible to achieve this goal as yet, the achievements in the realm of literacy and basic education have been significant. Recognizing the fact that it is the girl child who is compelled to leave school at an early age, special efforts are being made to increase enrolment and retention of these children in school. Combining a programme of non-formal education for the working children and supported with a massive adult literacy effort, India is geared to meet the target of 'Education for All' by the end of the current decade.

### *Rural Development*

Keeping in view the vulnerable status of women and children in rural society, particularly owing to their economic dependence on others, special provisions have been made to ensure that 40 per cent of all allocation for the Integrated Rural Development Programme (IRDP) and other mass employment programmes have been reserved for women. In order to help poor women working in the informal sector, a National Credit Fund has been started so that loans may be obtained by them at reasonable rates without the formal procedures of usual institutionalized banking. In addition, under programmes like Development of Women and Children in Rural Areas (DWCRA) efforts are being made to give rural women technical and management skills to build their own cooperative enterprises.

### *Special Initiatives*

A significant feature of the women's movement has been the network of associations and groups that have been formed, largely through the efforts of NGOs in India. These groups and associations have successfully organized women working in the informal sector and battled for improvement in their working conditions and for a fairer deal from their employers. Similarly, in the development of cooperatives, particularly in dairying, the contribution towards women's development has been significant.

## Child Health Programme in India

In 1951, India was the first country in the world to launch a family planning programme. Since then approaches aimed at reducing population growth have taken a variety of forms.

### *Major Milestones in Child Health*

The current status of these indicators is as follows:

| | |
|---|---|
| Infant mortality rate | 60 per 1,000 live births (SRS, 2003) |
| Neonatal mortality rate | 40 per 1,000 births (SRS, 2003) |

*Important Maternal and Child Health Indicators: Current Status Vs Goals*

| | Current | XV Year Plan | 2010 | MDG |
|---|---|---|---|---|
| IMR | 60 (SRS, 2000) | 45 | <30 | <30 |
| NMR | 26 (SRS, 2000) | 26 | <20 | <20 |
| MMR | 407 (NFHSI) | 200 | <100 | <100 |
| | Institutional deliveries | 47% | 80% | 80% |

## *Background*

Till 1977, the major health activity was family planning which was changed into Family welfare programme with Maternal and Child Health becoming an integral part of family planning programme with the vision that reduction in birth rate has a direct relationship with reduction in infant and child mortality.

The diarrhoea disease control programme was started in the country in 1978. The main objective of the programme was to prevent death due to dehydration caused by diarrhoea, diseases among children under 5 years of age due to dehydration. Health education aimed at rapid recognition and appropriate management of diarrhoea has been a major component of the Child Survival and Safe Motherhood (CSSM). Under the RCH programme ORS is supplied in the kits to all subcentres in the country every year.

National Health Policy 1983, envisioned significant reduction in IMR, NMR and CMR by 2000. All the child health programmes are directed towards achieving these goals.

Universal Immunization Programme against six preventable diseases, namely, diphtheria, pertusis, childhood tuberculosis, polio-myelitis, measles and neonatal tetanus was introduced in the country in a phased manner in 1985, which covered the whole of India by 1990. Significant progress was made under the Programme in the initial period when more than 90 per cent coverage for all the six antigens was achieved.

The UIP was taken up in 1986 as National Technology Mission and became operational in all districts in the country during 1989–90. UIP become a part of the Child Survival and Safe Motherhood (CSSM) Programme in 1992 and Reproductive and Child Health

(RCH) Programme in 1997. Under the Immunization Programme, infants are immunized against tuberculosis, diphtheria, pertussis, poliomyelitis, measles and tetanus. Universal immunization against 6 vaccine preventable diseases (VPD) by 2000 was one of the goals set in the National Health Policy (1983).

The acute respiratory infection (ARI) Control Programme was started in India in 1990. It sought to introduce scientific protocols for case management of pneumonia with cotrimoxazole. Initially 14 pilot districts were selected and later on new districts were included. A review of the health facility done in 1992 revealed that although 87 per cent of personnel were trained and the drug supply was regular yet there were problems in correct case classification and treatment. Since 1992, the Programme was implemented as part of CSSM and later with RCH. Cotrimoxazole tablets are supplied as part of drug kit for use by different category of workers for managing cases of Pneumonia. Under RCH–II, activities are proposed to be implemented in an integrated way with other child health interventions.

The Child Survival and Safe Motherhood Programme jointly funded by World Bank and UNICEF was started in 1992–93 for implementation up to 1997–98. The Child Survival and Safe Motherhood Programme were implemented in a phased manner covering all the districts of the country by the year 1996–97. The objectives of the programmes were to improve the health status of infants, child and maternal morbidity and mortality. The programmes seek to sustain high coverage levels achieved under the Universal Immunization Programme (UIP) in good performance areas and strengthen the immunization services of poor performing areas. The programme also provides for augmenting various activities under the Oral Rehydration Therapy (ORT) Programme, universalizing prophylaxis schemes for control of anaemia in pregnant women and control of blindness in children and initiating a programme for control of acute respiratory infection (ARI) in children. Under the safe motherhood component, training of traditional birth attendants (TBA), provision of asceptic delivery kits and strengthening of first referral units to deal with high risk and obstetric emergencies were taken up. The approved outlay for the CSSM Programme was ₹ 1,125.58 crores for the entire IDA credit facility of SDR period. The Programme yielded notable success in improving the health status of pregnant women, infants and children and also making a dent in IMF, MMR and incidence of vaccine preventable diseases.

### Reproductive Child Health (RCH) Programme

In order to effectively improve the health status of women and children and fulfil the unmet need for Family Welfare services in the country, especially the poor and underserved by reducing infant child and maternal mortality and morbidity, Government of India during 1997–98 launched the RCH Programme for implementation during the 9th Plan period by integrating Child Survival and Safe Motherhood (CSSM) Programme with other reproductive and child health (RCH) services. In addition, a new component for management of Reproductive Tract Infection (RTI) and Sexually Transmitted Infection (STI) has also been incorporated. The RCH Programme is partly funded by World Bank, UNICEF, UNFPA and European Commission, etc. Reproductive and Child Health Programme is in 5th year of its operation and is currently operational in entire country. The programme follows a differential strategy with inputs under the programme linked to the needs of the area coupled with the capacity for implementation. The programme was reviewed extensively not only in context of achievements during mid-term stage, but also in context of National Population Policy. Efforts were made to strengthen the routine immunization as well as PPI by launching a project for Immunization Strengthening with the World Bank assistance. The ongoing activities were accelerated and new schemes on Financial Envelop, Dais' Training, RCH Camps and RCH outreach services were started to address felt gaps. The implementation of Executive Committee (EC) assisted Sector Investment Programme has geared up, especially State/District level activities and urban RCH component.

Currently the initiatives that are being implemented by the Department of Family Welfare to achieve these goals are:

1. Control of deaths due to acute respiratory infection.
2. Control of deaths due to diarrhoeal diseases.
3. Provision of essential new-born care.
4. Vitamin A supplementation to children between the ages of 6 months to 3 years.
5. Iron folic acid supplementation to children under five years of age.
6. Implementation of exclusive breast feeding up to the age of 6 months and appropriate practices related to complementary feeding.
7. Integrated Management of Neonatal and Childhood Illnesses (IMNCI): It offers a comprehensive package for the management of

the most common causes of childhood illnesses i.e. sepsis, measles, malaria, diarrhoea, pneumonia and malnutrition. It is supported by appropriate strengthening of the health care system and promotion of positive health care practices of the community.

### Breastfeeding

#### Objectives

*Breastfeeding:* 'Exclusive breast-feeding of the first six months of life' to be propagated as it would have the following benefits:

- It is the ideal method of infant feeding.
- Is the single most cost-effective intervention for reduction of infant mortality.
- Delays return to fertility in the mother and hence acts as a natural contraceptive (Lactation Amennarrhoea Method, LAM).

#### Strategy

A breast-feeding partnership of the government with all major professional bodies and various NGOs has been formed. The Infant Milk Substitute (IMS) Act is being implemented:

(a) Baby Friendly Hospital Initiative

(b) Lactation Clinics

(c) Peer Counselling.

### Iron and Folic Acid Supplementation

#### Objectives

- Screening of children for anaemia wherever required and appropriate treatment of those found anaemic.
- Reducing prevalence of anaemia by 25 per cent and moderate and severe anaemia by 50 per cent in children (Tenth Plan).

2. Strategy

- Improve dietary intake to meet RDA for all macro- and micro-nutrients;
- Dietary diversification – inclusion of iron folate rich foods as well as food items that promote iron absorption;
- Food fortification, including introduction of iron and iodine-fortified salt and other iron-fortified items (e.g. attar in specific areas);
- Health and nutrition education to improve over all dietary intakes and promote consumption of iron and folate-rich foodstuffs.

*Infants*

- Exclusive breast-feeding for six months, and introduction of green leafy vegetables along with cereal/pulse/oilseed mix in the seventh month for the prevention of anaemia;
- Screening for anaemia in preterm, low birth weight infants and those with growth faltering and repeated episodes of infection; and
- Appropriate treatment for anaemic infants.

*Pre-school Children*

- advocacy with regard to dietary diversification for the prevention of anaemia;
- all growth retarded children and those with repeated infections have to have HB estimation carried out and those found to be anaemic are provided with appropriate treatment;
- In hookworm endemic areas, it is necessary to improve:
- sanitation and educate people not to walk barefoot;
- treat children with a history of passing worms with broad spectrum antihelmintics;
- screen all anaemic children for hookworm infestation and treat them.

The cooperation of the PRIs and women's' self-help groups, where-ever existent, may be sought to promote and monitor intake of IFA tablets in their community.

*Coverage*

- As per a survey carried out in 2002 by the National Nutrition Monitoring Bureau, under the ICMR, 67 per cent of the pre-school children were anaemic.
- 2,84,729 kits are distributed throughout the country each year under the RCH programme, each kit containing 13,000 tablets of paediatric IFA tablets.

*Implementation*

Through the health institutions under the government sector.

***Vitamin A Supplementation Strategy***

*Objectives*

- Decrease prevalence of Vitamin A deficiency form the current 0.7 per cent to 0.3 per cent

*Strategy*

*Infancy*

- Health and nutrition education is being taken up to encourage colostrums feeding, exclusive breast-feeding for the first six months and the introduction of complementary feeding thereafter.
- 1,00,000 International Unit (IU) dose of Vitamin A is being given at nine months.

*Childhood*

- Health education efforts to ensure adequate intake of Vitamin A rich food throughout childhood.
- Early detection and prompt treatment of infections.
- Vitamin A dose of 2,00,000 IU at 18, 24, 30 and 36 months of age.

*Sick Children*

- All children with xerophthalmia to be treated at health facilities.
- All children suffering from measles to be given one dose of Vitamin A if they have not received it in the previous one month.
- All cases of severe malnutrition to be given one additional dose of Vitamin A.

*Coverage*

- Vitamin A supplementation coverage rate (6–59 months) 2009. 44 per cent.
- 2,84,729 kits are distributed throughout the country each year under the RCH programme, each kit containing 6 bottles of 100 ml each.

*Implementation*

Through the health institutions and anganwadis under the government sector.

**Integrated Management of Neonatal and Childhood Illness (IMNCI)**

Integrated Management of Childhood Illness (IMCI) strategy, which has already been implemented in more than 100 countries all over the globe, encompasses a range of interventions to prevent and manage five major childhood illnesses, i.e. Acute Respiratory Infections, Diarrhoea, Measles, Malaria and Malnutrition. It focuses on preventive, promotive and curative aspects, and it gives a holistic outlook to the programme.

Government of India recognizes the need to strengthen child health activities in the country. In order to do so and introduce IMCI in the country, a Core Group was constituted which included representatives from Indian Academy of Pediatrics (IAP), National Neonatology Forum of India (NNF), National Anti-Malaria Programme (NAMP), Department of Women and Child Development (DWCD), Child-in-Need Institute (CINI), WHO, UNICEF, eminent Pediatricians and Neonatologists, and the representatives from Ministry of Health and Family Welfare, Government of India. The Adaptation Group developed Indian version of IMCI guidelines and renamed it as Integrated Management of Neonatal and Childhood Illness (IMNCI).

The major components of this strategy are:

- Strengthening the skills of the health care workers.
- Strengthening the health care infrastructure.
- Involvement of the community.

The first two components are the facility-based IMNCI and the third is the community-based IMNCI.

The major highlights of Indian adaptation are:

- Incorporation of neonatal care as it now constitutes two-thirds of infant mortality.
- Inclusion of 0–7 days.
- Incorporating National guidelines on Malaria, Anaemia, Vitamin A supplementation and Immunization schedule.
- Training schedule reduced from 11 to 8 days.
- Training begins with sick young infant upto 2 months.
- Proportion of training time devoted to sick young infant and sick child is almost equal.

The Government has initiated implementation of the IMNCI strategy in four districts each in nine selected states of Odisha, Rajasthan, Madhya Pradesh, Haryana, Delhi, Gujarat, Uttaranchal, Tamil Nadu and Rajasthan.

### The Road Ahead

India is a signatory to the Millennium Development Goals (MDGs). The fourth Millennium Development Goal is reduction of child mortality and the target for this is to reduce by two-thirds, between 1990–2015 the mortality rate of children under five. This is reflected in the Tenth Five-Year Plan (2002–07), which states that Infant Mortality Rate is to be reduced to 45/1,000 by 2007 and 28/1,000 live births by 2012.

# 18

# Reproductive Rights of Women

Human rights and reproductive health advocates increasingly are working together to advance women's and men's well-being. The modem human rights system is based on a series of legally binding international treaties that make use of principles of ethics and social justice, many of which are directly relevant to reproductive health care. By placing reproductive health in a broader context, a rights-based approach can provide tools to analyse the root causes of health problems and inequities in service delivery. By emphasizing fundamental values, most notably respect for clients and their reproductive decisions, a rights-based approach can shape humane and effective reproductive health programmes and policies. By taking advantage of the international human rights treaty system, a rights-based approach can challenge the status quo and pressure governments into working proactively for reproductive health.

### Human Rights in the Modern Era

The concept of reproductive rights is rooted in the modern human rights system developed under the auspices of the United Nations (UN). Since 1945, the UN has created internationally recognized standards for a range of human rights, including the right to health, and has established mechanisms to promote and protect those rights. In response to atrocities committed during World War II, the UN General Assembly adopted the Universal Declaration on Human Rights in 1948. International treaties (see Table 1, page 358) have since transformed the principles asserted in the declaration into legally binding obligations for nations that ratify the agreements. Parallel systems of human rights treaties and monitoring bodies also exist in some regions, including Africa, the Americas, the Arab states and Europe.

Transforming these legal obligations into a genuine political commitment to reproductive rights, however, required concerted and sustained pressure from women's advocates. The women's empowerment movement drew attention to human rights abuses stemming from women's subordinate position in society and pressured governments to change the circumstances of women's lives. In three landmark international meetings in the 1990s, the movement succeeded in forging a new consensus on reproductive rights and made them central concerns for health programmes and policies around the worlds.

The 1993 World Conference on Human Rights in Vienna affirmed that women's rights are human rights and should not be subordinated to cultural or religious traditions. The conference also marked a breakthrough for reproductive rights, acknowledging that human rights can and should be broadly applied to the areas of sexuality and reproduction. To realize their right to choose the number and spacing of their children unless they can afford transport to and user fees for family planning services (right to freedom from poverty and to work). They also must have access to informational materials and be able to read them (right to receive information and to education), and not fear a violent reaction from their partners (right to freedom from inhuman and degrading treatment).

### *Benefits of a Rights-Based Approach*

Human rights and health advocates can best achieve their common goal – improving people's well-being – by taking advantage of the complementary strengths of their two fields. Taking a rights-based approach to reproductive health offers many benefits:

- Human rights can provide core values and an ethical framework for public health practitioners.
- International treaty obligations increase the pressure on governments to provide adequate health services, fight violence against women and take other actions that improve public health.
- Framing a health problem like maternal mortality as a human rights or social justice concern, raises its visibility and can make it an urgent policy concern.

The 1994 International Conference on Population and Development in Cairo created a comprehensive framework to realize reproductive rights and health. Women's advocates persuaded governments to reject population policies focused solely on reducing fertility and to forge a new approach that focused instead, on meeting individual women's needs for a wide array of reproductive health services.

**Table 1**

*Universal Declaration on Human Rights in 1948 (International Treaties)*

| Human Right | Reproductive Health (RH) Obligations |
|---|---|
| Right to life and survival | • Prevent avoidable maternal deaths.<br>• End female foeticide and infanticide.<br>• Screen for cancers that can be detected early and treated.<br>• Ensure access to dual-protection contraceptive methods. |
| Right to liberty and security | • Eliminate female genital mutilation. |
| Of the person | • Obtain informed consent for all procedures, including HIV testing, sterilization and abortion.<br>• Encourage clients to make independent RH decisions<br>• Stop sexual trafficking. |
| Right to freedom from inhuman and degrading treatment | • Protect and care for survivors of sexual assault and domestic abuse and prosecute the perpetrators.<br>• Prohibit involuntary abortion and sterilization. |
| | • Eliminate rape as an instrument of war. |
| Right to marry and found a family | • Prevent early or coerced marriages.<br>• Provide access to infertility services to women and men.<br>• Prevent and treat reproductive tract infections that cause infertility. |
| Right to decide the number | • Provide access to a range of contraceptive methods. |
| and spacing of one's children | • Help people choose and use a family planning method.<br>• Provide access to safe abortion services, where legal. |

*Cont'd...*

*...Cont'd*

| | |
|---|---|
| Right to the highest attainable standard of health | • Provide access to affordable, acceptable and comprehensive RH services.<br>• Provide high-quality care.<br>• Allocate available resources fairly.<br>• Provide access to effective approaches to cervical cancer screening/early treatment. |
| Right to the benefits of scientific progress | • Fund research on women's as well as men's health needs.<br>• Provide access to emergency contraception.<br>• Provide access to antiretroviral treatment for AIDS.<br>• Provide access to obstetric care that can prevent maternal deaths. |
| Right to non-discrimination and respect for difference | • Offer RH services to all groups, including adolescents, unmarried women and refugees.<br>• Ensure that a husband's or parent's consent is not required for RH services.<br>• Offer services that meet women's and men's distinctive RH needs. |
| Right to receive, and impart information | • Make family planning information freely available.<br>• Offer. sufficient information for people to make good RH decisions |
| Right to freeway of thought, conscience and religion | • Do not limit RH services, such as emergency contraception, on religious grounds.<br>• Allow providers to refuse to offer contraceptive and abortion services on the grounds of conscience where referrals are possible and treatment in emergency situations is protected. |
| Right to privacy | • Ensure privacy for all services.<br>• Keep clients' information confidential. |

The 1995 Fourth World Conference on Women in Beijing confirmed and built on the link established in Cairo between women's reproductive rights and human rights already recognized by international treaties and national laws. The Beijing Platform for Action took a holistic, rights-focused view of health and the social, political and economic factors that affect it. It focused on governments' obligation to fulfil the right to health by creating the conditions that enable women to realize their right to health.

### *Fundamental Principles*

Many of the human rights defined in international treaties have implications for reproductive health care. They guide almost every aspect of the delivery of care, defining what services must be offered, to whom, and in what fashion. Three principles are key for reproductive health:

- Based on the rights to liberty, to marry and found a family, and to decide the number and spacing of one's children, individuals have the right to control their sexual and reproductive lives and make reproductive decisions without interference or coercion.
- The right to non-discrimination and respect for difference requires governments to ensure equal access to health care for everyone and to address the unique health needs of women and men.
- To fulfil people's rights to life and health, governments must make comprehensive reproductive health services available and remove barriers to care.

A rights-based approach to reproductive health is especially powerful because all human rights, including reproductive rights, are universal, inalienable, indivisible and interdependent. Universal because everyone is born with and possesses the same rights, regardless of where they live, their gender or race, or their religious, cultural or ethnic background. Inalienable because people's rights can never be taken away, no matter what they do, nor can an individual ever give up his or her rights. Indivisible and interdependent because all rights – civil, social, economic or political – are equal in importance and none can be fully enjoyed without the others.

The universal quality of human rights means that nations cannot cite cultural or religious traditions – which often place women in a subordinate position and validate harmful practices such as early marriage and female genital mutilation (FGM) – as an excuse not to respect and protect all of women's rights, including their reproductive rights.

The principle of indivisibility recognizes that women cannot realize their reproductive rights without realizing their broader human rights. Because regional systems are more sensitive to local cultural and religious concerns, their authority also tends to be accepted more readily by governments.

International and regional discourse on human rights is having an increasing impact at the national level. Government officials, legislators and judges in many countries often are basing their policies, laws, and court rulings on international and regional human rights treaties along with comments issued by treaty monitoring committees, and the programmes of action adopted at international conferences.

### *Role of National Governments*

The international treaty system imposes three obligations on national governments: to respect, protect, and fulfil human rights.

- Respect for rights means not interfering with people's ability to enjoy their rights, for example, by not prohibiting adolescents from getting contraceptives.
- Protecting rights means taking action against those who violate human rights, for example, by prosecuting the perpetrators of rape and domestic violence.
- Fulfilling rights means taking legislative, budgetary and judicial actions that allow people to fully realize their rights, for example, by building a public health infrastructure with enough facilities and providers to offer affordable and comprehensive reproductive health services throughout the country.

To meet their three obligations, national governments must adopt appropriate policies and laws. Many constitutions, bills of rights, and laws set binding standards for human rights, but their content and the degree of support for reproductive rights is influenced by national politics and varies widely.

To truly fulfil reproductive rights, governments also must address societal conditions that hinder women from enjoying their reproductive rights. Policies, laws and justice systems that empower women and promote gender equity are needed. For example governments can work to increase educational, economic, and political opportunities for women, and promote equitable, violence-free relationships between men and women.

Implementing these policies and laws poses a difficult challenge. Governments must allocate resources to enforce laws and policies and they also must hold officials accountable for their actions. In southern Africa, for example, governments have responded to the problem of violence against women by revising their laws but have failed to allocate money for enforcement or educate police officers, prosecutors, and judges about the law. As a result, many officials continue to make decisions based on personal beliefs about gender-based violence.

### Health Care System

Public health programmes are responsible for supplementing available private health services to ensure that everyone has access to a complete range of affordable, acceptable, and good-quality reproductive health information, services and commodities. This obligation requires action at the policy-making and upper managerial levels, for example, in building, equipping and staffing facilities or training personnel to offer reproductive health services. It also requires action at the local point of care, for example, in supervising the technical quality of care, arranging for privacy and maintaining reliable supplies of contraceptives. Health care providers who interact directly with clients carry special responsibilities, such as respecting confidentiality, helping clients make fully informed decisions and avoiding bias against certain services or clients.

*Clients and Community:* Health care clients and community members also can play a role in realizing their own reproductive rights. For example, clients may request privacy at clinics, ask providers for information and take the initiative in making reproductive health decisions. Clients also can hold providers and programmes accountable by complaining if, for example a provider breaches confidentiality regarding STI/HIV test results. Community members can influence reproductive rights by helping set the social norms that shape individual behaviour. Their attitudes determine, for example, whether it is socially acceptable for women to go alone to a clinic, for men to beat their wives or for girls to be circumcized.

- Rights education can empower health care clients and the community by instilling a sense of entitlement and establishing new social norms.
- Respecting human rights improves the effectiveness of health interventions: outcomes are better if adolescents are offered reproductive health services, if couples are encouraged to make an informed choice of family planning methods, and if sex workers are empowered, rather than coerced, to use condoms.
- A rights-based approach helps public health practitioners understand the societal factors, such as gender inequality that influence reproductive health and reach beyond the health sector to address them.

Public health methodologies also offer benefits to human rights advocates. Epidemiological studies can explain the causes of problems like avoidable maternal deaths and document their magnitude – unlike the case studies human rights advocates traditionally use to analyse rights violations. Statistical analysis of large data sets also can identify widespread problems, such as provider bias toward certain contraceptive methods that may be too subtle to attract the attention of rights advocates. Public health methodologies also are able to assess the impact of changes in policy and programmes on reproductive health indicators.

The reproductive health problem posed by violence against women demonstrates the synergies between the health and rights perspectives. Framing violence against women as a violation of human rights raises awareness and increases political will to address the problem. It holds governments accountable and broadens the response to include non-health sectors, like law enforcement and the judiciary. In Nicaragua, for example, activists used epidemiological research on the prevalence and effects of domestic violence to build support for legal reforms. It also increases appreciation of how poverty, education and social inequality contribute to levels of violence. The public health approach encourages the gathering of convincing evidence on the magnitude of the problem, its health consequences and risk factors; develops interventions to prevent violence and reduces harm when it occurs; and assesses the impact and cost-effectiveness of interventions.

### Obligations and Responsibilities

Although human rights treaties directly place obligations only on states and state officials, they indirectly create responsibilities for other organizations and individuals.

*International Organizations:* Each international human rights treaty provides for a committee to monitor the performance of ratifying nations. 'As part of a country reporting system, each nation periodically submits a report to the committee on their efforts to meet their treaty obligations. The committee discusses the report with country representatives and also hears testimony from UN agencies, nongovernmental organizations (NGOs), and, in some cases, individuals. At the end of this quasi-judicial process, the committee issues an official report highlighting areas of concern and recommending specific changes. These reports are submitted to the UN General Assembly'. The country reporting process gives the monitoring committees and civil society an opportunity to influence a government's actions through dialogue and the force of world opinion. The committees rely on the good faith of member states to comply with treaty obligations.

The treaty-monitoring committees also are responsible for interpreting broadly worded treaty provisions. In recent years, several committees have issued general comments or general recommendations that detail standards for governments to follow in meeting their treaty obligations regarding women's reproductive rights. By demonstrating how rights apply to particular reproductive health issues and by defining government obligations, these comments and recommendations have fostered compliance with the treaties.

Regional systems of human rights treaties and monitoring bodies have their own reporting and complaints procedures, which may set higher standards for human rights and their implementation than international agreements. They can address complaints more efficiently since they include courts that have the power to issue binding decisions on domestic abuse. Reproductive health programmes have tested many different approaches:

- The International Planned Parenthood Federation (IPPF) has designed and distributed posters on Client's Rights and Young People's Rights to encourage clients to claim their rights to confidentiality, privacy, information and other elements of good care.
- A cervical cancer prevention programme in San Martin, Peru, incorporated client rights and empowerment into an interactive educational session, with the goal of increasing women's self-esteem and hence their ability to overcome psychological and cultural barriers to screening.
- Community-based rights programmes in India cover reproductive rights along with literacy training, economic development, and other activities to empower women in every aspect of their lives. They have encouraged women to reject early marriages and seek health care without waiting for men's approval.

Reproductive rights education faces special obstacles. It is sometimes difficult to translate rights concepts into language that is relevant to a local culture, and communities used to thinking collectively may find the focus on the individual uncomfortable. Rights concepts also challenge long-established cultural and religious traditions, including patriarchal power structures and sexual taboos, and may ask people to act in ways that they find uncomfortable. Recognizing these difficulties, Cooperative for Assistance and Relief Everywhere (CARE) decided not to use the language of international treaties when it took a rights-based approach to ending the long-standing and culturally embedded tradition of female genital mutilation (FGM) in Ethiopia and Kenya. Instead, the projects asked the community to define rights and responsibilities and let their understanding guide programme strategies to bring about necessary social change.

## Monitoring Reproductive Rights

Process indicators-based approach to reproductive health, for three reasons. First, many reproductive rights focus on how health care is delivered. What matters, for example, is whether adolescents have access to and are allowed to make an informed choice of contraceptive methods, not which methods they choose and how effectively they use them. Second, the international treaty system recognizes that fulfilling many rights, including the right to health, will take time. In the short run, the treaty monitoring bodies ask nations to take reasonable, identifiable steps toward their realization. Third, data on many reproductive health outcomes in many countries is simply not available or not reliable.

Consequently, a rights-based evaluation of a programme to reduce maternal mortality should not focus on changes in maternal mortality rates and ratios alone. Programme managers also should assess whether states are providing needed maternal health services, including emergency obstetric care, which can help prevent maternal deaths. Important indicators include the number and distribution of health facilities providing obstetric care and the quality of those services.

## Conclusion

Effectively addressing reproductive health problems calls for an integrated, rights-based approach that draws on the fields of health, ethics, law, and human rights. By collaborating with experts in all these fields, reproductive health programmes can address the social, cultural, economic, legal, and policy factors that affect women's and men's reproductive health, as well as medical and public health concerns. By stressing fundamental human values, a rights-based approach also can energize efforts of reproductive health programmes to meet clients' needs and offer good quality care. With the tenth anniversaries of the Cairo and Beijing conferences fast approaching, it is time for reproductive health programmes to revisit the conferences' rights-based agendas and redouble their efforts to realize their health and human rights goals.

# 19

# Medical Ethics and Law in India

## Medical Profession

The prime object of the medical profession is to render service to humanity; reward or financial gain is a subordinate consideration. Whosoever chooses his profession, assumes the obligation to conduct himself in accordance with its ideals. A physician should be an upright man, instructed in the art of healings. He shall keep himself pure in character and be diligent in caring for the sick; he should be modest, sober, patient, prompt in discharging his duty without anxiety; conducting himself with propriety in his profession and in all the actions of his life.

No person other than a doctor having qualification recognized by Medical Council of India and registered with Medical Council of India/State Medical Council (s) is allowed to practice modern system of medicine or surgery. A person obtaining qualification in any other system of medicine is not allowed to practice modern system of medicine in any form.

### *Maintaining Good Medical Practices*

The principal objective of the medical profession is to render service to humanity with full respect for the dignity of profession and man. Physicians should merit the confidence of patients entrusted to their care, rendering to each a full measure of service and devotion. Physicians should try continuously to improve medical knowledge and skills and should make available to their patients and colleagues the benefits of their professional attainments. The physician should practise methods of healing founded on scientific basis and should not associate professionally with anyone who violates this principle. The honoured ideals of the medical profession imply that the responsibilities of the physician extend not only to individuals but also to society.

Registered medical practitioner shall maintain a Register of Medical Certificates giving full details of certificates issued. When issuing a medical certificate he/she shall always enter the identification marks of the patient and keep a copy of the certificate. He/she shall not omit to record the signature and/or thumb mark, address and at least one identification mark of the patient on the medical certificates or report.

### Exposure of Unethical Conduct

*A Physician should expose,* without fear or favour, incompetent or corrupt, dishonest or unethical conduct on the part of members of the profession.

*Payment of Professional Services:* The physician, engaged in the practice of medicine shall give priority to the interests of patients. The personal financial interests of a physician should not conflict with the medical interests of patients. A physician should announce his fees before rendering service and not after the operation or treatment is under way. Remuneration received for such services should be in the form and amount specifically announced to the patient at the time the service is rendered. It is unethical to enter into a contract of 'no cure no payment'. Physician rendering service on behalf of the state shall refrain from anticipating or accepting any consideration.

### Evasion of Legal Restrictions

The physician shall observe the laws of the country in regulating the practice of medicine and shall also not assist others to evade such laws. He should be cooperative in observance and enforcement of sanitary laws and regulations in the interest of public health. A physician should observe the provisions of the State Acts like Drugs and Cosmetics Act, 1940; Pharmacy Act, 1948; Narcotic Drugs and Psychotropic Substances Act, 1985; Medical Termination of Pregnancy Act, 1971; Transplantation of Human Organ Act, 1994; Mental Health Act, 1987; Environmental Protection Act, 1986; Pre-natal Sex Determination Test Act, 1994; Drugs and Magic Remedies (Objectionable Advertisement) Act, 1954; Persons with Disabilities (Equal Opportunities and Full Participation) Act, 1995 and Bio-Medical Waste (Management and Handling) Rules, 1998 and such other Acts, Rules, Regulations made by the Central/State Governments or local Administrative Bodies or any other relevant Act relating to the protection and promotion of public health.

## Duties of Physicians to Their Patients

### *Obligations to the Sick*

Though a physician is not bound to treat each and every person asking his services, he should not only be ever ready to respond to the calls of the sick and the injured, but should be mindful of the high character of his mission and the responsibility he discharges in the course of his professional duties. In his treatment, he should never forget that the health and the lives of those entrusted to his care depend on his skill and attention. A physician should endeavour to add to the comfort of the sick by making his visits at the hour indicated to the patients. A physician advising a patient to seek service of another physician is acceptable; however, in case of emergency a physician must treat the patient. No physician shall arbitrarily refuse treatment to a patient. However for good reason, when a patient is suffering from an ailment which is not within the range of experience of the treating physician, the physician may refuse treatment and refer the patient to another physician.

Medical practitioner having any incapacity detrimental to the patient or which can affect his performance vis-à-vis the patient is not permitted to practise his profession.

### *Display of Registration Numbers*

Every physician shall display the registration number accorded to him by the State Medical Council/Medical Council of India in his clinic and in all his prescriptions, certificates, money receipts given to his patients.

Physicians shall display as suffix to their names only recognized medical degrees or such certificates/diplomas and memberships/honours which confer professional knowledge or recognizes any exemplary qualification/achievements.

### *Use of Generic Names of Drugs*

Every physician should, as far as possible, prescribe drugs with generic names and he/she shall ensure that there is a rational prescription and use of drugs.

### *Highest Quality Assurance in Patient Care*

Every physician should aid in safeguarding the profession against admission to it of those who are deficient in moral character or education. Physician shall not employ in connection with his professional practice, any attendant who is neither registered nor enlisted under the Medical Acts in force and shall not permit such persons to attend, treat or perform operations upon patients wherever professional discretion or skill is required.

### *Patience, Delicacy and Secrecy*

Patience and delicacy should characterize the physician. Confidences concerning individual or domestic life entrusted by patients to a physician and defects in the disposition or character of patients observed during medical attendance should never be revealed unless their revelation is required by the laws of the State. Sometimes, however, a physician must determine whether his duty to society requires him to employ knowledge, obtained through confidence as a physician, to protect a healthy person against a communicable disease to which he is about to be exposed. In such instance, the physician should act as he would wish another to act toward one of his own family in like circumstances.

### *Prognosis*

The physician should neither exaggerate nor minimize the gravity of a patient's condition. He should ensure himself that the patient, his relatives or his responsible friends have such knowledge of the patient's condition as will serve the best interests of the patient and the family.

### *The Patient Must Not Be Neglected*

A physician is free to choose whom he will serve. He should, however, respond to any request for his assistance in an emergency. Once having undertaken a case, the physician should not neglect the patient, nor should he withdraw from the case without giving adequate notice to the patient and his family. Provisionally or fully registered medical practitioner shall not wilfully commit an act of negligence that may deprive his patient or patients from necessary medical care.

### *Engagement for an Obstetric Case*

When a physician who has been engaged to attend an obstetric case is absent and another is sent for and delivery accomplished, the acting physician is entitled to his professional fees, but should secure the patient's consent to resign on the arrival of the physician engaged.

## Duties of Physician in Consultation

### *Unnecessary Consultations Should be Avoided*

However, in case of serious illness and in doubtful or difficult conditions, the physician should request consultation, but under any circumstances such consultation should be justifiable and in the interest of the patient only, and not for any other consideration. Consulting pathologists/radiologists or asking for any other diagnostic lab investigation should be done judiciously and not in a routine manner.

### Consultation for Patient's Benefit

In every consultation, the benefit to the patient is of foremost importance. All physicians engaged in the case should be frank with the patient and his attendants.

### Punctuality in Consultation

Utmost punctuality should be observed by a physician in making themselves available for consultations.

### Statement to Patient After Consultation

All statements to the patient or his representatives should take place in the presence of the consulting physicians, except as otherwise agreed. The disclosure of the opinion to the patient or his relatives or friends shall rest with the medical attendant.

Differences of opinion should not be divulged unnecessarily but when there is irreconcilable difference of opinion the circumstances should be frankly and impartially explained to the patient or his relatives or friends. It would be opened to them to seek further advice as they so desire.

### Treatment After Consultation

No decision should restrain the attending physician from making such subsequent variations in the treatment if any unexpected change occurs, but at the next consultation, reasons for the variations should be discussed/explained. The same privilege, with its obligations, belongs to the consultant when sent for in an emergency during the absence of attending physician. The attending physician may prescribe medicine at any time for the patient, whereas the consultant may prescribe only in case of emergency or as an expert when called for.

### Patients Referred to Specialists

When a patient is referred to a specialist by the attending physician, a case summary of the patient should be given to the specialist, who should communicate his opinion in writing to the attending physician.

### Fees and Other Charges

A physician shall clearly display his fees and other charges on the board of his chamber and/or the hospitals he is visiting. Prescription should also make clear if the physician himself dispensed any medicine. A physician shall write his name and designation in full along with registration particulars in his prescription letter head.

(*Note:* In government hospital where the patient-load is heavy, the name of the prescribing doctor must be written below his/her signature.)

## Responsibilities of Physicians to Each Other

A physician should consider it as a pleasure and privilege to render gratuitous service to all physicians and their immediate family dependants.

### *Conduct in Consultation*

In consultations, no insincerity, rivalry or envy should be indulged in. All due respect should be observed towards the physician in-charge of the case and no statement or remark be made, which would impair the confidence reposed in him. For this purpose no discussion should be carried on in the presence of the patient or his representatives.

### *Consultant Not to Take Charge of the Case*

When a physician has been called for consultation, the Consultant should normally not take charge of the case, especially on the solicitation of the patient or friends. The Consultant shall not criticize the referring physician. He/she shall discuss the diagnosis treatment plan with the referring physician.

### *Appointment of Substitute*

Whenever a physician requests another physician to attend his patients during his temporary absence from his practice, professional courtesy requires the acceptance of such appointment only when he has the capacity to discharge the additional responsibility along with his/her other duties. The physician acting under such an appointment should give the utmost consideration to the interests and reputation of the absent physician and all such patients should be restored to the care of the latter upon his/her return.

### *Visiting Another Physician's Case*

When it becomes the duty of a physician occupying an official position to see and report upon an illness or injury, he should communicate to the physician in attendance so as to give him an option of being present. The medical officer/physician occupying an official position should avoid remarks upon the diagnosis or the treatment that has been adopted.

## Duties of Physician to the Public and to the Paramedical Profession

### *Physicians as Citizens*

Physicians, as good citizens, possessed of special training should disseminate advice on public health issues. They should play their part in enforcing the laws of the community and in sustaining the institutions that advance the interests of humanity. They should particularly cooperate with the authorities in the administration of sanitary/public health laws and regulations.

### *Public and Community Health*

Physicians, especially those engaged in public health work, should enlighten the public concerning quarantine regulations and measures for the prevention of epidemic and communicable diseases. At all times the physician should notify the constituted public health authorities of every case of communicable disease under his care, in accordance with the laws, rules and regulations of the health authorities. When an epidemic occurs a physician should not abandon his duty for fear of contracting the disease himself.

### *Pharmacists/Nurses*

Physicians should recognize and promote the practice of different paramedical services such as, pharmacy and nursing as professions and should seek their cooperation wherever required.

### *Unethical Acts*

A physician shall not aid or abet or commit any of the following acts which shall be construed as unethical:

### *Advertising*

Soliciting of patients directly or indirectly, by a physician, by a group of physicians or by institutions or organizations is unethical. A physician shall not make use of him/her (or his/her name) as subject of any form or manner of advertising or publicity through any mode either alone or in conjunction with others which is of such a character as to invite attention to him or to his professional position, skill, qualification, achievements, attainments, specialties, appointments, associations, affiliations or honours and/or of such character as would ordinarily result in his self-aggrandizement. A physician shall not give to any person, whether for compensation or otherwise, any approval, recommendation, endorsement, certificate, report or statement with respect of any drug, medicine, nostrum remedy, surgical, or therapeutic article, apparatus or appliance or any commercial product or article with respect of any property, quality or use thereof or any test, demonstration or trial thereof, for use in connection with his name, signature, or photograph in any form or manner of advertising through any mode nor shall he boast of cases, operations, cures or remedies or permit the publication of report thereof through any mode. A medical practitioner is, however, permitted to make a formal announcement in the press regarding the following:

1. On starting practice.
2. On change of type of practice.
3. On changing address.
4. On temporary absence from duty.
5. On resumption of another practice.
6. On succeeding to another practice.
7. Public declaration of charges.

Printing of self-photograph, or any such material of publicity in the letter head or on sign board of the consulting room or any such clinical establishment shall be regarded as acts of self-advertisement and unethical conduct on the part of the physician. However, printing of sketches, diagrams, picture of human system shall not be treated as unethical.

### Patents and Copyrights

A physician may patent surgical instruments, appliances and medicine or copyright applications, methods and procedures. However, it shall be unethical if the benefits of such patents or copyrights are not made available in situations where the interest of large population is involved.

### Running an Open Shop (Dispensing of Drugs and Appliances by Physicians)

A physician should not run an open shop for sale of medicine for dispensing prescriptions prescribed by doctors other than himself or for sale of medical or surgical appliances. It is not unethical for a physician to prescribe or supply drugs, remedies or appliances as long as there is no exploitation of the patient. Drugs prescribed by a physician or brought from the market for a patient should explicitly state the proprietary formulae as well as generic name of the drug.

### *Rebates and Commissions*

A physician shall not give, solicit, or receive nor shall he offer to give solicit or receive, any gift, gratuity, commission or bonus in consideration of or return for the referring, recommending or procuring of any patient for medical, surgical or other treatment. A physician shall not directly or indirectly, participate in or be a party to act of division, transference, assignment, subordination, rebating, splitting or refunding of any fee for medical, surgical or other treatment.

Provisions of para 6.4.1 shall apply with equal force to the referring, recommending or procuring by a physician or any person, specimen or material for diagnostic purposes or other study/work. Nothing in this section, however, shall prohibit payment of salaries by a qualified physician to other duly qualified person rendering medical care under his supervision.

### *Secret Remedies*

The prescribing or dispensing by a physician of secret remedial agents of which he does not know the composition, or the manufacture or promotion of their use is unethical and as such prohibited. All the drugs prescribed by a physician should always carry a proprietary formula and clear name.

### *Violation of Human Rights*

The physician shall not aid or abet torture nor shall he be a party to either infliction of mental or physical trauma or concealment of torture inflicted by some other person or agency in clear violation of human rights.

### *Euthanasia*

Practising euthanasia shall constitute unethical conduct. However, on specific occasion, the question of withdrawing supporting devices to sustain cardio-pulmonary function even after brain death, shall be decided only by a team of doctors and not merely by the treating physician alone. A team of doctors shall declare withdrawal of support system. Such team shall consist of the doctor in charge of the patient, Chief Medical Officer/Medical Officer in charge of the hospital and a doctor nominated by the in-charge of the hospital from the hospital staff or in accordance with the provisions of the Transplantation of Human Organ Act, 1994.

### *Misconduct*

The following acts of commission or omission on the part of a physician shall constitute professional misconduct rendering him/her liable for disciplinary action.

### *Violation of the Regulations*

If he/she does not maintain the medical records of his/her indoor patients for a period of three years as per regulation 1.3 and refuses to provide the same within 72 hours when the patient or his/her authorized representative makes a request for it as per the regulation.

If he/she does not display the registration number accorded to him/her by the State Medical Council or the Medical Council of India in his clinic, prescriptions and certificates, etc. issued by him or violates the provisions of regulation 1.4.2.

### *Adultery or Improper Conduct*

Abuse of professional position by committing adultery or improper conduct with a patient or by maintaining an improper association with a patient will render a Physician liable for disciplinary action as provided under the Indian Medical Council Act, 1956 or the concerned State Medical Council Act.

*Conviction by Court of Law:* Conviction by a Court of Law for offences involving moral turpitude/Criminal acts.

### *Sex Determination Tests*

On no account, sex determination test shall be undertaken with the intent to terminate the life of a female foetus developing in her mother's womb, unless there are other absolute indications for termination of pregnancy as specified in the Medical Termination of Pregnancy Act, 1971. Any act of termination of pregnancy of normal female foetus amounting to female foeticide shall be regarded as professional misconduct on the part of the physician leading to penal erasure besides rendering him liable to criminal proceedings as per the provisions of this Act.

### *Signing Professional Certificates, Reports and Other Documents*

Registered medical practitioners are in certain cases bound by law to give, or may from time to time be called upon or requested to give certificates, notification, reports and other documents of similar character signed by them in their professional capacity for subsequent use in the courts or for administrative purposes, etc. Such documents, among others, include the ones given at Appendix–4 of Medical Council of India Notification of Code of Medical Ethics. Any registered practitioner who is proved to have signed or given under his name and authority, any such certificate, notification, report or document of a similar character which is untrue, misleading or improper, is liable to have his name deleted from the Register.

A registered medical practitioner shall not contravene the provisions of the Drugs and Cosmetics Act and regulations made there under. Accordingly,

- Prescribing steroids/psychotropic drugs when there is no absolute medical indication;
- Selling Schedule 'H' and 'L' drugs and poisons to the public except to his patient; in contravention of the above provisions shall constitute gross professional misconduct on the part of the physician.
- Performing or enabling unqualified person to perform an abortion or any illegal operation for which there is no medical, surgical or psychological indication.
- A registered medical practitioner shall not issue certificates of efficiency in modern medicine to unqualified or non-medical person.

  (*Note:* The foregoing does not restrict the proper training and instruction of bonafide students, midwives, dispensers, surgical attendants, or skilled mechanical and technical assistants and therapy assistants under the personal supervision of physicians.)

A physician should not contribute to the lay press articles and give interviews regarding diseases and treatments which may have the effect of advertising himself or soliciting practices; but is open to write to the lay press under his own name on matters of public health, hygienic living or to deliver public lectures, give talks on the radio/TV/internet chat for the same purpose and send announcement of the same to lay press.

An institution run by a physician for a particular purpose such as a maternity home, nursing home, private hospital, rehabilitation centre or any type of training institution, etc. may be advertised in the lay press, but such advertisements should not contain anything more than the name of the institution, type of patients admitted, type of training and other facilities offered and the fees.

It is improper for a physician to use an unusually large sign board and write on it anything other than his name, qualifications obtained from a University or a statutory body, titles and name of his specialty, registration number including the name of the State Medical Council under which registered. The same should be the contents of his prescription papers. It is improper to affix a signboard on a chemist's shop or in places where he does not reside or work.

The registered medical practitioner shall not disclose the secrets of a patient that have been learnt in the exercise of his/her profession except in a court of law under orders of the Presiding Judge; in circumstances where there is a serious and identified risk to a specific person and/or community; and modifiable diseases.

In case of communicable/modifiable diseases, concerned public health authorities should be informed immediately.

The registered medical practitioner shall not refuse on religious grounds alone to give assistance in or conduct of sterility, birth control, circumcision and medical termination of pregnancy when there is medical indication, unless the medical practitioner feels himself/herself incompetent to do so.

Before performing an operation, the physician should obtain in writing, the consent from the husband or wife, parent or guardian in the case of minor, or the patient himself as the case may be. In an operation which may result in sterility the consent of both husband and wife is needed.

A registered medical practitioner shall not publish photographs or case reports of his/her patients without their permission, in any medical or other journal in a manner by which their identity could be made out. If the identity is not to be disclosed, the consent is not needed.

In the case of running of a nursing home by a physician and employing assistants to help him/her, the ultimate responsibility rests on the physician.

A physician shall not use touts or agents for procuring patients.

A physician shall not claim to be specialist unless he has a special qualification in that branch.

No act of in vitro fertilization or artificial insemination shall be undertaken without the informed consent of the female patient and her spouse as well as the donor. Such consent shall be obtained in writing only after the patient is provided, at her own level of comprehension, with sufficient information about the purpose, methods, risks, inconveniences, disappointments of the procedure and possible risks and hazards.

*Research:* Clinical drug trials or other research involving patients or volunteers as per the guidelines of Indian Council of Medical Research (ICMR) can be undertaken, provided ethical considerations are borne in mind. Violation of existing ICMR guidelines in this regard shall constitute misconduct. Consent taken from the patient for trial of drug or therapy which is not as per the guidelines shall also be construed as misconduct.

If a physician posted in rural area is found absent on more than two occasions during inspection by the Head of the District Health Authority or the Chairman, Zila Parishad, the same shall be construed as misconduct if it is recommended to the Medical Council of India/State Medical Council by the State Government for action under these Regulations.

A physician posted in a medical college/institution as teaching faculty or other posts shall remain in hospital/college during the assigned duty hours. If found absent on more than two occasions during this period, the same shall be construed as a misconduct if it is certified by the Principal/Medical Superintendent and forwarded through the State Government to Medical Council of India/State Medical Council for action under these Regulations.

## Punishment and Disciplinary Action

It must be clearly understood that the instances of offences and of professional misconduct which are given above do not constitute and are not intended to constitute a complete list of the infamous acts which calls for disciplinary action, and that by issuing this notice the Medical Council of India and or State Medical Councils are in no way precluded from considering and dealing with any other form of professional misconduct on the part of a registered practitioner. Circumstances may and do arise from time to time in relation to which there may occur questions of professional misconduct which do not come within any of these categories. Every care should be taken that the code is not violated in letter or spirit. In such instances as in all others, the Medical Council of India and/or State Medical Councils have to consider and decide upon the facts brought before the Medical Council of India and/or State Medical Councils.

It is made clear that any complaint with regard to professional misconduct can be brought before the appropriate Medical Council for disciplinary action. Upon receipt of any complaint of professional misconduct, the appropriate Medical Council would hold an enquiry and give opportunity to the registered medical practitioner to be heard in person or by a pleader. If the medical practitioner is found to be guilty of committing professional misconduct, the appropriate Medical Council may award such punishment as deemed necessary or may direct the removal altogether or for a specified period, from the register of the name of the delinquent registered practitioner. Deletion from the Register shall be widely publicized in local press as well as in the publications of different Medical Associations/Societies/Bodies.

In case the punishment of removal from the register is for a limited period, the appropriate Council may also direct that the name so removed shall be restored in the register after the expiry of the period for which the name was ordered to be removed.

Decision on complaint against delinquent physician shall be taken within a time limit of 6 months.

During the pendency of the complaint the appropriate Council may restrain the physician from performing the procedure or practice which is under scrutiny.

Professional incompetence shall be judged by peer group as per guidelines prescribed by Medical Council of India.

# 20

# First Aid and Disaster Health Care Management

First aid is the provision of initial care for an illness or injury. It is usually performed by a lay person to a sick or injured casualty until definitive medical treatment can be accessed. Certain self-limiting illnesses or minor injuries may not require further medical care past the first aid intervention. It generally consists of a series of simple and, in some cases, potentially life-saving techniques that an individual can be trained to perform with minimal equipment.

## Aims

The key aims of first aid can be summarized in three key points:

- *Preserve Life:* the overriding aim of all medical care, including first aid, is to save lives.
- *Prevent Further Harm:* also sometimes called to prevent the condition from worsening; this covers both external factors, such as moving a patient away from any cause of harm and applying first aid techniques to prevent worsening of the condition, such as applying pressure to stop a bleed becoming dangerous.
- *Promote Recovery:* first aid also involves trying to start the recovery process from the illness or injury and, in some cases, might involve completing a treatment, such as in the case of applying a plaster to a small wound.

First aid training also involves the prevention of initial injury, responsive safety and the treatment phases.

## Key Skills

Certain skills are considered essential to the provision of first aid and are taught ubiquitously. Particularly, the 'ABC's of first aid, which focus on critical life-saving intervention, must be rendered before treatment of less serious injuries. ABC stands for *Airway, Breathing,* and *Circulation.* The same mnemonic is used by all emergency health professionals. Attention must first be brought to the airway to ensure it is clear. Obstruction (choking) is a life-threatening emergency. Following evaluation of the airway, a first aid attendant would determine adequacy of breathing and provide rescue breathing if necessary. Assessment of circulation is now not usually carried out for patients who are not breathing, with first aiders now trained to go straight to chest compressions (and thus providing artificial circulation) but pulse checks may be done on less serious patients.

Some organizations add a fourth step of 'D' for *Deadly bleeding* or *Defibrillation,* while others consider this as part of the *Circulation* step. Variations on techniques to evaluate and maintain the ABCs depend on the skill level of the first aider. Once the ABCs are secured, first aiders can begin additional treatments, as required. Some organizations teach the same order of priority using the 3Bs: *Breathing, Bleeding,* and *Bones* (or '4Bs': *Breathing, Bleeding, Brain,* and *Bones).* While the ABCs and 3Bs are taught to be performed sequentially, certain conditions may require the consideration of two steps simultaneously. This includes the provision of both artificial respiration and chest compressions to someone who is not breathing and has no pulse, and the consideration of cervical spine injuries when ensuring an open airway.

## Preserving Life

In order to preserve life, all persons require having an open airway – a clear passage where air can move in through the mouth or nose through the pharynx and down in to the lungs, without obstruction. Conscious people will maintain their own airway automatically, but those who are unconscious (with a Glasgow Coma Scale (GCS) of less than 8) may be unable to maintain a patent airway, as the part of the brain which autonomously controls in normal situations may not be functioning.

If the patient was breathing, a first aider would normally then place them in the recovery position, with the patient leant over on their side, which also has the effect of clearing the tongue from the pharynx. It also avoids a common cause of death in unconscious patients, which is choking on regurgitated stomach contents.

The airway can also become blocked through a foreign object becoming lodged in the pharynx or larynx, commonly called choking. The first aider will be taught to deal with this through a combination of 'back slaps' and 'abdominal thrusts'.

Once the airway has been opened, the first aider would assess to see if the patient is breathing. If there is no breathing, or the patient is not breathing normally, such as atonal breathing, the first aider would undertake what is probably the most recognized first aid procedure – Cardiopulmonary resuscitation or CPR, which involves breathing for the patient, and manually massaging the heart to promote blood flow around the body.

**Promoting Recovery**

The first aider is also likely to be trained in dealing with injuries such as cuts, grazes or broken bones. They may be able to deal with the situation in its entirety (a small adhesive bandage on a paper cut), or may be required to maintain the condition of something like a broken bone, until the next stage of definitive care (usually an ambulance) arrives.

Conditions that often require first aid are:

- Altitude sickness, which can begin in susceptible people at altitudes as low as 5,000 feet, can cause potentially fatal swelling of the brain or lungs.
- Anaphylaxis, a life-threatening condition in which the airway can become constricted and the patient may go into shock. The reaction can be caused by a systemic allergic reaction to allergens such as insect bites or peanuts. Anaphylaxis is initially treated with injection of epinephrine.
- Battlefield First Aid – this protocol refers to treating shrapnel, gunshot wounds, burns, bone fractures, etc. as seen either in the 'traditional' battlefield setting or in an area subject to damage by large scale weaponry, such as a bomb blast or other terrorist activity.
- Bone fracture, a break in a bone initially treated by stabilizing the fracture with a splint.
- Burns, which can result in damage to tissues and loss of body fluids through the burn site.
- Choking, blockage of the airway which can quickly result in death due to lack of oxygen if the patient's trachea is not cleared, for example by the Heimlich Maneuver.

- Childbirth.
- Cramps in muscles due to lactic acid build up caused either by inadequate oxygenation of muscle or lack of water or salt.
- Diving disorders, drowning or asphyxiation.
- Gender-specific conditions, such as dysmenorrheal and testicular torsion.
- Heart attack or inadequate blood flow to the blood vessels supplying the heart muscle.
- Heat stroke, also known as sunstroke or hyperthermia, which tends to occur during heavy exercise in high humidity, or with inadequate water, though it may occur spontaneously in some chronically ill persons. Sunstroke, especially when the victim has been unconscious, often causes major damage to body systems such as brain, kidney, liver, gastric tract. Unconsciousness for more than two hours usually leads to permanent disability. Emergency treatment involves rapid cooling of the patient.
- Heat syncope, another stage in the same process as heat stroke, occurs under similar conditions as heat stroke and is not distinguished from the latter by some authorities.
- Heavy bleeding, treated by applying pressure (manually and later with a pressure bandage) to the wound site and elevating the limb if possible.
- Hyperglycemia (diabetic coma) and Hypoglycemia (insulin shock).
- Hypothermia, or Exposure, occurs when a person's core body temperature falls below 33.7°C (92.6°F). First aid for a mildly hypothermic patient includes rewarming, which can be achieved by wrapping the affected person in a blanket and providing warm drinks, such as soup and high energy food, such as chocolate. However, rewarming a severely hypothermic person could result in a fatal arrhythmia, an irregular heart rhythm.
- Insect and animal bites and stings.
- Joint dislocation.
- Poisoning, which can occur by injection, inhalation, absorption or ingestion.
- Seizures, or a malfunction in the electrical activity in the brain. Three types of seizures include a grand mal (which usually features convulsions as well as temporary respiratory abnormalities, change in skin complexion, etc.) and petit mal (which usually features twitching, rapid blinking, and/or fidgeting as well as altered consciousness and temporary respiratory abnormalities).

- Muscle strains and sprains, a temporary dislocation of a joint that immediately reduces automatically but may result in ligament damage.
- Stroke, a temporary loss of blood supply to the brain.
- Toothache, which can result in severe pain and loss of the tooth but is rarely life threatening, unless over time the infection spreads into the bone of the jaw and starts osteomyelitis.
- Wounds and bleeding, including lacerations, incisions and abrasions, Gastrointestinal bleeding, avulsions and sucking chest wounds, treated with an occlusive dressing to let air out but not in.

## Artificial Respiration

Artificial respiration is the act of simulating respiration, which provides for the overall exchange of gases in the body by pulmonary ventilation, external respiration and internal respirations. This means providing air for a person who is not breathing or is not making sufficient respiratory effort on their own (although it must be used on a patient with a beating heart or as part of cardiopulmonary resuscitation in order to achieve the internal respiration).

Pulmonary ventilation (and hence external respiration) is achieved through manual insufflations of the lungs either by the rescuer blowing into the patient's lungs, or by using a mechanical device to do so. This method of insufflations has been proved more effective than methods which involve mechanical manipulation of the patient's chest or arms, such as the Silvester method. It is also known as Expired Air Resuscitation (EAR), Expired Air Ventilation (EAV), and mouth-to-mouth resuscitation, rescue breathing or colloquially the kiss of life.

Artificial respiration is a part of most protocols for performing cardiopulmonary resuscitation (CPR) making it an essential skill for first aid. In some situations, artificial respiration is also performed separately, for instance in near-drowning and opiate overdoses. The performance of artificial respiration in its own is now limited in most protocols to health professionals, whereas lay first aiders are advised to undertake full CPR in any case where the patient is not breathing sufficiently.

Mechanical ventilation involves the use of a mechanical ventilator to move air in and out of the lungs when an individual is unable to breathe on his or her own, for example during surgery with general anaesthesia or when an individual is in a coma.

Insufflation, also known as 'rescue breath' or 'ventilation', is the act of mechanically forcing air into a patient's respiratory system. This can be achieved via a number of methods, which will depend on the situation and equipment available. All methods require good airway management to perform, which ensures that the method is effective. These methods include:

- *Mouth to Mouth:* This involves the rescuer making a seal between their mouth and the patient's mouth and 'blowing', in order to pass air into the patient's body Mouth-to-mouth insufflations.
- *Mouth to Nose:* In some instances, the rescuer may need or wish to form a seal with the patient's nose. Typical reasons for this include maxillofacial injuries, performing the procedure in water or the remains of vomit in the mouth.
- *Mouth to Mouth and Nose:* Used on infants (usually up to around one year old), as this forms the most effective seal.
- *Mouth to Mask:* Most organizations recommend the use of some sort of barrier between rescuer and patient to reduce cross infection risk. One popular type is the 'pocket mask'. This may be able to provide higher tidal volumes than a Bag Valve Mask.
- *Bag Valve Mask (BVM):* this is a simple device manually operated by the rescuer, which involves squeezing a bag in order to expel air into the patient.

## Disaster Management

National Rural Health Mission (NHRM), New Delhi provides medical training as part of its health programmes which includes first aid training to field level workers, Astha and Anganwadi Workers.

Reproductive and Child Health (RCH) Programme, New Delhi Under the RCH programme medical training is a part, this training includes first aid training for doctors.

National Disaster Management Authority (NDMA), New Delhi has issued guidelines for Medical Preparedness and Mass Casualty management and has constituted various committees to tackle the problem.

Government of India – UNDP Disaster Risk Management Programme, New Delhi. Programme in 169 multi-hazard prone districts of 17 Indian states focuses on providing community taskforces training in first-aid techniques for better prehospital care.

Indian Federation for Red Cross and Crescent Societies (IFRC), New Delhi. IFRC is involved in disaster preparedness and health care work and provides support to government for emergency support functions for medical and trauma counselling.

***Rahul Baneri, 'Amity Humanity Foundation, Noida' says:***

In a disaster, grassroots people are getting affected more than any other community is. Any organization or Government department can reach to them not before two or three hours, and thereafter, it takes some time to understand the whole situation and to initiate aid programme. Sometimes, they even need to establish shelter houses and organize the matter. This whole programme takes 5–6 hours before initiating practical programme. Therefore, it is important first to sentisitize the community and train them for some of the beginning steps. A few suggestions are mentioned below:

1. Community should be trained about some important steps like at the time of disaster what they should carry before leaving their place.
2. If the whole family are on the road or abandoned then where they should go.
3. If any small casualty happens (physically) then what should be the duty of other members of the family.
4. Most of the nervous breakdown cases creates chaos, so tips on emergency management should be initiated.
5. A particular interactive session between police, hospital staffs and local NGOs should be incorporated in the training programme.
6. All the civil societies can organize awareness programme for local school and college students as they can act as volunteer in an emergency.

***Shoib Akhter, 'Change Innovator's, New Delhi' says:***

I was recently going through various reports and documents on pre- and post-hospital care during emergencies. The points I want to share are mainly on Hospital Emergency Plans. A few of them, I could take from there are mentioned below. The hospital emergency plans should address these issues:

- *Care for Hospital Employees:* In an event involving weapons of mass destruction (WMD), the staffs needs to be assured of the physical security of the work environment. They also need to know that the hospital is addressing staff members' safety and well-being. Frequent communications with all internal hospital audiences is necessary. Screening may also be needed to assess how employees are affected by the stress and emotion of the situation.

- *Care for Employees' Families:* Establish a dependent-care plan for family members of staff. Ask staff about their families' needs. Inform staff that the hospital may need to lock down during an incident, but recognize that employees will not stay on the job if they think their loved ones are not being taken care of. Establish a separate telephone number for employees' families to call during emergencies.
- *Staff Education:* Encourage professional interaction among staff and between staff and public health agencies. Offer incentives to improve staff performance in disaster preparedness. Prepare fact sheets and use the hospital Intranet to educate staff about the clinical aspects of radiation e.g. signs and symptoms of contamination, and short- and long-term health effects. Incorporate radiological preparedness into existing mass casualty training and educational forums.
- *Staffing:* Determine roles and responsibilities for each member of the response team. Be ready to rotate communications' staff during emergencies. Be aware of overload; you cannot have the entire staff working at the same time. Employees need to get away from the stress once in a while to be effective when they return to the job. Ask other departments, such as the billing office, to support the emergency communications function. Ask medical, nursing and dental students to help. Draw upon the nuclear medicine department for technical expertise. Use volunteers, such as communications professionals from local universities.
- *Employee Notification:* Create a checklist for notifying and recalling staff during mass casualty events. Identify all audiences in the hospital and determine how to communicate with each. In addition to medical and professional personnel, consider part-time staff, volunteers, vendors and the board of directors. Assemble 24-hour contact information for all staff (home phones, cell phones, pagers, e-mail addresses). Determine who is responsible for calling these people.
- *Communications Systems:* Implement and test redundant communications systems to be established.

***Ravishwar Sinha, Independent Consultant Opines***

Linking trained first aid volunteers with existing public health and health care infrastructures. There is a shortage of properly trained volunteers in hospitals to handle medical emergencies. Many lives are lost during transportation or improper handling of the traumatized person. Enthusiasm of community is helpful but it needs to be supported with training for better results.

Initiatives like the National Rural Health Mission (NHRM), Reproductive and Child Health (RCH) and Universalization and expansion of the Integrated Child Health Services (ICDS) offers big opportunity of integrating the first aid training with their training programmes. This would not only add value to their day-to-day activities in the community but the skills gained by the field level workers such as Asha and Anganwadi workers and helpers, which are basically part-time workers/volunteers will also enhance their incomes and prestige in the communities they work in. This would add value to the original programmes also and would be an asset in times of disasters/emergency.

The schools and colleges are the other source of volunteers for integrating the First Aid training; it is also been happening in the National Cadet Corps and other institutions could also add value.

Educational institutes would also form emergency response teams; these could be linked to the local institutions of health and development and also engaged in the some projects in the community as volunteers. This would foster team work and would be an asset in case of emergencies.

Strengthening the pre-hospital care through capacity building of first responders from public services and on regularizing their trainings

The hospital infrastructure in the country whether government like in India and private that is growing are facing many challenges. The government programmes of NRHM, RCH and public private partnerships are supporting in overcoming the challenges. In the private sector, resources for meeting the needs both human and materials are a big constraint.

Some mechanism to garner and allot resources needs to be developed for this. As the emergencies and disaster are by the very definitions unpredictable, a locally need-based agreement should be in place for this. There are some in the government sector from very old British days and these have been not so very regularly supplemented.

The National Disaster Management Authority (NDMA) has initiated the steps to update and improve this aspect. This is very commendable.

Training is another component that needs to be strengthened to bring the available resources in sync.

### *Simple and Effective Approaches in Utilizing Community Volunteers in Mass Casualty Incidents*

In case of disasters that are more predictable like flood and famines, cyclones in costal areas, the community in a many cases has some coping mechanism in place from community memory and practices. There is need to be look into these in designing and putting into place community response teams. This, I believe, is part of the training needs outlined above.

Keeping the coherence of such teams some sort of periodical social service such as health camps, Public distribution system camps and organizing of melas/fairs should be done. Otherwise, I feel the interest of the team of volunteers would wane and in effect there would not be in position when needed most.

### *Garima Aggarwal, 'GoI–UNDP DRM Programme, New Delhi' Views:*

As rightly pointed out that mass casualty management is not possible without linking various health related facilities with each other and also linking them with administration; Under the GoI–UNDP DRM Programme, wherein focus has been largely to train first responders, i.e. primarily the community taskforces in first aid techniques, so that they can serve their communities before going to the hospitals.

In Delhi, first aid taskforces are being formed in schools, resident's colonies and offices and have been trained with the help of St John Ambulance Brigade.

The district administration has been maintaining database of the trained personnel as a part of Community Based Disaster Management planning process.

These Community Disaster Management plans have details of evacuation and response methods of the communities and also has Standard Operating Procedures [SOPs] for the first aid team. The first aid teams are expected to act as a first responder during any kind of local disaster until external help reaches. The taskforces have also been guided to help the teams of medical responders, which will come from the government and NGOs. For strengthening the coordination system, several times, mock-drills have been conducted at community, district and state level wherein taskforces have rehearsed their SOPs along with the local administration and hospitals and NGOs, etc. A separate Emergency Support Function (ESF) for Medical and Trauma Counselling has been formed at district level, which has team of doctors and paramedical staff belonging to various hospitals and supporting organizations like Delhi Civil Defiance, St. John Ambulance Brigade and Indian Red Cross Society, etc.

The team leaders of Medical and Trauma Counselling ESF has to coordinate with the State level ESF for meeting requirements of manpower and resources. The team leader of State level ESF will also take updates from the field teams and team leaders. The mechanism has also been tested through mock drills.

However, Government of Delhi is conscious about handling large-scale disasters like earthquake and the effectiveness of the existing health support system.

Therefore, in April 2007, Delhi had organized a workshop for the representatives of major hospitals under State and Central Government and private hospitals. More than 70 hospitals were called together and sensitized about the importance of hospital preparedness plans and also preparation of mass casualty system which shall include management of causalities, injuries, transportation of injured people to nearby hospitals through heli-ambulances, etc. Critical issues during disasters like media management system and disposal of carcasses and dead bodies, etc. were also discussed in detail. At the last, a road map was prepared and district administration was encouraged to prepare district-level mass casualty plans with the involvement of hospitals and clinics. District administration was also suggested to prepare inventory of resources, medicos/chemist shops and trained medical and paramedical staff and also to link the community taskforces with the emergency response system by conducting regular mock drills.

# Bibliography


Babb, D.A., 'Use of Traditional Medicine by HIV Infected Individuals.' *Psycho Health Med* 12, 2007, pp. 314–320.

Barry, Anne-Marie and Chris Yuill, *Understanding Health: A Sociological Introduction*. New Delhi: Sage Publications, 2002.

Berkman, L.F. and Kawachi, I. "A Historical Framework for Social Epidemiology", in Berkman, L.F. and Kawachi, I., eds. *Social Epidemiology*, New York: Oxford University Press, 2000, pp. 3-12.

Bird, Chloe E., Peter Conrad and Allen M. Fremont, *Handbook of Medical Sociology* (Fifth Edition). Upper Saddle River, NJ: Prentice Hall, 2000.

Blaxter, Mildred, *Health*. UK, Cambridge: Polity Press, 2004.

Bloom, Samuel William, *The Word as Scalpel: A History of Medical Sociology*. New York: Oxford University Press, 2002.

Brown, Phil, *Perspectives in Medical Sociology* (Fourth Edition). Long Grove, IL: Waveland Press, 2008.

Bury, Michael and Jonathan Gabe, *The Sociology of Health and Illness: A Reader*. UK: Routledge, 2003.

Cockerham, William C., *Readings in Medical Sociology*. New Jersey: Prentice Hall, 1997.

——, *The Blackwell Companion to Medical Sociology*. UK: Oxford and Malden, MA: Blackwell, 2001.

——, *Medical Sociology* (Ninth Edition). New Jersey: Pearson Prentice Hall, 2003.

Cockerham, William C. and Ferris Joseph Ritchey, *Dictionary of Medical Sociology*. Westport, Connecticut: Greenwood Press, 2007.

Connor, Linda and Geoffrey Samuel, *Healing Powers and Modernity: Traditional Medicine, Shamanism, and Science in Asian Societies*. Westport, Connecticut: Greenwood Publishing Group, 2001, pp. 3–4.

Conrad, Peter et al., *Handbook of Medical Sociology*. New Jersey: Prentice Hall, 2000.

Conrad, Peter, *The Medicalization of Society: On the Transformation of Human Conditions into Treatable Disorders*. Baltimore, MD: Johns Hopkins University Press, 2007.

——, *The Sociology of Health and Illness: Critical Perspectives*. New York: , 2008, pp. 1–55.

'Country Comparison: Life Expectancy at Birth.' *CIA: The World Factbook*. Central Intelligence Agency, 2009. <https://www.cia.gov/library/publications/the-worldfactbook/rankorder/2102rank.html> (5 November 2009).

Dak, T.M. *Sociology of Health in India*. Jaipur: Rawat Publications, 1991.

Das Gupta, Monica et al., *Women's Health in India*. Delhi: Oxford University Press, 1998.

Datar, A. et al., 'Health Infrastructure and Immunization Coverage in India.' *Indian Journal of Medical Research* 125, 2007.

DiCenso A., G. Guyatt, A. William, L. Griffith, "Intervention to Reduce Unintended Pregnancies among Adolescent: Systematic Review of Randomized Controlled Trials", *BMJ*, 324, pp. 1420-1432, 2002.

'Epidemics: Malaria, AIDS, Other Disease: Post-colonial Africa.' *Encyclopedia of African History*. <http://www.credoreference.com/entry/routafricanhistory/epidemics_malaria_aids_other_disease_postcolonial_africa> (November 2009).

Fredrickson, J. and A. Kanabus, 'Impact of HIV/AIDS on Africa.' <http://www.avert.org/aids-impact-africa.htm> (November 2009).

Gallagher, Eugene B. and Janardan Subedi, *Global Perspectives on Health Care*. New Jersey: Prentice Hall, 1995.

Gilbert J. Botvin and Kenneth W. Griffin, "School-based Programmes to Prevent Alcohol, Tobacco and Other Drug Use", *International Review of Psychiatry*. Journal of American Medical Association, 2007.

Haggett, Peter. *Encyclopedia of World Geography: South America*. Tarrytown: Andromeda Oxford Ltd., 2002, p. 672.

Helman, Cecil, *Culture, Health and Illness* (Fifth Edition). London, England: Hodder Arnold, 2007.

Hermalin, Albert, *The Well-being of the Elderly in Asia: A Four-country Comparative Study*. Ann Arbor, MI: , 2002, pp. 1–3.

'HIV and AIDS Estimates and Data.' World Health Organization, 2007, pp. 214–233. <http://data.unaids.org/pub/globalreport/2008/jc1510_2008_global_report_pp211_234_en.pdf> (December 2009).

Johnston, Rosalind. Averting HIV and AIDS. 2009. Averting HIV and AIDS. 26 November 2009. p. 173. <http://www.avert.org/southamerica.htm> (1 December 2009).

Kendall, Patricia L. and George G. Reader, 'Contributors of Sociology to Medicine', in Freeman, et al. *Handbook of Medical Sociology*, Englewood Cliffs NJ: Prentice Hall, 1972.

Law, Jacky, *Big Pharma: Exposing the Global Healthcare Agenda*. New York: Carroll and Graf, 2005.

Levy, Judith A. and Bernice A. Pescosolido, *Social Networks and Health* (First Edition). Amsterdam, The Netherlands; Boston, MA: JAI, 2005.

Lewis, Milton James and Kerrie L. Macpherson, *Public Health in Asia and the Pacific: Historical and Comparative Perspectives*. London: Routledge, 2005, pp. 222–235. <http://books.google.com/books?id=pr14oqopge8c&printsec=frontcover&dq=public+health+in+asia+and+the+pacific#v=onepage&q=&f=false>

Lindemann, Mary, *Medicine and Society in Early Modern Europe*. Cambridge: Cambridge University Press, 1995.

Littman, Robert J., 'The Plague of Athens: Epidemiology and Paleopathology.' *Mount Sinai Journal of Medicine* 76, 2009, pp. 456–467.

Marshall, Gordon. 'Sociology of Health and Illness.' *A Dictionary of Sociology*, 1998. <http://www.encyclopedia.com> (30 November 2009).

Mechanic, David, *Inescapable Decisions: The Imperatives of Health Reform*. New Brunswick, NJ: Transaction Publishers, 1994.

Medical Council of India. Code of Ethics Regulations, 2002. <http://www.mcindia.org/know/rules/ethics.thml>

Micollier, Evelyne, *Sexual Cultures in East Asia: The Social Construction of Sexuality and Sexual Risk in a Time of AIDS*. London: Routledge, 2004, pp. 98–101. <uac&printsec=frontcover&dq=sexual+cultures+in+east+asia#v=onepage&q=&f=false>

Miller, Henry I., 'Understanding Swine Flu.' *Wall Street Journal*, 28 April 2009.

Misra, Rajiv et al., *India Health Report*. New Delhi: Oxford University Press, 2003.

Morgan, Myfanwy, 'Managing Hypertension: Beliefs and Responses to Medication among Cultural Groups.' *Sociology of Health and Illness* 10 (4), 1998.

Mumtaz, Z. and S.M. Salway, 'Gender, Pregnancy and the Uptake of Antenatal Care Services in Pakistan.' *Sociology of Health and Illness* 29 (1), 2007, pp. 1–26.

Nagla, Madhu, *Medical Sociology*. Jaipur: Printwell Publishers, 1988.

Nosikov, Anatoliy, *The European Health Report 2002*. World Health Organization Regional Office Europe, 2002.

Otsuka, Ryutaro and Stanley J. Ulijaszek, *Health Change in the Asia-Pacific Region: Biocultural and Epidemiological Approaches*. Cambridge: , 2007, p. 4, 136 and pp. 7–9. <http://books.google.com/books?id=0rkmrnhph6yc&printsec=frontcover&dq=health+change+in+the+asia-pacific#v=onepage&q=&f=false>

Packer, Lester, Choon Nam Ong and Barry Halliwell, *Herbal and Traditional Medicine: Molecular Aspects of Health*. Boca Raton, FL: , 2005, pp. 2–5.

Palmerlee, D., S. Bao and C. Beech, *South America on a Shoe String*. USA: Lonely Planet, 2004, pp. 1056–1057.

Park, K., *Park's Text Book of Preventive and Social Medicine* (Sixteenth Edition). Jabalpur: M/S Banarsidas Bhanot Publishers, 2000.

——, *Park's Text Book of Preventive and Social Medicine* (Twentieth Edition). Jabalpur: M/S Banarsidas Bhanot Publishers, 2005.

PATH (Program for Appropriate Technology in Health). 'A Rights-Based Approach to Reproductive Health.' *Outlook* 20 (4), 2003.

Phillips, David, . London: Routledge, 2000, pp. xiv-xv.

Porter, Dorothy, *Health, Civilization, and the State: A History of Public Health from Ancient to Modern Times*. New York: Routledge, 1999.

Porter, Roy and Vivian Nutton, eds., *The History of Medical Education in Britain*, Amsterdam: Rodopi, 1995.

Powers, John, 'The Spread of Confucianism.' <http://science.jrank.org/pages/9703/humanity-asian-thought-spread-confucianism.html.> (1 December 2009).

Punamaki, Raija-Leena, 'Reasons for Consultation and Explanations of Illness among Finnish Primary-care Patients.' *Sociology of Health and Illness* 17 (1), 1995.

Rogers, Anne and David Pilgrim, *A Sociology of Mental Health and Illness* (Third Edition). Maidenhead, England: Open University Press, 2005.

Roizman, Bernard, *Infectious Diseases in an Age of Change*. Washington, DC: National Academy Press, 2005, pp. 67–68.

Rosenstock, Irwin M., Strecher, Victor J. and Becker, Marshall H., "Social Learning Theory and the Health Belief Model", *Health Education and Behavior* 15 (2): 178-183, 1988.

Rozario, Santi and Geoffrey Samuel, *The Daughters of Hariti: Childbirth and Female Healers in South and Southeast Asia*. London: , 2002, pp. 1–2.

Saari, Peggy, 'Medicine and Disease: Who was the First Doctor in History?', in Julie L. Carnagie (ed.), *History Fact Finder*. UXL-GALE, 2001. enotes.com. 2006. (2 November 2009).

Scambler, Graham and Paul Higgs, *Modernity, Medicine, and Health: Medical Sociology Towards 2000*. London and New York: Routledge, 1998.

Scombler, Graham, *Sociological Theory and Medical Sociology*. London and New York: Tavistock Publications, 1987.

Srinivasan, R., 'Health Care in India, Vision 2020: Issues and Prospects, 2009.' <www.planning commission.nic.in/rep>

Starr, Paul, "The Limits of Privatization," in Steve Hanke, ed., *Prospects for Privatization* (Academy of Political Science, 1987): 124-137. Reprinted in Dennis J. Gayle and Jonathan N. Goodrich, eds. *Privatization and Deregulation in Global Perspective* (Quorum, 1990). Reprinted in a revised and expanded form as a report of the Economic Policy Institute, Washington, D.C, 1988.

Taylor, Steve and David Field, *Sociology of Health and Health Care*. Oxford, England: Wiley-Blackwell, 2007.

Timmermans, Stefan and Steven Haas, 'Towards a Sociology of Disease.' *Sociology of Health and Illness* 30 (5), 2008, pp. 659–676.

Training of Doctors: The Goodenough Committee's Report. *Br Med J,* 1944.

Turner, Bryan M., *The New Medical Sociology: Social Forms of Health and Illness*. New York: W.W. Norton, 2004.

WHO, Definition and Diagnosis of Diabetes Mellitus and Intermediate Hyperglycemia, Geneva: World Health Organization, 2006.

'WHO World Health Statistics 2008.' <http://www.who.int/whosis/whostat/2008/en/index.html> (December 2009).

White, Kevin, *An Introduction to the Sociology of Health and Illness*. New Delhi: Sage Publications, 2002, pp. 4–5.

Willcox, Merlin, Gerard Bodeker and Philippe Rasoanaivo, *Traditional Medicinal Plants and Malaria*. United States of America: CRC Press, 2004.

World Learning Study Abroad. <http://www.sit.edu/studyabroad/ssa_cih.htm> (3 December 2009).

Yang, Guoshu, *Progress in Asian Social Psychology: Conceptual and Empirical Contributions*. Westport, Connecticut: Greenwood Publishing Group, 2003, pp. 11–12 and 294–295.

# Index